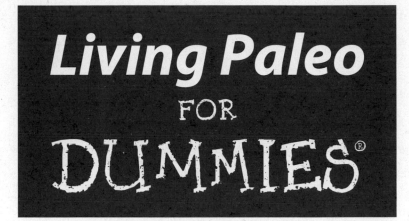

Living Paleo FOR DUMMIES®

by Melissa Joulwan and Dr. Kellyann Petrucci

WILEY

John Wiley & Sons, Inc.

Living Paleo For Dummies®

Published by
John Wiley & Sons, Inc.
111 River St.
Hoboken, NJ 07030-5774
www.wiley.com

WILEY

About the Authors

Melissa Joulwan is the author of *Well Fed: Paleo Recipes for People Who Love to Eat* (Smudge Publishing, LLC) and the author of the recipes and Meal Map included in the *New York Times* Bestseller *It Starts With Food: Discover the Whole30 and Change Your Life in Unexpected Ways* (Victory Belt Publishing). Her recipes have appeared in *Paleo Magazine,* and she was a featured chef for U.S. Wellness Meats and Lava Lake Lamb. She also teaches Paleo cooking classes at the Whole Foods Culinary Center.

Melissa has been following a strict Paleo diet since 2009, when she underwent a thyroidectomy. In the aftermath of the surgery and recovery, she became particularly interested in how diet affects hormones, body composition, mood, and mental well-being. Her experiences are chronicled on the popular, award–winning blog *The Clothes Make The Girl* (www.theclothesmakethe girl.com), where she writes daily about the Paleo lifestyle, recipes, fitness training, yoga, meditation, and motivation.

Melissa is also a community ambassador for *Experience Life* magazine, a contributor to health and fitness periodicals, and a frequent presenter at Paleo conferences.

Dr. Kellyann Petrucci earned her bachelor's degree from Temple University, hosted her alma mater's Department of Public Health Intern Program, and mentored students entering the health field. She earned her master's degree from St. Joseph's University and her Doctor of Chiropractic degree from Logan College of Chiropractic/University Programs, where she served as the Postgraduate Chairperson. Dr. Kellyann did postgraduate coursework in Europe. She studied Naturopathic Medicine at the College of Naturopathic Medicine, London, and she is one of the few practitioners in the United States certified in Biological Medicine by the esteemed Dr. Thomas Rau, of the Paracelsus Klinik Lustmühle, Switzerland.

In Dr. Kellyann's many years in a thriving nutritional-based practice and consulting, she's helped patients build the strongest, healthiest body possible. She learned early on that looking and feeling amazing came down to learning simple, principle food values that made astonishing differences in people's lives. She realized that deep nutrition wasn't about fancy powders, ancient elixirs, or the latest creams; it was about reprogramming the body to get back to the basics and eat the way people were designed to eat. She found the principles of living Paleo to be the key for those who want to lose weight, boost immunity, and fight aging. Dr. Kellyann has seen so much success from those eating Paleo that she feels a moral obligation to spread the message of eating real food.

Dr. Kellyann is the coauthor for the health and lifestyle book *Boosting Your Immunity For Dummies* (Wiley). She also created the successful kids' health and wellness program Superkids Wellness and developed the PaleoSmart System and International Wellness Consulting.

You can find free nutritional videos and a weekly dose of news, tips recipes, and inspiration on her website www.DrKellyann.com.

Dedication

From Melissa: I dedicate this book to my husband, Dave, for always approaching the dinner table with an open mind and an open heart; you're my favorite taste-tester. And to my parents, Tom and Roni Joulwan, thank you for letting me be weird, for teaching me how to play in the kitchen, and for proving that love and food can be happily intertwined.

From Dr. Petrucci: I dedicate this book to my boys: my husband Kevin and my little guys John and Michael. There were a lot of "no's" and "no shows" during the creation of this book, and they were always positive and did what it whatever it took to make my dreams flourish. Kevin, thanks for all of the paleo meals you created for us while in the throes of my writing. It wasn't always easy wearing so many of the household hats, and you done good! And I can't forget the eager faces of my little boys, with their bright eyes and sparkly smiles, asking me, "What page are you on now?" (every ten minutes) and saying, "Really, Mom, you're going to be in a bookstore?" You injected every tireless writing day with a burst of sunshine. I will never take for granted a single day I share with my boys! And for my parents, John and Ellie, who have always taught me that if I make value-based decisions, the world will unfold as it should, when it should. Thank you Dad for teaching me how to be an entrepreneur. And Mom, you're such a beautiful artist. Thank you times ten for always embracing and enriching my creativity. I also dedicate this book to my sister, Dr. Kathleen Petrucci, and her husband Glenn. Kathy, I respect your grit and good-spirited high energy more than you'll ever know. I love sharing the "twin syndrome" with you. I'm so glad I have you and Glenn to chew the paleo fat with! To my brothers, Joseph and John Michael, who have added so much joy and laughter to my life, thank you for forever making my life rich! And to Dr. Jennifer Bonde, who will always be my dearest friend on the planet. She may not be my biological sister, but she is a sister of the heart. I'm so glad my life's journey has you in it! Finally to Pamela and Andrew Carroll, I admire your determination to find solutions and your love of the power of paleo. I value all of our exchanges and find it heartwarming watching you skillfully sharing your passion with others.

Authors' Acknowledgments

From Melissa: First, a big hug of thanks and a sincere nod of respect to my coauthor, Dr. Kellyann, for inviting me along on this adventure. I also send deep gratitude to the readers of *The Clothes Make The Girl* for encouraging me to write *Well Fed,* which put me on the path to this book. Heartfelt thanks to Jen Sinkler, all-around excellent human and exemplary fitness model, for demonstrating the exercises and proving that strong is beautiful. And to Melissa and Dallas Hartwig of Whole9, I'm forever grateful that you taught me how to "just eat" real food so I could find my way back into the kitchen.

From Dr. Petrucci: Thank you to my talented coauthor, Melissa Joulwan, for taking a leap of faith and for all of the heart-to-hearts along the way; I respect her talents a great deal. I also feel deep gratitude and will be forever thankful to my agent, Bill Gladstone, of Waterside Productions for giving me my first "break." I'm grateful he not only believed in me, but encouraged me to roll the dice and go for it. And to Margot Hutchinson of Waterside Productions who made fantastic deals happen along the way and truly cares about my future — you're a good egg, Margot! Also, thank you to all the masterful pros at John Wiley & Sons: Acquisitions Editor Tracy Boggier, who worked like mad to shepherd and organize this title, and to the Project Editor Tim Gallan who kept the quality up, and the stress low. Thanks Tim. To Scott Frishman (a.k.a. Tell It), thank you for all of the guidance. And thanks to Rick Frishman for making the magic happen in so many of our lives. To all of the doctors, coaches, and business leaders that I have learned from in the last 30 years, your messages and inspiration will always be pieces of my life's quilt.

Publisher's Acknowledgments

We're proud of this book; please send us your comments at http://dummies.custhelp.com. For other comments, please contact our Customer Care Department within the U.S. at 877-762-2974, outside the U.S. at 317-572-3993, or fax 317-572-4002.

Some of the people who helped bring this book to market include the following:

Acquisitions, Editorial, and Vertical Websites

Senior Project Editor: Tim Gallan

Senior Acquisitions Editor: Tracy Boggier

Copy Editor: Jennette ElNaggar

Assistant Editor: David Lutton

Editorial Program Coordinator: Joe Niesen

Technical Editor: Rachel Nix

Recipe Tester: Mike Tully

Nutritional Analyst: Patti Santelli

Editorial Manager: Michelle Hacker

Editorial Assistants: Rachelle S. Amick, Alexa Koschier

Art Coordinator: Alicia B. South

Cover Photo: © Kensuke Okabayashi

Cartoons: Rich Tennant (www.the5thwave.com)

Photographer: Bob McNamara

Composition Services

Project Coordinator: Sheree Montgomery

Layout and Graphics: Jennifer Creasey, Joyce Haughey

Proofreaders: Melissa Cossell, Dwight Ramsey, Sossity R. Smith

Indexer: Riverside Indexes, Inc.

Publishing and Editorial for Consumer Dummies

    Kathleen Nebenhaus, Vice President and Executive Publisher

    David Palmer, Associate Publisher

    Kristin Ferguson-Wagstaffe, Product Development Director

Publishing for Technology Dummies

    Andy Cummings, Vice President and Publisher

Composition Services

    Debbie Stailey, Director of Composition Services

Contents at a Glance

Recipes at a Glance

Table of Contents

Introduction

· ·

You've probably heard a lot of names for what we call living Paleo: the Paleo lifestyle, the cave man diet, eating primal, and the real food diet. All these terms describe roughly the same way of eating. It's nutrition based on the idea that for optimal health, both mentally and physically, we should try to eat like our hunter-gatherer ancestors. In practical terms, that means focusing on whole foods that are processed as little as possible and avoiding foods, like grains and dairy, that cause inflammation inside your body.

When you remove inflammatory foods from your meals, you reduce your risk for diseases of civilization, such as heart disease, diabetes, and cancers. You also have more energy, look younger, lose weight, get stronger, and sleep more soundly. In short, you enjoy your life more.

Living Paleo isn't a "diet" in the traditional sense, though we do ask you to give up certain foods — sometimes just for 30 days and, in some cases, indefinitely. Although that may sound intimidating, this book shows you the reasons you should avoid certain foods for optimal health and fitness. We also provide plenty of practical tips to make the transition as easy as possible for you and your family. From how to stock your kitchen cupboards to healthy travel to reversing disease and exercising wisely, you'll find everything you need to adopt the Paleo lifestyle.

About This Book

Adopting the Paleo diet may seem overwhelming at first, so this book is organized in a way that makes the benefits of living Paleo easy to understand. We explain the foundation of Paleo principles and show you how adapting some of the lifestyle characteristics of our hunter-gatherer ancestors can vastly improve your modern quality of life.

We break down the "yes" and "no" lists of Paleo foods so you know exactly where to begin your new nutritional lifestyle, and we help you understand just how much to eat to reach your goals. Whether you're trying to lose weight, reverse a medical condition, or improve your athletic performance, this book provides the information you need to succeed.

Understanding the underlying science of the Paleo diet can help keep you on track when cravings or temptations arise, so we explain the nutritional aspects of the Paleo lifestyle and answer your questions about fiber, vitamins, minerals, supplements, and more. But living Paleo goes beyond the food that you put on your plate, so we also explore how you can learn from our cave-man ancestors to improve your sleep, enhance your playtime, and improve your fitness, while enjoying the modern conveniences that make your life easier.

If you're more interested in practical application than scientific theories, we've got you covered there, too, with chapters that outline how to revamp your kitchen for the Paleo lifestyle as well as tips for traveling — for work or pleasure — without kissing your good habits goodbye.

And finally, we include plenty of delicious, satisfying recipes to help you and your family make the transition to living Paleo. The recipes will keep you well fed from breakfast through dinner with healthy snacks in between; we also provide easy meal ideas that don't require a recipe at all to create your own Paleo-friendly "fast food"; and we even include a few dessert recipes for those special occasions when you want something a little sweeter than usual.

Conventions Used in This Book

We use the following conventions throughout the text to make things consistent and easy to understand:

- All web addresses appear in monofont.

- When this book was printed, some web addresses may have needed to break across two lines of text. If that happened, rest assured that we haven't put in any extra characters (such as hyphens) to indicate the break. So when using one of these web addresses, just type in exactly what you see in this book, pretending as though the line break doesn't exist.

- **Boldface** highlights keywords in bulleted lists and the action parts of numbered steps.

What You're Not to Read

We've written this book so you can find information easily and quickly. Each chapter covers one aspect of living Paleo and includes specific details and practical tips to help you understand how to incorporate it into your new life-style. If you don't have the time (or the desire) to read every word, you can skip the text in the sidebars, the shaded boxes you see throughout the book. They provide detailed examples or information to supplement the primary points explained in the chapters.

You don't need to read every single paragraph of this book to begin to enjoy the benefits of living Paleo. Feel free to skip around to the stuff that interests you most.

Foolish Assumptions

As we wrote this book, we made the following assumptions about you:

✔ You want to change your diet, lose weight, improve your fitness, or manage some type of medical condition and have heard about the Paleo diet.

✔ You have control over your food choices and those of your family, and you want to help your loved ones enjoy a healthy, Paleo lifestyle, too.

✔ You want to stop eating processed and unhealthy foods to feel younger, healthier, more vibrant, and happier.

✔ You're interested in learning how food affects you physically and mentally, but you don't want to get bogged down in too much scientific detail.

✔ You're open to the idea of making lifestyle changes — avoiding certain foods, making sleep a priority, adopting a fitness program — to enhance your quality of life.

How This Book Is Organized

We've divided this book into five parts to make the different topics more manageable and easier to digest. Each part deals with certain aspects of living Paleo and discusses the relevant issues, including nutrition, how to get started, fitness, social situations, shopping, travel, and recipes. You don't have to read straight through the book from cover to cover; you can pick a chapter of interest and read it to find out everything you need to know about that issue.

Part I: The Power of Paleo

Living Paleo is all about taking the advantages of the hunter-gatherer lifestyle and adapting them to your modern life. In the first chapter, we explain how living Paleo can affect your body and mind as well as dramatically change the way you look and feel. Chapter 2 addresses the "food rules" of living Paleo, and Chapter 3 provides helpful tips for getting started.

Part II: Embracing the Paleo Lifestyle

Understanding how our hunter-gatherer ancestors lived and moved is the key to revamping our modern lives to better fit our heritage. The first few chapters of this part explain Paleo nutrition as well as aspects of the cave-man lifestyle, such as adequate sleep, sun, and exercise, that contribute to higher quality of life. In Chapter 7, we explain how to give your kitchen a Paleo makeover, and Chapter 8 outlines the 30-Day Reset, which will help you jumpstart your new Paleo lifestyle.

Part III: Paleo Recipes for Success

As you understand why eating Paleo foods is the best choice for you and your family, you need new recipes to put satisfying meals on the table. This part includes a collection of delicious, comforting recipes that will fill every meal (and your stomach) with healthy, energizing foods. Along with a chapter to help you reconnect with the experience of eating, we include recipes for everyday entrees, easy one-pot meals, side dishes, sauces and seasonings, and even snacks and treats.

Part IV: Making Paleo Practical in a Modern World

We live in a world of deadlines, responsibilities, and technology that present challenges never faced by the hunter-gatherers of our history. In these chapters, we show you how to overcome common obstacles to adopting the Paleo lifestyle, including some mental roadblocks that might get in your way. In Chapters 16 and 17, you discover how to eat while dining in restaurants, traveling, and celebrating special occasions without sacrificing your Paleo habits. Chapter 18 explains how you can help your family members make the transition to living Paleo with minimum fuss and muss.

Part V: The Part of Tens

Like all *For Dummies* books, this one includes the fun and exciting Part of Tens. Here, we list ten foods to always have in the kitchen. We also show you ten no-equipment exercises you can do just about anywhere.

Icons Used in This Book

To make this book easier to navigate, we include the following icons that can help you find key information about living Paleo.

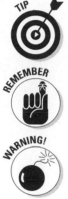

This icon indicates practical information that can help you in your quest for improved health or in your progress in adopting the Paleo lifestyle.

When you see this icon, you know that the information that follows is important enough to read twice!

This icon highlights information that could be detrimental to your success if you ignore it. We don't use this one much, so pay attention when we do.

Where to Go from Here

This book is organized to be read in the way that makes the most sense to you — feel free to jump around to the information that's most relevant to you right now. You can use the table of contents to find the broad categories of subjects or use the index to look up specific information.

Do you want to know more about the "food rules" of the Paleo diet so you can get started on the Paleo path? Start with Chapter 2. Are you ready to clean out your kitchen? Turn to Chapter 7. Worried about the nutritional aspects of living Paleo? Chapter 4 provides an in-depth look at the nutritional underpinnings of the Paleo lifestyle. Feeling hungry but want to make wise food choices? Feel free to jump right into the recipes in Chapters 10 through 14.

If you're ready to commit to the Paleo lifestyle, you may want to jump right into the 30-Day Reset by reading Chapters 3 and 8.

And if you're not sure where to begin, read Part 1. It gives you the basic information you need to understand why and how living Paleo can help you improve your health and quality of life.

Part I
The Power of Paleo

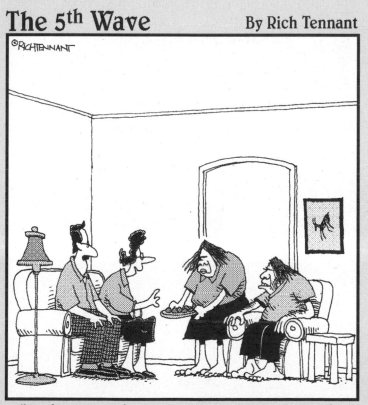

The 5th Wave   By Rich Tennant

"So how long have you been living Paleo?"

In this part . . .

In practical terms, living Paleo begins with eating a Paleo diet. In this part, we look at the "yes" and "no" foods of eating Paleo, along with the benefits of adopting some of the aspects of the hunter-gatherers' lifestyle. We take a close look at how you can gear up for living Paleo, including an overview of the 30-Day Reset that can help you jump-start your success.

Chapter 1

What Is Paleo?

In This Chapter

▶ Explaining the foundations of the Paleo diet and why it works

▶ Looking and feeling better following the Paleo lifestyle

▶ Understanding the science behind living Paleo

*P*aleo is the answer. If you've suffered with weight problems or health issues, you're in for a treat. Every aspect of your health improves when you incorporate Paleo principles into your life. Your body starts to transform right before your eyes, and, suddenly, your outlook is optimistic.

Your eyes brighten, your skin takes on a completely different sheen, and your wrinkles start to fade. You begin to shed body fat as you watch your stomach get flatter and flatter. Your muscle tone improves, your hair gets silky, your teeth seem stronger. Your mood elevates, and you begin to notice that you feel happier. Your body begins to calm, releasing anxiety and tension. You start to forget what it feels like to have aches and pains, and your entire body seems to lose the bloated feeling it's been carrying around for far too long. You begin to be more than just *present* in life; you begin to start really *living* life. For some, it's the first time in a very long time.

You'd be hard-pressed to find a more excited group of people than those who have transformed their lives to living Paleo. What you find in the pages of this book is that an easy-to-follow nutritional blueprint actually exists and works — and when you adopt this plan, everything gets easier.

In this chapter, you discover some foundational Paleo principles, including the answers to questions about how the Paleo diet came to be, the foods that make up the Paleo diet, the science behind Paleo success, and how living Paleo will soon have you looking and feeling better than ever.

Living Paleo takes you from a place of hopelessness to hope. So what are you waiting for? Dig in!

The Foundations of the Paleo Lifestyle

Living Paleo takes the mystery out of eating. It's simplicity at its finest, which is one of the reasons eating Paleo foods works well for so many. When you eat simply (but deliciously), you get results.

So many eating plans, programs, and products give you lots of rules and may even require special foods, which makes understanding these plans and staying committed to them even harder. The biggest missing element in other plans is the core ingredient for long-term success — *health*. Most programs don't move you toward health either biologically or behaviorally. If your cells aren't getting healthier and behavior is only expected to change in strict ways for the short term, the entire purpose is lost. You don't discover how to eat and live for the *rest of your life*.

Paleo is different; Paleo is based on simple, easy-to-understand nutritional principles. Eating Paleo takes away all the confusion and is natural to implement. It's something you can get on plan with and stick with for a long time.

Paleo is the abbreviation for *Paleolithic*. The Paleo diet refers to foods consumed during the Paleolithic era, the time from about 2.5 million years ago up to 10,000 BC. During this time, early man was called a *hunter-gatherer*.

A lot of people start the Paleo diet to get a killer body. And living Paleo is a great way to move toward your ideal body, but what most people experience is even more powerful. Living Paleo literally changes their lives for the better. If you've had aches and pains, fatigue, skin issues, menstrual problems, chronic inflammation, digestive complaints, weight gain, depression, fertility problems, autoimmune struggles, diabetes, or cardiovascular disease, you're going to love living Paleo.

The hormone modulating, anti-inflammatory, nutrient-dense properties of the Paleo lifestyle help regulate all the systems and functions of the body. Your body resets at a higher functioning level, so you'll not only look better eating Paleo, but you'll also feel better. Living Paleo supports the healing and prevention of many chronic diseases. And thanks to the nutrition-packed foods of the Paleo diet, you start sporting a much stronger cellular system and with that comes healing and transformation.

In the following sections, we walk you through what makes the Paleo diet a lifestyle you can follow, from looking at the foods you eat to understanding how your body was designed to live.

Enjoying foods that make up the Paleo diet

When you think Paleo foods, think grass roots — simple, back to nature, foods filled with nutrients that bring you back to life. Paleo foods are what you're *designed* to eat. They're the foods that your body digests and absorbs efficiently. Paleo foods have the most positive impact on all the structures and functions of your body.

The foundational Paleo foods include lean meats, seafood, vegetables, fruits, nuts, seeds, and naturally occurring healthy fats. Our hunter-gatherer ancestors survived on these foods. In the Paleolithic era, no industrialized foods or planting crops existed. Our ancestors didn't have access to grains, sugars, starches, legumes, dairy, processed foods, or oils — and autopsies show that they were better for it. (See Chapters 2 and 4 for details on what foods qualify as Paleo foods.) They may not have had the convenience of a one-minute meal, but our ancestors had far higher levels of health and didn't suffer from the modern-day diseases we do today.

Changes in everyday foods and in food processing have fundamentally altered modern diets. Paleo foods differ nutritionally in several ways, such as their ability to do the following:

- Balance blood sugar and keep your overall sugar load down
- Create a fatty-acid balance (omega-6 to omega-3 balance)
- Balance macronutrients (proteins, fats, and carbohydrates)
- Contain trace nutrient density (minerals)
- Promote and maintain acid-base balance (how acid and alkaline you are)
- Add robust amounts of fiber to your daily plate (for intestinal health)

The fact that modern-day foods aren't working is rather obvious. People are sicker and fatter than ever and are more confused about what to eat and how to live than in any other time in history. But living Paleo cuts through the confusion and clarifies what foods move you toward health.

When you begin eating Paleo, your body sheds all its unhealthy cells. You peel away layers of fat; you become leaner, stronger, and healthier.

Paleo success stories: Theresa

Meet Theresa, 49, Artist, Hopewell Township, New Jersey:

"I was skeptical to start Paleo because I was concerned about giving up some foods, like whole grains. I have three daughters, so it was really important to me to always have good nutrition in the house. I was so caught up in the food pyramid that I just couldn't believe it was wrong. However, the stories I heard about the success with Paleo were so compelling, I decided to give it a try for just a month. I was surprised how good I felt! I decided to keep eating Paleo because I felt so good (and lost 4 inches around my waist)!

"About 6 months later, I went to my doctor for my annual physical and had my blood work done. I always had excellent blood work results. I was so happy it was exactly the same — all good! The big surprise came, though, when my doctor asked me how my reflux and stomach pains were. Well, I had *completely* forgotten about them because they disappeared once I started eating Paleo. It's still hard for me to get my head around the fact the food pyramid wasn't the nutritional bible I thought it was. The best part of making the switch is that my daughters now pay attention to how food makes them feel after they eat, and they now make healthy choices on their own."

Taking a cue from our ancestors

Our bodies haven't changed much since before agricultural society. Our body's needs now are similar to what they were during Paleolithic times, before the dawn of agriculture.

Humans are shaped and molded by over a hundred thousand generations. What our bodies were designed to eat then, we're designed to eat now. In other words, our genes are still stuck in the hunter-gatherer's time, even though we're living in the modern world. Our genes simply haven't caught up to the modern-day divergence.

So how did our ancestors live? They enjoyed a balanced life of working, playing, relaxing, and worshipping. The men hunted, and the women cared for the children and gathered berries. Families lived close together in bands and enjoyed the relaxation of the evening as the meat the men hunted hung on tree branches. The kids laughed, played, and sang by the fire, and adults enjoyed conversation as they made plans for the next day. They felt closeness to one another and everyone had purpose. Despite their real life stresses, they were happy, healthy people.

About 10,000 years ago, the birth of *agriculture* changed the way people lived. Hunter-gatherers became attracted to a new way of life based on a routine and settled existence that centered around agriculture and the breeding of animals.

The tidal wave of change happened again a few hundred years ago with the *Industrial Revolution*. The impact that this technological progress has had on human biology is huge. Some of these advancements have provided safety and convenience; we can all agree those things are mostly good. But some of these man-made environmental changes have caused a pandemic of human suffering and disease that was unknown to our ancestors.

Autopsies show that the hunter-gatherers were some of the healthiest people to walk the earth. Using their lifestyle as our template, we can strike a balance between modern-day living and our grass-roots beginning.

Living the way we were designed

If you've tried other eating plans and haven't been successful long term or if you've been trying to get well and are making little headway, you're probably carrying the wrong road map. Here's why: The missing link is probably that you're not eating the foods that you're *designed* to eat.

Our genes have changed very little since Paleolithic times. In fact, according to medical anthropologist S. Boyd Eaton, MD, 99.99 percent of our genes were formed before the development of agriculture. This is big. That means that our hunter-gatherer ancestors programmed our genes. How they ate is our nutritional blueprint, how they moved is the blueprint for our physiology, and how they lived is the blueprint for the lifestyle we should strive to lead.

The death of a cave man

Okay, you may be thinking that these hunter-gatherers were healthy, but didn't cave men (hunter-gatherers) die too young to get the diseases we do today? And if they died so young, were they really that healthy in the first place?

Our ancestors did die earlier than we do *on average,* but they died of problems that we have since found solutions to handle. They died mainly of infection, trauma, and complications in childbirth. In fact, the average is kind of marred because of the large number of infant mortality rates. Many hunter-gatherers actually did have life spans into their 70s, which is close to modern-day expectancies.

When our ancestors died, it wasn't because of the ailments — heart disease, cancer, diabetes, and a host of other degenerative diseases — that plague us today. In our culture today, even young kids are showing signs of degenerative diseases and are suffering with diabetes at astounding rates.

There's no denying that despite our modern medical advances, our ancestors died from more emergent causes, while our current culture dies from more lifestyle-related, degenerative diseases. We can definitely learn something from our remarkable ancestors, and using some aspects of their life is a road map that works!

We don't need to live life as a science experiment, trying to reenact everything our ancestors did or see the world through Paleo goggles. We just need to understand how our genes were programmed and try to model that as close as we can. When you model the Paleo lifestyle, your struggles will be over.

As humans, our bodies are the result of an optimal design shaped and molded by nature. To look and feel your absolute best, you have to do what your body is designed to do. *Living Paleo For Dummies* is your reference guide to show you how to live according to your nature.

Understanding that Paleo is a lifestyle, not a diet

Living Paleo is about getting you healthy. When your cells are healthy, everything falls into place. You feel better, look better, and lose weight. What makes Paleo different than everything else is that the nutrient-dense foods are just one piece of the puzzle. The way you live *outside* of the kitchen has as much to do with how you look and feel as the foods you eat.

Traditional diets provide food rules, and that's where they end. You follow the rules, hope to get results, and hope that the results stick. This pattern is often the recipe for disappointment and frustration because eventually the rules stop, and your life takes over. You haven't made lifestyle changes that carry the lasting results.

A good analogy is trying to learn a new language. If you approach the new language by just trying to learn the rules for pronunciation and grammar, the language is difficult to learn and challenging to make it stick. If, however, you immerse yourself into the lifestyle and culture, learning the language takes on a whole new energy. You learn quicker, and it becomes more meaningful, so it sticks. Living Paleo immerses you in healthy living beyond just food, so it becomes meaningful, long-lasting, and very effective.

Paleo considers why you eat, when you eat, how you eat, and other factors in your life that influence how you feel, such as amount and quality of sleep, stress levels, sunlight, movement, supplementation, and your thoughts (see Chapter 5). It's a lifelong change that's fairly simple to make and has lasting, positive consequences, unlike a diet that's meant as a short-term solution to lose a few pounds, which ultimately leads to frustration and hopelessness.

In the end, your habits and patterns are responsible for how you look and feel. Living Paleo gives you the lifestyle patterns and strategies that go well beyond a flash-in-the-pan diet. You figure out how to make the lifestyle changes that have lasting, positive effects.

Paleo success stories: Sarah

Meet Sarah, 42, Business Owner, Pennington, New Jersey:

Sarah knows busy. She's a mother of two; she and her husband own an information technology business with offices in New York City and Princeton, New Jersey. Between the travel, her family commitments, business commitments, and everything else required by a mom with a career, Sarah's life is pretty intense. Her busy life caused her to eat a lot of grab-and-go convenience foods. When she started having terrible digestive issues that grew worse, became plagued with headaches,

felt sluggish, and was gaining weight, she knew something had to change. She found Paleo.

Sarah felt changes immediately. Within days, her bloating disappeared. To her total delight, the intestinal discomfort that was almost debilitating disappeared. Her skin improved, her energy picked up, and she felt like a new person. Sarah says, "I can't say enough about Paleo. It has completely changed my life. I feel better and look better in my 40s than I ever have. If you're suffering with anything, you owe it to yourself to give Paleo a try."

Genetically, you can live for 120 years. The key is creating healthy lifestyle patterns so your body expresses health and vitality and doesn't express disease or obesity. That's what living Paleo is all about.

Here are some of the lifestyle patterns of living Paleo (we include chapter references in parentheses where you can find out more):

- Putting real foods first (Chapters 2 and 4)
- Supporting yourself with nutritional supplementation when you need the boost and avoiding supplementing when you don't need to (Chapter 4)
- Getting sleep that matters (Chapter 5)
- Reaping the benefits of sunlight (Chapter 5)
- Managing stress effectively (Chapter 5)
- Living healthy in a toxic world (Chapter 5)
- Moving in a way that creates a powerful strong body that fights aging and disease (Chapter 6)
- Understanding and embracing the wellness paradigm (Chapter 5)
- Creating thoughts that serve you (Chapter 3)
- Contributing to feeling a sense of purpose (Chapter 5)
- Developing skills to handle setbacks or roadblocks along the way (Chapter 15)

The Prescription for Modern Ailments

Modern-day ailments have become pandemic. Everyone knows someone who's wrestling with diabetes, cancer, or autoimmune diseases. To be in one's 60s and not be on medication is remarkable. Even worse, the diagnosis of chronic childhood diseases has almost quadrupled over the past four decades.

Think about it. With all the modern drugs and all the surgeries, we're not getting any better. You can't possibly look at the data on our supposed healthcare care model and think that what we're doing is working. In fact, in a two-part series published in the *Annals of Internal Medicine,* Dr. Elliot Fisher, professor of medicine at Dartmouth University, came to the following conclusion: "Our study suggests that perhaps ⅓ of medical spending is now devoted to services that don't appear to improve health or quality of care — and may makes things worse."

What that means is staggering. Here's some perspective: We're spending annually about $1.4 trillion on healthcare a year that's proven to be ineffective! So that's $4 billion per day down the drain! Then there's the issue of not only having ineffective treatments but also having adverse effects from the treatments. Either way you look at it, *it's not the answer.*

So the question becomes, what *is* the answer? How do we get well and stay well? By understanding how we really got into this mess in the first place. We're not sick because of bad genes or rotten luck. Most of our modern-day ailments were born out of *bad choices.* If we want to get well and stay well and avoid the circus of healthcare, we have to get in the right paradigm and learn to make *smart choices.*

Putting real food first, like eating Paleo foods that you're designed to eat, is one of the smartest things you'll ever do to get well and stay well. The following sections explore other benefits of living Paleo.

Losing weight on the Paleo diet

If your goal is to lose weight, you've come to the right place. When you eat Paleo, your body naturally loses body fat until you've reached your ideal weight. When you get healthy, everything in your body recalibrates, including your weight. What's so great about eating Paleo is that you lose stored fat because you're actually using that stored fat for energy. Your body transforms in a way it may never have before, and you begin to look — and feel — lean and toned.

Here are some of the reasons you lose weight by eating Paleo:

- ✔ You're eating foods with a high-nutrient density without all the garbage calories.
- ✔ You lose the bloat (dump excess water retention).
- ✔ You reduce food sensitivities.
- ✔ You eat foods that help you maintain a healthy blood sugar.
- ✔ You eat foods that regulate your hormones along with the signals associated with hormones.
- ✔ You burn stored fat, thanks to the proteins and fat in the food you eat.
- ✔ You feel more satiated because of the healthy fats you're eating.
- ✔ You eat nutrient-dense foods, creating healthy cells, and weight loss is a natural byproduct.
- ✔ You have more energy eating Paleo, so you tend to move more and have more efficient workouts.
- ✔ You use stored fat for energy instead of sugary carbohydrates, which is a more efficient fat-burning pathway.
- ✔ You eat foods with a high fiber content, which encourages weight loss.

Living Paleo is about getting you to optimal health and keeping you there. The weight loss is a wonderful bonus!

Clearing up gut and skin issues

Eating Paleo is like an internal spring cleaning. You feel healthy from the inside out. All the grains, sugars, starches, legumes, and poorly prepared, processed, and denatured foods have created havoc in your intestines. Over time, this means inflammation and *leaky gut.*

What is leaky gut? Well, as you may have guessed, *gut* refers to your intestines, which are this incredible 25-feet tubular structure that has such an important role in your body. Your intestines pull the good stuff out of your foods (nutrients) to ensure that all the structures and functions of your body are working. It's also where about 80 percent of your immunity is stationed.

Here's where the *leaky* part fits in. Your intestinal walls are lined with these armed guards (immune cells). As long as these cells and good bacteria are there lying over your intestines, you're good to go. Nothing can get in or out.

Your body is in a health lockdown. Now, when your gut becomes damaged or perforated by the inflammation caused by the foods you eat or the medications you take, it becomes leaky and porous — *intestinal permeability.* The structures of the intestines become damaged, and your armed guards are killed in action. You can't absorb your nutrients the same. Undigested food and bacteria flow into your body where they don't belong and aren't recognized. When undigested food and bacteria flows into your bloodstream, your body screams "attack!" like it would with any foreign invader. Your body literally attacks itself instead of protecting itself, as it's designed to do, and you get autoimmune problems, chronic disease, unexplained fatigue, intestinal distress, and hypersensitivities. Not a whole lotta fun.

Those tiny little porous holes can certainly do a lot of rebel raising! Interestingly enough, a damaged gut causes skin problems as well. A direct link exists between intestinal health and the health of your skin. If you have acne, rashes, eczema, psoriasis, or poor skin tone, a leaky gut may be the culprit. If you want beautiful skin, it's an inside job, and it starts with putting real food first.

The upside here is a leaky gut isn't hard to fix. It's completely reversible, and when eating Paleo foods, you're well on your way!

Getting a good night's sleep

One of the most motivating factors to give Paleo a spin is the improvement to your sleep cycle. After you're adjusted to Paleo and you've hit your Paleo stride, you'll find your sleep is deeper and more restful.

For a lot of people, quality sleep is hard to come by. Maybe you have trouble falling asleep or you wake in the middle of the night, unable to drift back to sleep. Either way, eating Paleo completely changes the quality and duration of your sleep.

Got bacteria?

Your gut is filled with bacteria. They key is to make sure the bacteria you're carrying around in your intestines are mostly healthy, "good" bacteria. You need these bacteria as a protective guard. Many modern-day foods lack nutrients and fiber, are filled with toxins, and are lacking these healthy bacteria (probiotics). Because of depleted soil from poor farming practices, a high consumption of denatured foods, and poor food choices (not eating fruits and vegetables), we consume much less of this bacteria than our ancestors did, which is unfortunate because these bacteria are helpful to our immune system, prevent pathogens (bad bacteria) from colonizing, and provide nutrients for your intestines. Another reason Paleo foods are healthy for your long-term well-being: Paleo foods provide the nutrition and healing so these healthy bacteria keep hanging round.

Here are some of the reasons you sleep like a baby when you start living Paleo:

- ✔ You're getting foods loaded with minerals, which are grounding and calming to your body.

- ✔ When your blood sugars are more balanced, like they are with Paleo foods, you don't get that blood sugar dip in the middle of the night, causing your body to release hormones to restore blood sugar, which disturbs sleep.

- ✔ A lot of Paleo foods contain B vitamins, which are great for calming nerves and balancing the nervous system for restful sleep.

- ✔ Some Paleo foods, like eggs, turkey, nuts, fish, and some fruits, contain an essential amino acid called *tryptophan,* which helps promote sleep.

- ✔ When eating Paleo, your body naturally regulates hormones and signals associated with hormones that, in turn, help you sleep better.

- ✔ When you create healthy cells like you do when eating Paleo, all the systems and functions in your body run smoother, including sleep cycles.

- ✔ You have more energy eating Paleo so you run your battery down naturally with activity, rather than with sugary foods and carbohydrate crashes, leading to more restful sleep.

Sleep is no joke. You discover how important it is to your health and your weight in Chapter 5.

If you have sleep issues, let Paleo be your all-natural sleep aide. It works — and there's no nasty side effects!

Stabilizing blood sugar

What may be most astonishing about eating Paleo is its powerful ability to manage blood sugar, which is one of the most compelling and worthwhile reasons to make the switch. In Chapters 3 and 8, we discuss how important managing your blood sugar really is in all areas of your health and well-being. Managing blood sugar is essential to how it relates to disease, your energy levels, and how youthful you look and feel.

People with diabetes or pre-diabetes or who feel a little out of kilter with their blood sugar benefit tremendously when eating Paleo. By eating mainly non-starchy vegetables and fruit with minimal starchy food altogether, you can dramatically lower blood sugar load. Lean proteins and healthy fats round out the Paleo diet to even further control blood sugar.

High blood sugars are a thing of the past when eating Paleo. Work with a healthcare provider who knows you and your situation and prepare to be amazed!

Paleo success stories: Drew

Meet Drew, 56, Horticulturist, Bensalem, Pennsylvania:

Drew has been happily married for 32 years, and he and his wife raised three great kids. Drew loves his life, and you'll often find him working happily in his garden or coaching his basketball team. There was just one problem: Drew's blood sugars were creeping up at an alarming rate. His wife, a seasoned nurse, was beside herself with concern. They would have tried anything. Thank goodness they tried Paleo.

Before Drew started eating Paleo, his blood sugar reached an all-time high of 358! In just four months of eating a 100 percent Paleo diet, his blood sugar plummeted to an amazing 90 to 100 range. Drew is one of the most excited and amazed Paleo people you'll ever meet. This is where great support comes in because his wife was very much involved in creating great Paleo foods and being there in any way she could. The end result was amazement to Drew's family physician, his family, and his friends.

Reducing chronic inflammation

When you think inflammation, you probably think "ouch!" Because the inflammation you've probably heard about or experienced firsthand is the kind of inflammation that makes you feel all-over aches, pains, swelling, fatigue, or just plain discomfort.

One kind of inflammation is actually a good thing; it's called *acute inflammation*, or short-term inflammation. This inflammation is a natural part of your body's healing process and one of the "trump cards" your body hands out to give you a healing push. When you get an illness, like the flu, or physical trauma, like a shoulder injury, your body starts going into action immediately by calling on your immune system for healing. The inflammation that ensues is there to protect the damage already done and make sure it doesn't get any worse.

So how does this good thing (your healing push) get out of hand and cause you trouble? If your intestines have those pesky little perforations that we call leaky gut (see earlier section "Clearing up gut and skin issues"), foods are going to squeak through the holes to the other side of your intestinal wall into your bloodstream where they don't belong and aren't recognized. When your body goes into overdrive to fight off these foreign invaders, you have chronic inflammation.

Whatever overloads your immune system can cause this overreaction and inflammation. Here are some of the immune system stressors:

- Unhealthy foods (packaged, processed, or foods denatured in any way)
- Foods containing gluten
- Toxic overload (everything from environmental toxins to toxic cleaning products)
- Excessive stress
- Overload of medications or antibiotics
- Sleep deprivation
- Too much exercise training

You can see from this list that many of these immune stressors are lifestyle choices, including the foods you eat. When you eat Paleo foods, you make a huge difference in _controlling_ and _preventing_ the long-term inflammation that can lead to a lot of misery.

Here are some of the conditions that are caused by chronic inflammation:

- Arthritis
- Asthma and allergies
- Autoimmune diseases, like celiac disease
- Cardiovascular disease
- Diabetes
- Intestinal inflammatory disease, like Crohn's disease
- Thyroid dysfunction

Eating Paleo does an outstanding job at keeping your immune system strong and inflammation at bay. You can see how important eating the anti-inflammatory Paleo foods really are!

Why Start Paleo Living?

Most people are intrigued when they're introduced to Paleo. It's hard not to be when you see so many people enthused and getting results. When you see or hear from friends and family or read about how you can lose weight, clear up skin issues, get better sleep, stabilize blood sugar, reduce chronic inflammation, and literally de-age, you pay attention!

Paleo success stories: Kathleen

Meet Kathleen, 42, Business Owner, Yardley, Pennsylvania:

"The results I got when I first started eating Paleo amazed me. I thought I ate pretty healthy. I have always exercised, and I buy all my foods from a natural foods store. But I always felt tired and bloated, which would get worse as the day went on. I was like that for so long, I thought it was 'the norm.' Certainly not related to my food, because all my foods were supposed to be healthy. Well, I guess they weren't for me because immediately after one Paleo meal, I knew something was different. I got no bloating whatsoever, and I felt energized instead of tired. My bowel movements went from looking like little pebbles to a healthy formed stool, and my stomach felt like it was getting flatter and flatter with every meal. I definitely got results immediately, like someone gave me some kind of secret formula or something! I will never eat any other way; I feel too good!"

But, like anything else, when you start something from scratch, you may be skeptical. Living Paleo will not only make you healthier and leaner in the long term, but you'll feel immediate results that back it up.

Look and feel better within 24 hours

Sounds too good to be true, we know. But some people feel better immediately after starting to eat Paleo foods. If you're eating a lot of foods that are inflammatory to your system or if you've been depleted in nutrients, you may perk up immediately.

One of the most common complaints people have is bloating or intestinal discomfort after eating. Switching to Paleo will give you the *wow!* effect. You'll find relief — some will feel it immediately. Eating Paleo is such a perfectly suited balanced diet that many people feel better after one meal!

Lose weight through good health, not fads and get-slim-quick schemes

Paleo isn't a fad diet, red carpet diet, or a slim-down-quick system. Paleo focuses completely and utterly on the health of your cells and all the structures and functions of your body. That's it. Weight loss just so happens to be a side effect of health and vitality — it's against natural law not to be. So what you're getting with Paleo is a side effect bonus of sorts, which just so happens to be fat melting away for lasting weight loss. With Paleo, all your systems regulate, balance, recalibrate, and begin to work at a higher functioning level, which all promote weight loss.

Many of the weight loss programs or products on the market have just a single-minded goal, which is to get the weight off. Period. Unfortunately, this goal often means poor-quality foods are recommended as part of the plan, with short-term results. You don't change the relationship you have with foods, so you don't really learn anything moving forward. Also, if you're not eating real, clean, balanced foods, you're not resetting your body for success.

When your focus is on getting healthy and staying healthy, like with eating Paleo, you lose weight naturally. And just watch your body de-age!

The Science Behind Paleo

Yes, the excitement and results of living Paleo are awesome. But knowing that some of the most respected leaders in the field, as well as some of the most brilliant researchers, have found evidence to why Paleo foods work well is a great reassurance. So just in case raving fans aren't enough, we include some research in this section to help you further see the value of living Paleo.

Here are some facts from leading Paleolithic researchers S. Boyd Eaton, MD, and M. Konner, PhD, cited in the *New England Journal of Medicine* ("Paleolithic nutrition: a consideration of its nature and current implications." 1985: N. Eng. J. Med. 321, 283–289):

- ✔ "The human genetic constitution has changed relatively little in the past 40,000 years."

- ✔ "The development of agriculture 10,000 years ago has had a minimal influence on our genes."

- ✔ "The Industrial Revolution, agribusiness, and modern food processing techniques have occurred too recently to have any evolutionary effect at all."

- ✔ "Physicians and nutritionists are increasingly convinced that the dietary habits adopted by Western society over the past 100 years make an important etiologic contribution to coronary heart disease, hypertension, diabetes, and some types of cancer."

- ✔ "These conditions have emerged as dominant health problems only in the past century and are virtually unknown among the few surviving hunter-gatherer populations whose way of life and eating habits most closely resemble pre-agricultural human beings."

Here's some compelling research from Dr. Loren Cordain (*The Paleo Diet* [Wiley]), professor in the Health and Exercise Science Department at Colorado State University and one of the top global researchers in the area of evolutionary medicine:

- ✔ "DNA evidence shows genetically humans have hardly changed at all (to be specific, the human genome has changed less than 0.02% in 40,000 years)."

- ✔ "Nature determined what our bodies needed thousands of years before civilization developed, before people started farming and raising livestock."

- ✔ "In other words, built into our genes is a blueprint for optimal nutrition — a plan that spells out the foods that make us healthy, lean and fit." (The *blueprint* is Paleo foods.)

Finally, Rainer J Klement and Ulrike Kämmerer discuss the striking benefits and prevention of cancer with a Paleo diet in *Nutrition & Metabolism* ("Is there a role for carbohydrate restriction in the treatment and prevention of cancer." October 2011. 8[75]):

- ✔ "Cancer is *very* rare among uncivilized hunter-gatherer societies."

- ✔ "The switch from the 'caveman's diet' consisting of fat, meat, occasionally roots, berries and other sources of carbohydrates to a nutrition dominated by easily digested carbohydrates derived mainly from grains as a staple food, would have occurred too recently to induce major adoptions in our gene encoding and metabolic pathways." (In other words, our bodies don't have the genetic wiring for adapting to grains.)

- ✔ "[In a cave man–like diet,] carbohydrate restriction is not only limited to avoiding sugar and other high glucose foods, but also to a reduced intake of grains. Grains can induce inflammation in susceptible individuals due to their content of omega-6 fatty acids, lectins, and gluten."

- ✔ "Paleolithic-type diets, that by definition exclude grain products, have been shown to improve glycemic control and cardiovascular risk factors more effectively than typically recommended low-fat diets rich in whole grains. These diets are not necessarily low carbohydrate diets, but focus on replacing high glycemic index modern foods with fruits and vegetables, in this way reducing the total glycemic [sugar] load. *This brings us back to our initial perception of cancer as a disease of civilization that has been rare among hunter-gatherer societies until they adopted our western lifestyle.*"

Many anthropologists and healthcare providers recognize that the hunter-gatherers represent a *reference standard* for modern-day nutrition and a model way of eating to get well and stay well. When you see the results *and* the research, you begin to understand why.

Chapter 2

Modern Foods and Your Inner Cave Man

*Y*ou're about to realize that the Paleo diet — with the throwback name and cave-man roots — is far more natural, easy to follow, and delicious than you may at first imagine. Paleo eating is all about *enjoying* natural foods. So forget about feeling like you're on a diet or focusing on giving up favorite foods, because when you make the transition to the Paleo diet, something kind of magical happens.

This chapter is devoted to helping you clear the clutter and confusion about how and what to eat on the Paleo plan. You figure out which foods are Paleo-approved and which ones need to be banished from your kitchen — but in exchange for the ones taken away, you get the green light on some surprisingly healthful foods that you can include in your everyday diet. In this chapter, you also discover how to build your perfect Paleo plate and see how Paleo-approved foods can make you more energetic, help you think more clearly, and make you feel better than ever.

Getting Familiar with the "Yes" and "No" Foods of the Paleo Diet

Eating Paleo is a lifestyle approach to nutrition, not a short-term diet. Although eating Paleo will help you lose weight and will increase your muscle mass, both of which lead to a leaner physique, the Paleo "diet" is about even more than that. Before you can enjoy all the benefits of the Paleo diet, though, you have to understand a few Paleo-food rules.

The "yes" and "no" lists for Paleo eating include foods that help you with two major accomplishments: reducing inflammation inside your body and slaying the sugar demon that can trick you into making poor food choices, which can make you overweight and undernourished as well as leave you tired, cranky, and craving more sugar.

In Chapter 4, we discuss all the nutritional aspects of Paleo-approved foods. In the following sections, we fill you in on the foods that will make up the majority of your meals (and those you should leave out) so you can see right now that eating Paleo isn't about deprivation or denial; Paleo eating is really about feeding your body and mind with real, whole foods that supply essential building blocks, energy, vitamins, and minerals.

We start with the good news — the Paleo "yes" list.

100% Paleo-approved: Checking out the Paleo "yes" list

The Paleo "yes" list is made up of nutrient-dense foods — proteins, vegetables, fruits, and fats — that any human, at any time in human history, would recognize as food. With these four basic nutrients, outlined in the following sections, you can power your body with all the healthy fats, vitamins, and minerals it needs to be lean, strong, and healthy. To kick these Paleo foods up a notch, we provide some staples and pantry items that make preparing Paleo foods easy, fun, versatile, and absolutely delicious. We also clue you in on some Paleo-approved drinks that will keep you healthy and keep the sugar demon away.

Powerful Paleo proteins

The Paleo diet focuses on animal proteins from high-quality sources. Surely, you'll find a lot of your favorites on this list:

- Beef
- Bison
- Chicken
- Duck
- Eggs
- Elk
- Fish

- Goat
- Lamb
- Nitrite- and gluten-free deli meats
- Nitrite- and gluten-free sausages
- Organ meats
- Pork
- Pheasant

- Quail
- Shellfish
- Turkey

- Veal
- Venison
- Wild boar

Nutrient-rich vegetables

A rainbow of vegetables makes your plate look appetizing and packs a major nutritional punch. Eat at least two servings of the following vegetables at every meal, and enjoy as much variety as possible:

- Artichoke
- Arugula
- Asparagus
- Beets
- Bell peppers
- Bok choy
- Broccoli
- Brussels sprouts
- Cabbage
- Carrots
- Cauliflower
- Celery
- Chile peppers
- Cucumber
- Eggplant
- Endive
- Escarole
- Garlic
- Greens (beet, collard, mustard, and turnip)
- Green beans
- Kale
- Kohlrabi

- Leeks
- Lettuce (all types)
- Mushrooms
- Nori (seaweed)
- Okra
- Onion
- Parsnip
- Pumpkin
- Radish
- Shallots
- Snow peas
- Spaghetti squash
- Spinach
- Sugar snap peas
- Summer squash (zucchini, yellow summer squash, crookneck, marrows, straightneck, scallop, and cocozelles)
- Sweet potatoes/yams
- Tomatoes
- Tomatillos
- Turnips
- Winter squash (butternut and acorn)

Satisfyingly sweet fruits

Fruit delivers its nutrition with a side serving of sweetness, so vegetables should always be the first produce priority — but one or two servings of fruit per day are satisfying and nutritious; choose any from the following list. As your body becomes balanced and your internal environment becomes cleaner and stronger, you may be able to add more fruit, but at the beginning of your transition to Paleo, sticking to one or two servings is your best strategy.

Limit your consumption of dried fruit; it's easy to overeat and lacks the nutrition of fresh fruits, while concentrating the sugars. Fruit juice should also be avoided because it provides all the sugar of the fruit, without the fiber and satiety of eating.

- Apple
- Apricot
- Banana
- Blackberries
- Blueberries
- Cantaloupe
- Cherries
- Clementine
- Cranberries
- Date
- Fig
- Grapefruit
- Grapes
- Honeydew
- Kiwi
- Kumquat
- Lemon
- Lime
- Lychee
- Mandarin
- Mango
- Nectarine
- Orange
- Papaya
- Peach
- Pear
- Pineapple
- Plum
- Pomegranate
- Raspberries
- Strawberries
- Tangerine
- Watermelon

Tasty essential fats

Fats ensure that you feel satisfied after a meal and are vital to the function of your body and brain — plus they taste really, really good. So go ahead and eat some of the following healthy fats with every meal to ensure proper absorption of nutrients and to please your taste buds.

> ✔ Avocado
>
> ✔ Clarified butter (organic, grass-fed only)
>
> ✔ Coconut (butter, fresh, flakes, oil, and milk)
>
> ✔ Nuts and nut butters (almonds, Brazil nuts, cashews, chestnuts, hazelnuts, macadamia nuts, pecans, pistachios, and walnuts)
>
> ✔ Olives and olive oil
>
> ✔ Seeds (pumpkin, sesame, sunflower, and pine nuts)

Pantry powerhouses for extra flavor

Herbs and spices add zing to your meals and can take you on a world tour of cuisines. All herbs and spices are Paleo-approved; just be sure to check labels for problematic ingredients — you want *pure* spices and extracts with no added sugars or chemicals. (See more on deciphering labels in Chapter 7.)

Here are more Paleo-approved goodies to keep in your pantry (we share details for how to stock your Paleo-friendly kitchen in Chapter 7):

> ✔ Almond meal
>
> ✔ Broth and stock (beef, chicken, seafood, and vegetable)
>
> ✔ Canned tomatoes and tomato paste
>
> ✔ Coconut aminos (replacement for soy sauce)
>
> ✔ Coconut flour
>
> ✔ Curry paste

Paleo-approved liquids for hydration

Wouldn't you prefer to eat your calories in delicious food rather than mindlessly drink them in a sugary beverage? Drinks like sodas, sports drinks, and fruit juices are basically liquid carbohydrates in a bottle. You can unknowingly take in 20 teaspoons of sugar and 300 calories without even thinking about it! And packaged drinks almost always include artificial sweeteners and chemical additives that do you no favors.

Here's the "yes" list of Paleo-approved drinks:

> ✔ Water (preferably filtered)
>
> ✔ Black coffee
>
> ✔ Tea (black, herbal, green, and white — check labels for added sugars)

Paleo no-nos: Watching out for foods on the "no" list

Now that you've had a look at the lengthy list of foods you *can* enjoy, it's time to swallow the potentially bad news of the "no" list. You may find some of your favorites on this list, but in Chapter 4, you discover why we believe these foods are harmful to your health and well-being.

The foods on the "no" list can wreak havoc on your health and sabotage your weight-loss goals. They create hormonal imbalances, trigger inflammation, and make you age more quickly.

Say "goodbye" to grains and gluten

Grains contain toxic *antinutrients* — substances that prevent your body from absorbing the nutrients it needs and that create autoimmune and digestive irritation — and inflammatory proteins like gluten. They damage your gut lining and cause irritation throughout the body. Many of these grains also cause the body to release insulin, which triggers fat storage. Grains are not only nutritionally unnecessary but even downright harmful. For many people, they're also problematic for their high carbohydrate content, but even fans of healthier starches generally recommend eating starchy tubers like sweet potatoes rather than grains.

In a paper published in *The American Journal of Clinical Nutrition* in 2005, Dr. Loren Cordain examined 13 nutrients most lacking in the diet . He then ranked seven food groups — whole grains, milk, fruits, vegetables, seafood, lean meats, and nuts/seeds — for each of these 13 vitamins and minerals in 100-calorie samples. He ranked the food 7 to 1, where 7 was the most nutrient-dense and 1 was the lowest. He summed up all the ranked scores to determine the most nutrient-dense foods.

Fresh vegetables were a clear winner, followed by seafood, lean meats, and fruits. Whole grains and milk came in last. Therefore, whenever you choose grains rather than these other foods, your vitamin and mineral content is actually lowered. (For more research, check out Dr. Cordain's website at www.thepaleodiet.com.)

Clearly, our diets don't need grains to be healthy or to provide us with the nutrients we need. Better, more efficient ways exist. So all grains — and the baked goods, flours, and pastas made from them — are at the top of the "no" list.

- ✔ Amaranth
- ✔ Barley
- ✔ Buckwheat
- ✔ Bulgur
- ✔ Corn
- ✔ Millet
- ✔ Oats
- ✔ Quinoa

- Rice
- Rye
- Sorghum
- Spelt
- Teff
- Wheat

Pitch the processed foods

Foods that come in brightly colored boxes or crinkly, vacuum-sealed bags are generally not Paleo-approved. Candy, baked goods, junk food, and prepackaged meals are usually loaded with chemicals, additives, sugar, and other ingredients you'll find on the Paleo "no" list. Eating Paleo means eating real, natural food, so foods produced in a lab or a factory are out.

Let go of the legumes

Although beans have a reputation for being healthful, they contain many of the same antinutrients that grains do. Even with pre-soaking, sprouting, or fermenting, beans are a high-carbohydrate food that triggers insulin release and are difficult for your body to digest. Keep away from the following legumes:

- Black beans
- Broad beans
- Garbanzo beans (chickpeas)
- Lentils
- Lima beans
- Mung beans
- Navy beans
- Peanuts and peanut butter
- Peas
- Pinto beans
- Soybeans, including tofu, tempeh, natto, soy sauce, miso, edamame, and soy milk
- White beans

Snow peas, sugar snap peas, and green beans are the exception to the no-beans rule because those vegetables are green and are more pod than pea.

Ditch the dairy

We humans are the only species that drink the milk of another animal, and we're the only species that continue to drink milk past the weaning period. Cow's milk is designed to help calves grow quickly so they can sprint away from predators, not for humans to consume throughout their lives. In addition, processed cow's milk contains growth hormones, bacteria, and antibiotics and also produces a strong insulin response. Paleo practitioners don't "got milk." The following dairy products are on the Paleo "no" list:

- Cheese
- Cream
- Half-and-half

- ✔ Milk
- ✔ Sour cream
- ✔ Yogurt

One exception to the no-dairy rule is clarified butter from a cow that's organically and grass-fed. This type of butter is an excellent source of healthy fat. (See Chapter 14 for instructions on clarifying butter.)

Wipe out white potatoes

White potatoes are like the useless, black sheep of the vegetable family, and they deserve a shady reputation. Because of their high sugar and starch content, they produce a big insulin response, and they also contain antinutrients that can cause intestinal distress. Be extra careful not to eat potatoes that appear to be turning green because it's an indication of an increased level of *solanine* and *chaconine*. These substances occur in nature to ward off insects, disease, and predators by making the food bitter, which also makes them toxic to you. So if your potatoes taste bitter or are starting to turn green, definitely take them off the menu!

Say "no" to added sugar

Eliminating all sugar from your diet is impossible. After all, the carbohydrates in healthy vegetables and fruits are, essentially, sugar. For optimal health and weight loss, you need to eliminate *added* sugars from your diet, including sugar in all its (deliciously sweet) forms and artificial sweeteners, such as the following:

- ✔ Agave
- ✔ All other packaged, boxed, or packets of artificial sugars
- ✔ Aspartame (NutraSweet or Equal)
- ✔ Brown sugar
- ✔ Corn syrup
- ✔ High-fructose corn syrup
- ✔ Maltodextrin
- ✔ Maple syrup
- ✔ Molasses
- ✔ Raw sugar
- ✔ Rice syrup
- ✔ Sucralose (Splenda)
- ✔ Sugar cane
- ✔ Stevia
- ✔ White sugar

Sugar is sugar is sugar, but after your 30-Day Reset (see Chapter 3), you can enjoy organic, raw honey from time to time. All types of sugar, including high-quality honey, produce an insulin response in your body. But once in a while, a little honey can be a sweet treat as part of a healthy Paleo diet.

Ignore the industrial and seed oils

These oils are often billed as "healthy," but they're not naturally occurring fats, so they require significant processing to become edible. They're prone to turning rancid and creating free radicals in your body, making them very inflammatory.

- Canola oil
- Corn oil
- Cottonseed oil
- Margarine
- Palm kernel oil
- Partially hydrogenated oil
- Peanut oil
- Safflower oil
- Soybean oil
- Sunflower oil
- Trans fats
- Vegetable shortening

Avoid (most) alcoholic beverages

Common sense tells you that drinking alcohol, particularly spirits or beer that contain gluten, isn't going to make you healthier. So generally speaking, alcohol is on the "no" list.

But don't despair. An occasional glass of wine may be a good thing. Find out more in the section "Making happy hour truly happy," later in this chapter.

The Truth about Common Foods

Some of our favorite foods are the source of confusion, especially on morning TV shows and magazine covers. Is it sugar or fat that's making us fat and unhealthy? Do eggs dangerously raise our cholesterol? Wait, doesn't saturated fat cause heart disease? Is alcohol a bad idea, or should I drink a glass of red wine every day?

We tackle these issues one by one in the following sections to show you that sugar and its associated insulin cycles are the demons of the food world. We also discuss how the right fats can actually make you leaner and healthier. In fact, eggs are an excellent source of protein, and you can eat them to your heart's (and health's) content. And, yes, an occasional glass of wine can be part of a Paleo lifestyle.

Slaying the sugar demon

Thanks to processed foods and soft drinks, sugar consumption has reached dangerous proportions. If you're like a typical American, you consume about

165 pounds of sugar every year. Two decades ago, the average American ate just 26 pounds of sugar per person per year. All that sugar has led to an epidemic of lifestyle ailments, including diabetes, cancers, obesity, and heart disease.

But don't think your lack of willpower is solely to blame. Sugar's behavior in the body is insidious and makes resisting the temptation of a sweet treat very difficult. Eating sugar releases insulin in the bloodstream to reduce your level of blood sugar. This increase in insulin can make your blood sugar fluctuate too low, so your brain triggers your body to eat more sugar. The diabolical being who rules this cycle is know as the *sugar demon* (and, yes, he really does exist!).

If you've been trapped in the sugar cycle, you know it can be pretty unpleasant. Physical hunger and mental temptation gnaw at you, compelling you to make poor food choices, which lead to more unhealthy food choices again later. You feel edgy and cranky before eating, energized for a short time while eating, then sluggish and sleepy after a meal.

The Paleo diet helps you break this cycle to vanquish the sugar demon. To be your leanest, healthiest self, you must break out of the sugar cycle. The most successful way to do that is by eating Paleo-approved foods that stabilize your insulin, reduce inflammation, and increase your food satisfaction. (See Chapter 3 for details on how to slay the sugar demon once and for all!)

Making the case for high-quality fats

Fat doesn't make you fat. Go ahead and chew on that for a few minutes.

The media has told you for decades that the key to a leaner body is a low-fat diet and that saturated fats are the cause of heart disease. Both of those assertions are wrong.

Fat, including saturated fat, is essential to your health and, as it turns out, to building a lean, strong body. To access the fat stored in your body for energy, you need to consume fat in your meals, so your body can then burn stored fat for energy.

Dietary fat is also crucial in helping your body absorb fat-soluble vitamins, such as vitamins A, D, E, and K. And let's be honest about taste: A little bit of fat makes food more palatable, so you feel more satisfied after eating. A diet that's too low in fat can lead to food cravings that compel you to overeat or make poor food choices.

Additionally, when your body doesn't regularly receive high-quality fat in meals, it can retaliate with dry skin, hair loss, bruising, intolerance to cold, and, in extreme cases, loss of menstruation.

Don't get us wrong: We're not giving you a free pass to dive face first into a bowl of butter. Instead, we're encouraging you to free yourself from a fear of fat. Choose high-quality fats from the "yes" list (see the earlier section, "100% Paleo-approved: Checking out the Paleo 'yes' list") in appropriate quantities to make your meals taste great while doing good things for your body. (Later in this chapter, we outline how much fat is the right amount for you.)

Fitting fruit into the Paleo plan

Fruit provides beneficial plant compounds, fiber, and antioxidant power; however, you must eat fruit in moderation. Fruits contain fructose, which is just another form of sugar, so consuming too much fruit can cause weight gain and may cause blood sugar swings.

When you're just beginning to fight the sugar demon and starting to live Paleo, remember to not let your fruit take over your plate. Reach for vegetables more often than fruits, and keep your fruit intake to about one or two servings per day.

All fruits aren't equal on the health scale. Some have a higher sugar content than others. The more sugar present, the higher the insulin release, and the more insulin that's released, the more fat that will be stored.

Here are a few things to keep in mind about fruit:

- ✔ Melons and tropical fruits, like bananas, mango, and pineapple, include higher amounts of natural sugar.

- ✔ Fruits that are darker in color — blueberries, raspberries, strawberries, blackberries, and cranberries — have higher amounts of antioxidants and less sugar.

- ✔ Eating fruit that's in season is your best bet for nutrition and an appropriate amount of sugar.

Realizing that eggs are A-Okay (and cholesterol isn't so bad)

Eggs are just about the perfect food. They're filled with vitamins and minerals, including choline and biotin. *Biotin* helps your body turn the foods you eat into energy, and *choline* helps move cholesterol through your bloodstream. They're both an excellent source of fatty acids and sulfur-containing proteins, which make the walls around your cells healthy.

Many people have eliminated eggs from their shopping list because of worries about high cholesterol and heart disease, and the egg yolk, in particular, has been demonized for the natural cholesterol it contains. But the yolk is the prize of the egg. It's loaded with healthy omega-3 fatty acids and nutrients.

The cholesterol fuss is based on the assumption that if you eat cholesterol, you raise your blood levels of cholesterol. But that's simply not true. In fact, egg yolks contain the B vitamin choline, which is a concentrated source of *lecithin* (a natural fat transporter), and naturally keeps cholesterol from entering the bloodstream.

Cholesterol isn't all bad. Your body needs cholesterol to make bile, which breaks down fats. And your brain cells need cholesterol to deliver your body's messages where they need to go.

Almost everyone produces less cholesterol in their bodies based on how much they consume in food — studies show that dietary cholesterol doesn't have much of an affect on blood cholesterol. Moreover, cholesterol isn't a good indicator of heart disease. Dietary cholesterol has very little impact on blood cholesterol.

Making happy hour truly happy

Even we can't dismiss some of the positive aspects of alcohol — there's an appropriate time to enjoy a moderate amount of alcohol to unwind or to celebrate. Aside from the positive aspects of socializing, some types of alcohol are associated with a lower risk of cardiovascular disease, and they may also reduce the risk of infection with the bacteria that causes ulcers.

Here are a few key factors to help you decide whether you should pop a cork:

- Alcohol is a toxin to the liver.
- Alcohol is a drug, which means it's addictive.
- If losing weight is your goal, remember that your liver can't help you with fat burning if it's busy detoxifying alcohol.

Before you pour yourself a glass of something intoxicating, consider your goals and your overall eating habits, and then make smart choices about which type of alcohol you drink.

Steer clear of grain-based drinks that can also include gluten, such as the following:

- Beer
- Bourbon
- Gin (some brands are processed with grain-based alcohol)

- ✔ Grain-based vodka
- ✔ Whiskey

To celebrate on special occasions, feel free to choose one of these:

- ✔ Potato vodka
- ✔ Red wine
- ✔ Rum
- ✔ Sparkling wine
- ✔ Tequila
- ✔ White wine

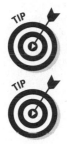

To manage your body's insulin response to the sugars found in alcohol, mix spirits, like tequila or vodka, with soda water, ice, and a squeeze of lemon or lime juice. Avoid fruit juices that are liquid sugar, and avoid tonic water, which is also high in sugar.

When uncorking wine, choose the driest (least sweet) wines possible. The driest reds include Pinot Noir, Cabernet Sauvignon, and Merlot; the driest whites are Sauvignon Blanc and Albarino.

Our hunter-gatherer ancestors occasionally let their hair down when they were exposed to alcohol by eating fermented grapes. But they didn't sit around the fire doing shots. You can't maintain a high level of health if you drink alcohol frequently or in large quantities. The pleasant buzz that alcohol provides also places stress on your liver, creates a strong insulin response, and dehydrates your cells. Enjoy cocktails in moderation.

During your 30-Day Reset, abstain from alcohol completely. Doing so ensures that you break free of the sugar demon and can make clear-headed food choices. (For more on the first 30 days of living Paleo and the 30-Day Reset, see Chapter 3.)

Figuring Out How Much You Can (And Should) Eat

Knowing how much to eat is essential to your success in your dietary goals. If you don't eat enough food, your body may lack the nutrition it needs. You can start breaking down muscle or slow your metabolism. But if you eat more than you need, you can gain weight or feel fatigued — and that leads to frustration.

Living Paleo makes it easier than ever to assess how much you need to eat, and when you eat foods from the Paleo "yes" list (see the earlier section "100% Paleo-approved: Checking out the Paleo 'yes' list"), feeling satisfied while giving your body everything it needs to thrive is easy. Your weight will normalize, and you'll feel more vibrant and energetic than ever before. After you develop the ability to know how much food your body needs, which we help you figure out in the following sections, many of your struggles will be behind you.

Understanding why a calorie isn't just a calorie

Conventional thinking abides by the theory that people become overweight because they habitually eat more calories than they can burn off. Under this theory, those extra calories lead to an individual becoming overweight and, eventually, obese. It's a simple equation of calories in, calories out. The amount of calories you eat *does* matter, but there's much more to it than that. Here are two key points you must understand:

- ✔ **All calories aren't created equally.** The most fattening foods in the grocery store aren't the ones that are highest in calories. The most fattening foods you can eat are the foods that wreak havoc on your blood sugar and insulin levels: poor-quality carbohydrates.

- ✔ **The *amount* of total calories you consume is less important than the *quality* of the calories you eat.** When you eat concentrated sources of carbohydrates that cause a strong insulin response, you gain weight.

Some examples of carbohydrates that trigger this unfavorable insulin response include grains, dairy, fruit juices, soda, alcohol, potatoes, and corn — these are all found on the "no" list (see the earlier section "Paleo no-nos: Watching out for foods on the 'no' list").

When you eat carbohydrates from the "yes" list (see the section "100% Paleo-approved: Checking out the Paleo 'yes' list," earlier in this chapter), you regulate your insulin and store less fat. Paleo-approved carbohydrates, like leafy greens and other vegetables, are bound up by fiber, so they elicit a low insulin response and your blood sugar remains low.

Even though a calorie isn't just a calorie, it's still important to eat just the right amount. Luckily, you come equipped with a natural means to figure out just how much you need to eat on any given day — and living Paleo will help you tap into that innate calorie meter so you feel satisfied and energetic.

Trying the eat-until-satisfied approach

It seems simple enough: Eat until you're satisfied.

Eating until you're satisfied, however, doesn't mean eating until you're full. If you're a numbers person, *satisfied* is about 70 percent of full — and that means you're not hungry, but you're not stuffed. You feel at ease and satiated, but not stuffed.

It may take some time to get accustomed to this feeling, but after you internalize this concept, knowing when to stop eating gets easier. You can figure out how to really listen to your body's signals, and this awareness leads to eating that feels natural and instinctive.

But for you to receive your body's messages, it needs to send you the right signals. To produce the hormones that are in charge of sending messages to your brain, you have two jobs: (1) You have to get enough sleep, and (2) you have to eat enough food. Lack of sleep leads to a spike in the appetite, thus, stimulating the hormone ghrelin and declining the hormone lectin, which tells you when you're full. You also have to make sure you're eating enough food so you're producing enough lectin in the first place!

Your mom's advice was solid: Eat slowly and chew your food. It's not just about good table manners; you need to give your brain time to get the signal from your body that you're full, and that takes about 20 minutes. If you eat too fast, you'll miss the signal. But with smaller bites and leisurely meals that include fiber- and nutrient-dense foods, you'll feel fuller faster. And that's good for your waistline and your health.

Measuring your food at a glance

Portion distortion is common. Most people never realize how much they're eating in a day. We recommend that, until you get in the swing of things, you pay attention to the portion sizes of what you're eating. After the first 30 days, understanding correct portions becomes second nature, and you automatically know how much should be on your plate. The goal here is to reset your visual imaging.

The amount of food you choose to eat every day is determined by three variables:

- Your hunger level
- Your energy level
- Your exercise/activity level

To build each meal, you need to take those three variables into account and fill your plate with an appropriate portion size of Paleo foods.

With the following at-a-glance guidelines, you can stay on track, whether you're eating in a restaurant, traveling for work or pleasure, or dining with friends — no embarrassing or annoying tools involved. You'll develop a useful lifetime skill that will help you quickly eyeball how much food to grab.

- **Protein:** A serving of meat, fish, or poultry should be about the size and thickness of your palm. (That's about 3 to 4 ounces for women, 5 to 6 ounces for men.) Each meal should include a serving of protein.

  A serving of eggs is as many as you can easily hold in your hand. (That's about two or three for women, three or four for men.) For egg whites, double the amount of whole eggs.

- **Vegetables:** A serving of vegetables should be at least the size of a softball. You can't eat too many vegetables, so fill your plate with at least two or three softballs' worth.

- **Fruit:** A serving of fruit is half an individual piece (for example, half an apple, half an orange) or a tennis ball size serving of berries, grapes, or tropical fruits. (That's about half a cup.)

  Eat no more than two servings of fruit per day, and break them up across meals and snacks to distribute your sugar intake. Eating multiple servings in one sitting will release more insulin than if they're broken up throughout the day.

- **Fat:** A serving of liquid fat should be about the size of a super ball, or typical bouncy ball. (That's about 1 tablespoon.) Each meal should include one to two servings of fat.

  A serving of nuts, seeds, coconut flakes, and olives is about one closed handful. A serving of avocado is one-quarter to one-half of the avocado. A serving of coconut milk is one-third to one-half of the can.

Supercharging Your Body with the Power of Paleo Foods

We love to use the term *supercharge* when it comes to Paleo. When living Paleo, it feels as if someone plugged you back into your energy source! All of a sudden, the magic starts to happen. You feel thinner, your skin looks better, and your eyes glisten. Hormonally, things just start to "shift." You sleep better, PMS disappears, acne goes away, wrinkles fade, and you actually feel like exercising. You feel like playing with your kids; you feel like cooking that meal for your family. Your life goes from a bunch of "I have to" to a bunch of "I want to!"

There are reasons for this change. Your body begins to come alive, often flooded with nutrition for the first time in years. You're also eating energy-producing foods. Many people have had such a nutritionally devoid diet for so long that they don't even remember what it's like to feel consistently good for long stretches of time! They haven't had food that's alive, so their body perks up in every way when it starts to get what it needs.

Other reasons Paleo works for so many is because people know they're eating in a way that their body is designed, but they're also getting healthier by being more alkaline, releasing toxins, and eating notoriously low-allergen foods. We discuss the power of Paleo in the following sections.

Getting the nourishment you need

Paleo foods create *nutritional sufficiency* — the point when your body is balanced with all its vitamins, minerals, and essential fats. Many people live in the state of *deficiency,* not getting the nourishment they need, because they aren't getting their macronutrients in the right quantity or the right quality.

The hunter-gatherers' nutrition came from macronutrients but in different quantities and a much higher quality than today's typical consumption. Their foods came from wild game, fish, vegetables, fruits, and nuts. Here's the breakdown of our ancestors' macronutrients:

- Protein: 20 to 35 percent
- Carbohydrates: 25 to 40 percent
- Fat: 30 to 45 percent

The modern diet, on the other hand, consists of marbled grain-fed conventional meats, grains, sugar and artificial sweeteners, and rancid fats:

- Protein: 15 to 20 percent
- Carbohydrates: 45 to 55 percent
- Fat: 35 to 40 percent

Creating healthy cells

When people think about nutrition, it's usually from a biological perspective — how the structures in your body (such as organs) process biochemical and bio-available nutrients. These vitamins and other nutrients are essential to your health and well-being.

But food also has an electrical component, based on its mineral composition. Your food basically has a life force from this electrical component. Cellular metabolism is dependent on biochemical reactions, but it also depends on the capacitance (the ability to store a charge) of the body.

Everything in life has a vibration or frequency attached to it. Seemingly solid objects are molecules, atoms, and particles floating, vibrating, and rotating. Our world is definitely vibrational, so our food has different energies, or charges, attached to it, just like any object.

When your food is healthy, vibrant, and alive (like healthy meats, vegetables, fruits, and healthy fats), they hold a better charge. When your food is processed, over cooked, microwaved, or depleted of nutrients, the charge is weak.

Eating Paleo naturally encourages healthier nutrition from both a biochemical and a molecular standpoint. Health comes down to the cells, and our living Paleo plan will create healthy cells. Incorporating fresh raw vegetables that are filled with energy and life into your daily diet can increase cellular health.

Balancing your pH

One of the most challenging health issues people have today is that they don't have a pH that's conducive to health. Your pH is the acid-base balance of your body — literally, how acidic or alkaline you are. It's as important as your body temperature. Just as your body works to keep a tight control on temperature, it does the same in regard to pH.

Unfortunately, most people are on the acidic side of the pendulum, which is a major stressor to the body. Your body will be in a constant fight to keep healthy and regulate your level by taking minerals, like calcium and magnesium, from your bones and dumping them into your bloodstream.

How do you get acidic? Dietary choices, such as processed foods, dairy, grains, and sugary drinks, cause acidity in your body. You may be on the acidic side if you have any of the following symptoms:

✔ Aches and pains

✔ Arthritis

✔ Fatigue

✔ Headaches

✔ Inflammation

✔ Low immunity

✔ Muscle cramps

✔ PMS

✔ Skin disorders

If you want to test your pH, you can find test strips at any pharmacy. These strips test your acidity by using a urine or saliva sample. A normal reading is about 7.4. Anything below that, and you start to get into the more acidic range.

Identifying food allergies and sensitivities

How do you know whether you have a food allergy or sensitivity? Right off the bat, be aware that a difference exists between a full-blown food allergy and a food sensitivity. If you have a true food allergy, even a tiny bit of the offending food can cause a quick, severe reaction, called *anaphylaxis.* Some of the symptoms are swelling, tingling, breathing problems, and sudden low blood pressure. This is a life-threatening condition.

Food sensitivities, on the other hand, come on slowly, and you can eat some of the offending food and be fine. You won't get a sudden severe reaction, however, you do experience discomfort and symptoms over time. When you have food sensitivities, one of the biggest problems is that your body is repeatedly exposed to a food that causes increased stress on the immune system. This constant exposure can trigger autoimmune diseases and, eventually, affect other body organs. This exposure can cause rapid aging and discomfort.

How do you know whether you have food sensitivities? Here are some of the symptoms:

- Acne
- Arthritis
- Attention deficit disorder
- Autoimmune problems
- Bloating
- Depression
- Fatigue
- Food cravings
- Irritable bowel
- Migraines
- Sinus drainage
- Skin disorders
- Skin rashes
- Stomach cramps
- Weight gain

To find out whether you have a food sensitivity, try an elimination/provocation test: Eliminate the suspected foods from your diet for 30 days. If you feel better, you may in fact be sensitive. Slowly (and carefully) add them back in one at a time to see which one may be the culprit. A great time to implement this test is during the 30-Day Reset (see Chapter 3).

Following are the most common food allergens:

- ✔ Eggs
- ✔ Fish
- ✔ Milk
- ✔ Peanuts
- ✔ Shellfish
- ✔ Soy
- ✔ Tree nuts
- ✔ Wheat

Isn't it great to know that half the list doesn't even include Paleo-approved foods! The reason for that is because living Paleo has very low sensitivity foods, making it a great eating plan for those with a lot of food sensitivities.

Chapter 3

Gearing Up for Paleo

*L*iving Paleo is probably a new way of life for you. Whenever you approach anything new, getting some tips and strategies to help you along your journey is a great way to ensure success. That's what this chapter is all about — gearing you up with all the essentials to help you live Paleo!

In this chapter, we talk about the first 30 days to start off your Paleo lifestyle, the 30-Day Reset. We show you specifically why these first 30 days are so important and what you can expect.

For those of you who say, "Don't tell me about the results; show me," we've got you covered. Certain physical markers help you track your results numerically. These numbers tell you whether your body shape is improving, whether you're getting stronger, whether your acid-alkaline balance is optimal, whether inflammation is going down, and whether your blood pressure, cholesterol, and blood sugar are all improving.

Finally, we help you capture your personal transformation from before you started living Paleo to after you have the plan underway to help mark your "big picture" result. After all, you'll definitely want to celebrate the results we know you'll have!

Your success and achievement living Paleo are simply a result of learned skills. Anyone who's willing to put in the time and effort can understand and master these skills. Look to this book as your personal coach to keep you on track and to give you viewpoints that may be different from what you once thought. This chapter is your guide to help you start living Paleo.

Beginning Your Paleo Journey

Trying anything new isn't easy, and we're here to guide you through your transition into living Paleo with the topics we discuss in the following sections. The very first step in your Paleo life is to work on reprogramming. We show you how to navigate your emotions and self-talk toward the positive so you get the outcome you desire.

Understanding and adopting the 30-Day Reset is a topic that we're excited to share with you because we know it will make your life easier in the long run. After you get physically ready and understand the *why* behind the 30-Day Reset, it's time to commit and start your Paleo journey. You'll soon begin to achieve the ultimate in health and in weight loss.

Unplug and reprogram

Here's a statistic that will blow your mind: 95 percent of the thoughts that run through your head on a daily basis come from your subconscious mind. What's more amazing is that most of your belief system (subconscious mind) is formed by the time you're about 18. You're basically a smorgasbord of all your past inputs, whether you're exposed to them intentionally or not. This smorgasbord consists of inputs from your parents, friends, relatives, schooling, religious experiences, the media, what you watch, what you read — anything you've been exposed to.

As you move forward, make sure you have powerful thoughts, program yourself for future success, and don't go back to old habits that won't serve you. Concentrate on breaking free from any past negative experiences you may have had with food, and choose your own thoughts and actions to lead you to success. Use your mind to strengthen you, not weaken you.

Where do you begin? Start by developing a strong belief system. Whether you realize it, you talk to yourself all the time. In doing so, you either build yourself up or put yourself down. That's where affirmations come in.

Affirmations are healing "self-scripts" that help you visualize the life you want. They help you let go of thoughts you've been carrying around for years. Affirmations actually push out these thoughts and pull powerful, positive thoughts into your subconsciousness. Affirmations are a great tool to give you mental power.

How do you use affirmations, you ask? First, using red ink, journal what you want or who you want to be. (Seeing something in red helps it stick in your mind.) You can refer to many books to help develop your list of affirmations, or you can make up your own. Then, say your affirmations out loud every day. Say them in the morning before your mind has time to fight back; say them with intention and move while you say them; say them with clarity and don't speed through them; write them and say them as if they're already happening, such as " I am lean, strong, and healthy. I am starting my living Paleo plan with ease." When you start doing this daily, soon these affirmations become ingrained in your cells, and they become your identity.

Don't overlook this step because you feel a little uncomfortable or it seems just too easy to really make a difference. When you train your mind to dismiss any failure of thought, you'll be shocked how different your life plays out. Try it for 30 days and see for yourself!

Anytime is a good time to start journaling affirmations. For some, a great time to give this mental exercise a whirl is during the 30-Day Reset. Doing so helps you keep your mind focused and your spirit uplifted.

Embrace the 30-Day Reset

After you start reprogramming your mind for success, the next step is to reprogram your body for success. This reprogramming is the 30-Day Reset.

The purpose of this reprogramming is to reset your internal system in such a way that you push your body's compost button and clear out anything unwanted. It's like giving your body a super good cleaning. When your body isn't working hard to deal with what it doesn't need, it focuses on getting you more of what you do need. You get healthier, stronger, and leaner. You can think of it this way: Where there's waste, there's weight. By taking the time to clear out your body's waste, your body composition begins to change and your energy skyrockets.

During these 30 days, you begin to break unhealthy food habits. How much you eat, what you choose to eat, and the pleasure you connect with food is often times an end result of a habit you've created. You may not even realize that what you're doing isn't healthy or isn't getting you to where you want to be. These 30 days help you address these concerns and begin to reprogram your habits.

Another vitally important objective of the 30-day reset is to diminish food cravings and food addictions. A very common food addiction is sugar. Escaping sugar is hard to do if you've ever bought or eaten anything packaged, boxed, wrapped, or processed. Added sugar is found in many foods (even unsuspecting foods like bread, "health" cereals, or "all-natural" snacks).

The more you eat sugar, the more you come to depend on and crave sugary foods. Soon, this addiction controls your food choices more than imaginable. Most people have no idea that they're addicted to sugar or that they're making food choices based on this addiction. We refer to breaking this habit as "slaying the sugar demon" (see the section "Battling the sugar demon," later in this chapter). The 30-Day Reset period begins to break you of the sugar demon and other food cravings you may have. During these 30 days, you train your mind, body, and senses to approach food in a way that's most beneficial to you.

Make the 30 days about you. No matter how crazy-busy your life is, do your best to make these 30 days about what you need to be successful. Explain to the people in your tribe that these 30 days are foundational to your goals and ask them to support you in any way they can. Even if it's just a hug!

Decide, commit, and go!

This is where the rubber meets the road. Before you do anything that's worth doing, you've got to make the decision to commit. You commit by first deciding that you're going to follow through fully, and then you make this commitment real by taking your calendar and scheduling in the 30 days like you would anything that's important to you. When you schedule something, it takes on life and becomes more than an idea or a thought; it becomes a plan, an action.

Why the first 30 days are so strict

You may be wondering how the 30-Day Reset is different than just eating Paleo. It's different because we ask you to be completely strict with both your food choices and proportions (see Chapter 2) — no cheating, no swaying. We ask you to stick to the Paleo Big Three (lean proteins, Paleo-approved vegetables and fruits, and healthy fats; see Chapter 4) for the 30 days.

We know the 30-Day Reset will revitalize you and flood your body with good nutrition. This reset will change your biochemistry, and you'll start to desire different foods as your taste buds start to come alive again and your senses are heightened back to a normal state. After these 30 days, or when you're ready, you can start having fun with some of the Paleo recipes (Paleo pancakes, muffins, treats, and so forth). You can also have some flexibility and step outside of eating Paleo once in a while when you're ready and have good grounding. But for 30 days, we ask that you hunker down and stick to a strict Paleo plan with your long-term benefits in mind.

After you make the decision to go forward with the 30-Day Reset and you've scheduled it in, move forward and don't look back. Make sure you're doing your affirmations to give you the mental muscle you need. (For more on affirmations, refer to the earlier section "Unplug and reprogram.")

The best step you can take after you start doing your affirmations and you've scheduled in your 30 days is to get yourself organized in the other important place — the kitchen (see Chapter 7). When you put all these pieces together, you're gearing up for a great 30 days that will change the rest of your life.

Building the Foundation for Success: The 30-Day Reset

The 30-Day Reset is the foundation of our program. Ensuring that we equip you with all you need to know about these 30 days is essential. When you get past these 30 days, everything gets easier. Everything starts to fall into place. The magic starts to happen.

In the following sections, we share why we pick 30 days (and not 23 or 28, for example) for the first part to this plan. Also, we explore what's happening to your cells during the 30-Day Reset that makes such startling improvements happen for you. We then provide a master plan to help you walk through your days with certainty. Half the battle of doing anything new is facing the unexpected. We show you what you can expect during your transformation so you can prepare in the best possible way.

The brain versus the tongue (what you know you should eat versus what you crave) is an interesting battle, but it's easy to decode and deal with when you know that's what's happening. We explain the ins and outs of this battle and what it means for you during these 30 days.

Developing a habit with 30 days

The reason we picked the number 30 is because it's a good start to developing a habit. We know dropping some of your favorite foods and cutting out packaged, processed foods with sugar isn't an easy battle. In fact, you may want to cry in your ice cream bowl for a while.

You may not be completely automatic in your responses after 30 days; however, this time frame will go a long way in starting you off in the right direction.

It has most likely taken you a long while to develop your eating habits, and it will take some time before you can erase those old habits and form new ones. We've seen this 30-Day Reset happen for many people. Just know that after 30 days, most everyone feels considerably better, and cravings are greatly diminished. The longer you've depended on sugary foods, the more difficult it may be to retrain your taste buds to natural sweetness again.

It also takes about 21 days for your intestinal cells to turn over, which helps you get through this process a little easier as your body renews with good raw material.

Renewing your system

In the preceding section, we talk about the fact that you're developing new eating habits and cutting cravings during these 30 days. Those changes are able to happen because you're renewing your system and making it stronger and healthier.

During the 30-Day Reset, you're improving the caliber of your cells. Keep in mind that you're only as healthy as your cells. When you eat foods that are denatured, packaged, and processed, you're poisoning your cells. When people are lean and healthy and have a youthful vibrant appearance, they have cells that are free of waste.

By eating the cleansing Paleo-approved foods, waste leaves through the following *detox organs:*

- ✔ **Kidney:** Toxins leave through adequate fluid intake.
- ✔ **Liver:** The liver eliminates or neutralizes toxins as they pass.
- ✔ **Lungs:** Toxins leave as you exhale.
- ✔ **Intestines:** Toxins leave through stool elimination.
- ✔ **Skin:** Toxins leave through sweating.

As you eat foods full of nutrition and drink plenty of water (see Chapter 5 for water requirements), the toxins start to flood out of your body and nutrients enter. Your cells start to regenerate and exude health.

You can do a few things during this time to move waste along. Here are some suggestions to help rid your body of toxins:

- ✔ **Get sweaty.** Sweat is a great carrier of waste. Sweating through exercise or sauna is a great way to eliminate toxins. The toxins leave through your kidneys, so be sure to drink extra fluids while you sweat.

✔ **Jump.** Mini trampolines called *rebounders* squeeze waste matters from cells as you bounce lightly. Rebounding is one of the healthiest exercises you can do for your cells and for elimination of toxins.

✔ **Brush.** Dry brushing cleanses your skin, which is important because your skin is your largest organ and an eliminator of toxins. Through dry brushing, waste is lifted, which allows your body to take in more oxygen through the skin. It also stimulates the lymphatic system, which is your body's drainage system, so you have clear pathways to eliminate effectively. Brush your legs and arms first then your upper torso in circular strokes. Dry brush before exercise or showering for best results. Be sure to purchase a natural bristle brush, which you can find in most stores for about $8 to $10.

✔ **Eat.** Add some raw vegetables to your plate daily. This is a great way to move food through your colon and help your intestines in the elimination process.

✔ **Breathe.** Yoga breathing is so simple but very powerful. Because your lungs are eliminative organs as well, when you exhale, you release toxins. Most people usually take shallow breaths, but when you take the time to inhale and exhale deeply, you get more oxygen in and toxins out. Yoga is a fantastic addition to the 30-Day Reset and beyond for detoxification as well as health benefits. (For more on the benefits of yoga, see Chapter 6.)

The process of ridding your body of this waste is like magic to your body. When you start giving your cells less toxins and begin flooding them with nutrition, you can see and feel the difference in your weight, energy levels, skin, and overall health. Your cravings start to diminish and your body naturally desires healthier foods as your taste begins to change.

Mastering the plan

Now that you know the *why* behind the 30-Day Reset, you're ready to begin implementation. For the most successful journey possible during your 30 days, here are some sample guidelines to follow:

1. **Make the decision to move forward with the 30-Day Reset.**

   Grab a calendar and mark off the 30 days. Don't wait too long! Don't give yourself time to back out — just mark it down and get going.

2. **Tell people in your tribe what you're up to.**

   Ask for their support during this time, and explain that you need to put more focus on yourself for the next 30 days. Make sure they know how important this is to you. Another bonus to doing this is that as soon as you tell people, it helps you be more accountable to the plan, which will push you along when you need the strength to keep going.

3. **Start your positive reprograming through affirmations.**

Remember to try to do these internal self-scripts first thing in the morning and say them loud and clear. A good plan is to say your affirmations in the morning as soon as your feet hit the floor. Hang them in your bathroom or somewhere you're sure to see them. You may want to try journaling at night. Journal your thoughts in a positive tone as if they're already happening, such as "I am feeling healthier, thinner, and more vibrant than I ever have." (For more on affirmations and journaling, see the section "Unplug and reprogram," earlier in this chapter.)

4. **Clear the decks.**

Go through your kitchen with a trash bag and get rid of foods that aren't part of your 30-day plan. Stock your kitchen with all the wonderful Paleo-approved foods, which we discuss in Chapters 2 and 4. For tips on how to clean out and restock your kitchen, check out Chapter 7.

5. **Get organized.**

Make sure you have the ingredients and the equipment you need to plan the foods you want. Get as many resources as you can get your hands on to help you prepare meals or give you snack ideas. Try to keep it as simple as possible when you first start. The recipes in this book will give you some great ideas! Keep your sample grocery list found in Chapter 7 handy so you'll always know what to buy.

In addition to the steps in the master plan, you can do the following things to keep your spirits up and promote a healthy mind and body:

✔ **Move every day.** The more you move, the more you'll start feeling the healing affects of your 30-Day Reset. High-intensity exercise, walking, yoga — no matter what you do, it helps toxins leave your body and keep your mind clear. Make sure you adjust your food accordingly. (Check out Chapter 2 for guidelines on what to eat before and after a workout.)

✔ **Set aside 20 minutes for meditation every day.** You have a lot of options to help you meditate, but the important thing is to be still, calm, and quiet for 20 minutes each day. This practice will start to balance and rejuvenate you. (See Chapter 6 for more info.)

✔ **Get a weekly massage and chiropractic adjustment.** This is a great way to start calming your nervous system and to help your body detox. When your nervous system works better, your organs work better; when your organs work better, they detox more readily and effectively. (See Chapter 6.)

At the end of your 30 days, celebrate! You just accomplished a major milestone. Give yourself a pat on the back.

Understanding your body's transformation

You may feel pretty lousy during the first few weeks transitioning to Paleo. But with this book, you're equipped with so much knowledge about implementing these first 30 days that you're way ahead of the game.

Some people experience mental fuzziness, fatigue, headaches, moodiness, shakiness, and are just plain out of it. What's happening is your body is conquering carbs, and it takes a while for your body to adjust. While your body may be looking better, sometimes it takes a while for the rest of you to catch up. Some coin these symptoms as "the carb flu," which is the nasty transition that your body goes through when going from a high-carb to a lower-carb diet. Even though living Paleo isn't considered a low-carb diet, it's naturally lower in carbs so your body is making that transition.

What's happening during this process is your body needs glucose (sugar) for the brain, muscles, cells, and so on. Until you started living Paleo, glucose was easy to access from all the sugary carbohydrates you may have been eating. Now your body has to create glucose from fats and proteins, which isn't as easily done. It will happen, though, soon enough, and you'll start feeling better and your body will run more efficiently because of it.

Try some extra healthy fats like coconut and lots of water to calm the effects of the carb flu.

Some people feel few symptoms during this transition period; others get a heavy dose. But just remember: It's worth it on the other side, so hang tight!

Battling the sugar demon

When you're going through the first 30 days, you're breaking food habits and cravings. The toughest of these to break is cravings for sugary foods. The sugar demon will constantly tap you on the back, trying to get you to eat your bagel, pasta, or bowl of cereal. This guy will try to justify why it's no big deal to have a bowl of oatmeal or a sandwich.

Your mind will rationalize why you need to stop what you're doing and hit the bagel barn. What your brain thinks it wants isn't always what your body needs, and you need the strength to have a clear understanding of what's happening.

How do you know whether you have a sugar addiction? If eating sugar makes all your symptoms magically go away for a while or if you can't go long without sugary foods, you're probably addicted.

When you have a craving, your body is usually looking for a quick burst of something to make it feel better. Often, that "something" is a brain chemical called *serotonin*. This chemical affects mood, specifically happiness and well-being. The higher the levels, the happier you feel. When serotonin levels drop, your body screams out for a change. It's looking for that feel-good chemical to alter its present brain chemistry. That's one of the reasons so many people are in the vicious cycle of eating sweets and high-carb foods. Often times, people self-medicate with sugary carbohydrate foods, looking for something to make them feel good and change their state of mind.

The following factors can lower serotonin levels:

- **Stress:** One of the biggest reasons so many people who are stressed out have a weight problem is that they're looking for ways to pull their serotonin back up, and sugary carbohydrates often fit the bill.

- **Lack of sunlight:** Sunlight plays a role in the synthesis and regulation of serotonin. If you work in an office or are indoors a lot, the lack of sunlight can cause your serotonin levels to drop.

- **Natural aging:** This natural process can drop serotonin.

To really help your cravings on an ongoing basis and to rid yourself of the sugar demon once and for all, you have to be in the practice of maintaining your serotonin levels. Always strive for healthy ways to elevate your serotonin levels. To balance serotonin, do the following:

- **Eat Paleo foods.** This is one of the best things you can do for your serotonin levels. The high-fiber fruits and vegetables, Paleo proteins, and non-processed foods are all foods your brain loves. Paleo-approved foods are the perfect intervention for low serotonin levels.

- **Exercise.** Exercise is an amazing tool for altering brain chemistry and serotonin levels. For more on incorporating Paleo exercises into your life, see Chapter 6.

- **Think good thoughts.** Try to focus on keeping your thoughts happy and positive. This habit will do your serotonin levels a lot of good! Thinking positively is a very powerful tool for keeping your mood naturally elevated.

The sugar demon (or sugary cravings) is *not* hanging around because you lack willpower or because you're weak. People who manage to be content with wrapping their protein in lettuce instead of bread aren't stronger, nor do they hold some special gift of willpower. Most likely, they've managed to slay their sugar demon. Their body is no longer screaming for sweets, and they truly are content doing without. When you follow the steps we've given you, you'll also be free of this demon and at peace with your lettuce wraps.

After you go through your 30-Day Reset, you'll feel the sugar demon start to distance itself. Before long, you'll be rid of that bugger once and for all! The key is to stay onboard and understand what's happening to your body. The more knowledge you have through living Paleo, the harder it will be for the sugar demon to talk you into a trip to the bakery.

The Big Seven: Tracking Your Progress with Health Markers

Professor Peter Drucker, a well-known management consultant said, "what gets measured, gets managed." That's the philosophy behind the big seven health markers, which we discuss in the following sections. Tracking your progress with these health markers gives you the actual data behind your success or shortcoming. It takes the guesswork out of the picture. The best part: If you're not on the right path, tracking data allows you to make a mid-course correction and correct a variable early on.

- **Body composition** refers to the ratio between your lean body mass and your fat body mass. For many people looking to start the living Paleo plan, losing fat is a major goal. Measuring your body composition uncovers how much body fat you have and how much you're actually losing.

- Developing some muscle mass has many advantages. Measuring your **strength** tells you in what direction you should strategize your fitness goals.

- **Blood pressure** is a basic number that's so easy to track and can help you catch early signs of heart disease.

- Your **blood sugar markers** are significant to your health, particularly because so many people have blood sugar handling problems. Understanding how your body processes sugar can tell you how your food choices have been affecting you on a metabolic level.

- Inflammation and inflammatory diseases are at an all time high. You can check inflammation through **C-reactive protein** as a marker for disease.

- **Cholesterol and triglycerides** are common — and important — numbers to check on a regular basis.

- As we discuss in Chapter 2, **pH (acid-base balance)** is a key component to any health program and ties in with everything you do.

Body composition

If you took two people of the same height and weight and compared them, their bodies may look completely different due to their differing body composition. *Body composition* is the ratio between how much lean body mass you have and how much fat mass you have. It's your ratio of fat to muscle.

Body composition is the reason your clothes often fit differently after you start living Paleo. Your ratio of lean body mass is going up, while your fat mass is going down. For many people, decreasing body fat is an important outcome of living Paleo, so knowing how to test your body composition is an essential test.

You can test for body composition in several ways. The two most practical and assessable are *body fat calipers* and *bioelectrical impedance (BIA)*:

- ✔ **Body fat calipers:** Calipers are used to measure skin folds. The calipers pinch several areas of the skin to measure the thickness of the fat layer under the skin. Measurements are then plugged into an equation to compute body fat. You see this method done at a lot of fitness centers. If you test your body fat this way, make sure you get your before and after measurements done by the same person, using the same points and the same algorithm (formula to figure out body fat percentage).

  A waistline of more than 40 inches in men and more than 35 inches in women can be an indication of heart disease.

- ✔ **BIA scale:** This scale is a useful way to check body composition from home. BIA works by sending an undetectable current through your body. Fluids within your body carry an electrical current, however, fat can't. The current measures the resistance to the electrical signal as it passes through water found in muscle and fat. The more fat in your body, the more resistant the current. It's safe and is accurate enough to get a good benchmark number. All you do is step on the scale, so it's very easy.

  For the most accuracy with a BIA scale, wake up in the morning, drink a glass of water (exact same amount and temperature each time you do the test), wait 30 minutes, go to the bathroom, and then test. However, because the current is going through only your upper or lower body (depending on the scale), it's not 100 percent accurate, but it's the easiest way to get a number that's close enough. Plus what you're mainly looking for is to use that number as a benchmark to see whether you're progressing. BIA scales with higher accuracy are the Tanita scales (www.tanita.com/en).

Strength

Strength comes from putting on more muscle. Having lean muscle mass makes your body run much more efficiently. In fact, the stronger you are, the longer you're likely to live because you decrease your chance of many diseases. Putting on muscle is like taking a pill against metabolic diseases. It's great for your bone density, and you'll stay healthier and look younger. What more incentive could there possibly be?

To see whether you're getting stronger, you need to see how much you can push or lift. A great strength test is the leg press machine. We love this exercise because you use many major muscle groups. Test your *three-rep max:* After warming up, lift as hard and as heavy as you can for three repetitions and rest, and then repeat this cycle for a total of three times. Jot down the absolute heaviest you can push. Repeat monthly to see your progression.

You can do this test with any strength exercise if you don't have access to a leg press. Just make sure you're lifting as much as you possibly can and that you can't lift another pound by the end of the three reps.

If you don't want to test by lifting or pushing heavy weights, you can do a grip strength test, which requires a small hand-held device called a *dynamometer.* You grip the meter as hard as you can, and it records your strength.

Whichever strength test you choose, just make sure you're seeing progression. When you begin a strength program, you'll be surprised how much you see your body start to sculpt. Adding muscle makes your body healthier, and you look better. Win-win!

Blood pressure

Your blood pressure is measured by the amount of blood your heart pumps and the amount of resistance to blood flow in your arteries. Your blood pressure will be high when your body is pumping blood through narrower arteries. You can think of it like this: It's easy for blood to go through a wide-open space, but it's harder to go through a small narrow space, so your body has to work harder. That's when your blood pressure goes up.

Blood pressure should be checked regularly for one clear-cut reason: Heart disease is a silent killer. You may have no indication whatsoever that you're facing a problem. The good news is many of the reasons we get high blood pressure are totally within our control to change. If you've been diagnosed with high blood pressure, you should invest in a home model meter. You can buy a good quality meter for about $50 to $100 in any drug store or major shopping outlet.

Here are blood pressure guidelines:

- **Normal blood pressure:** Less than 120/less than 80
- **Prehypertension:** 120–139/80–89
- **Hypertension stage 1:** 140–159/90–99
- **Hypertension stage 2:** 160 or more/100 or more

Blood sugar markers

Two simple blood tests tell you how your body handles sugar. They're called *fasting insulin* and *hemoglobin AIC.* These two tests together tell you how your body is processing sugar both long-term and short-term.

- ✔ **Fasting insulin:** If you've been eating processed foods over the years, your body may have developed resistance to insulin. Insulin resistance can also happen naturally as you age. The fasting insulin test is a predictor of insulin resistance and other metabolic diseases that have become such a problem with so many people. It's a quick blood draw, but as the name indicates, you must fast the night before the test.

  When you eat the wrong kind of carbohydrates, blood sugar increases dramatically. Insulin gets pumped out constantly until, finally, your body stops listening to the messages. This excess insulin can cause your body's signals to get confused, causing a resistance to insulin, which can lead to all kinds of problems, like diabetes and obesity. So you can see the value in the fasting insulin test!

- ✔ **Hemoglobin AIC:** This test is more of a trend analysis of what's happening to blood glucose over a period of four to six weeks' time. This test has great stability because the variability of test levels aren't affected by stress or illness because it's not just a snapshot in time.

Another reliable and inexpensive way to test for blood sugar if you want to test in your own home is to use a glucometer, which you can purchase from your local pharmacy. This test is called a *postprandial* (post meal) *blood sugar test,* meaning you test your blood after eating. The American Association of Clinical Endocrinologists recommends that your post meal blood sugar goes no higher than 140 mg/dl.

The consequences of high blood sugar are pretty severe; you can experience diabetic complications, such as nerve damage, visual problems, or stroke. These tests are easy, so take the time to check your numbers as a base line.

You're going to love seeing how, when you start eating the foods you were designed to have, your numbers improve a great deal. It really does give you the certainty to know that you're on the right track.

C-reactive protein

C-reactive protein is protein found in the blood that, when elevated, is an indicator of inflammation in the body. This inflammation may be a predictor of heart disease. Inflammation can damage the inner lining of the arteries and make a heart attack more likely.

When your body continues to stimulate proinflammatory immune cells that may not be needed, you can get chronic inflammation. The following are some of the signs and symptoms:

✔ Allergies and sensitivities

✔ Body aches and pain

✔ Skin problems

✔ Stiffness

✔ Swelling

✔ Weight gain

Checking for C-reactive protein is a great idea when you consider some of the problems that chronic inflammation can cause:

✔ Alzheimer's

✔ Arteriosclerosis

✔ Cancer

✔ Diabetes

✔ Heart disease

✔ High blood pressure

✔ Parkinson's

✔ Osteoporosis

The great news is the living Paleo eating plan and recipes are all completely non-inflammatory foods. So if you do have chronic inflammation, the living Paleo plan is a great place to start! Paleo-approved foods are also natural inflammatory busters, so eating Paleo is a great preventative lifestyle as well.

Cholesterol and triglycerides

Fats and their related compounds are called *cholesterol*. Liquid fats are *oils*, and solid fats are simply *fat*. Fats in food are called *dietary fats*. Fats aren't bad for you. In fact, they're an important part of feeling and looking your best. Getting fats in the right balance is the key.

Triglycerides are the most common kind of fat that comes from food. You make this fat to burn for energy. When you eat more calories than you need, extra calories change into triglycerides and are stored in fat cells for when your body needs energy. Lifestyle is one of the most common causes of high triglycerides, and sugary carbohydrates are a major player.

The following sections go into detail about both cholesterol and triglycerides and how to keep the right levels in your system.

Checking out your cholesterol

Despite common belief, cholesterol is actually a good thing! You need this fatty substance for your brain, the production of hormones, and *cellular membranes* (the stuff that lines your cells). Dietary cholesterol doesn't significantly affect cholesterol levels in the blood or risk for heart disease. (Find more on cholesterol and diet in Chapter 2.)

Your body needs cholesterol to be healthy. Cholesterol is found in the walls of your cells, in your fatty tissues, in your organs, in your brain, and in your glands. Here's what cholesterol does for you:

- Protects your cells
- Helps your nerve cells get information from one place to another
- Provides the building block for vitamin D
- Enables your gallbladder to make the digestive juice bile
- Gives you the raw material on which you build hormones

You make cholesterol in your liver. You also get cholesterol from foods that come from animals: meat, poultry, fish, and eggs.

The fear of cholesterol stems from the potential for fatty deposits to cause a restriction of blood flow. Your heart needs oxygenated blood flow; without it, you're susceptible to a heart attack. And if you don't have enough blood flow to the brain, you can get a stroke. However, you can combat these fears by eating the right foods (such as all the foods on the Paleo-approved list in Chapter 2) and strengthening your blood vessels.

The best way to prevent fatty deposits from lining your vessels is not to stop eating anything with cholesterol. A better strategy is to eat foods that are nutrient-dense so you maintain your immune function and strengthen the integrity of your blood vessels. Eating Paleo-approved foods, which include foods like grass-fed meats with a favorable omega-6 to omega-3 ratio, makes it easy. These foods are non-inflammatory and naturally raise your good cholesterol.

Your good cholesterol is called HDL. Think of it as "happy" and your bad cholesterol, LDL, is "lacking." The goal is to eat foods that increase the good stuff and reduce the bad. Paleo, grass-fed proteins and healthy fats do just that. Paleo fruit and vegetables are great for strengthening your vessels.

Getting the skinny on triglycerides

Triglycerides are the fats that are constantly circulating in your bloodstream. When your triglycerides are elevated, it's an indication that some kind of metabolic problem, such as Type 2 diabetes, coronary heart disease, or obesity, may be occurring.

Here's the kicker: Eating too much of the wrong type of carbohydrates (grains, potatoes, sugary drinks, and so on) causes elevated triglycerides, which happens because the liver converts excess carbohydrates into triglyceride for storage. If you're producing too much triglyceride, your body stores more.

Elevated triglycerides are completely a lifestyle issue that's well within your reach to remedy. When you start living Paleo, lifestyle health issues usually start to melt away.

Finding out your levels

Finding out your cholesterol and triglyceride levels is simply a matter of getting a blood test from your physician. If levels are high, blood can become clogged by plaque deposits, leading to coronary heart disease. The best defense? Living Paleo foods and exercise; the perfectly balanced fats in Paleo foods and the functional Paleo movements keep your coronary artery disease risk low.

For a more advanced cholesterol screening, find a physician in your area who uses Genova Diagnostics. This advanced testing, called CV Health, will not only give you all the valuable numbers you need for cholesterol and triglycerides but will also give you the size of the cholesterol particles in your blood, which is imperative. Ask your doctor whether he works with this lab. If not, you can call Genova Diagnostics (check out www.gdx.net) to find a doctor in your zip code who works with their lab.

pH (acid-base balance)

We talk about acid-base balance in Chapter 2. Testing for your body's pH is easy, inexpensive, and very telling of your body's state of health. When your acid-base balance is healthy, you look and feel much younger. That's why living Paleo is such a brilliant life plan to follow.

Most people are on the acidic side of the acid-base pendulum. When you consume processed foods and sugary drinks and experience all the stress that an inverted way of eating, living, and thinking bring, you get acidic. Negative emotions (like anger and resentment) and negative lifestyle habits (too much screen time, smoking, or alcohol) play a role in your body's acidity as well — it's not just about food; it's about the way you live day to day.

Capturing Your Personal Before and After Makeover

One of the most important things you can do for yourself is to capture your brilliance and bravery. The one comment we hear so often is, "I really wish I had a picture of myself before I started Paleo." You will transform — and you'll want to capture your transformation. Here are a few tools you can use to keepsake your transformation:

- **Photos:** Take a picture of yourself standing against a plain background and wearing something revealing like a bathing suit. If you want the date documented, hold a newspaper or magazine in your hand. Be sure to get a photo from all angles. Don't settle for a poor quality photo and just be done with it. Take the time to get some good shots of yourself. You will be so glad you did.

- **Blind measurements:** Another fantastic tool is something we call *blind measurements*. Here's how it works: You take a piece of yarn and wrap it around the body part you want to measure. Cut the yarn when you're done and label the piece of yarn with the date and the body part you measured. In four to six weeks, take that same piece of yarn and measure the same body part to see the difference. Whatever excess yarn you have, cut it off and keep it in a baggie. You keep all these little pieces of yarn left over as a visual reminder of your success. You end up with something more valuable than just a number. You have these tangible pieces of yarn to remind you of all the inches you ditched!

- **The emperor's new clothes:** Your clothing will start to fit pretty differently as you progress on your living Paleo path. You can find plenty of newfound Paleo people out there shopping for new clothes. It kind of goes with the territory; you can almost set your watch by it. Relish in this moment because odds are you won't be digging in those green bags for your old clothes any time soon.

Part II
Embracing the Paleo Lifestyle

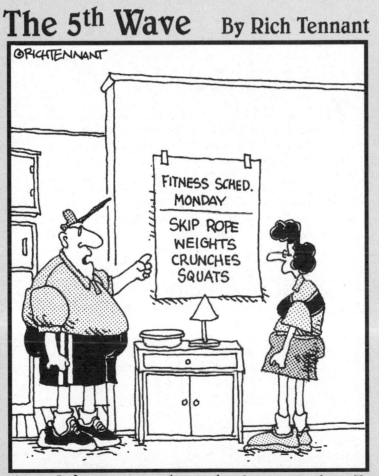

The 5th Wave   By Rich Tennant

@RICHTENNANT

FITNESS SCHED.
MONDAY

SKIP ROPE
WEIGHTS
CRUNCHES
SQUATS

"I __AM__ following the schedule! Today I
skipped the rope, then I skipped the
weights, then I skipped the crunches."

In this part . . .

The lifestyle of our hunter-gatherer ancestors was more relaxed, more nutritious, and more in touch with nature than our modern lives. In this part, we explore Paleo nutrition and address essentials, like sunshine, water, sleep, and stress management, to see how they impact your health and well-being. We also demonstrate how to add Paleo movement into your life and how to stock your kitchen for success. Finally, we delve into the 30-Day Reset that will help you make the Paleo transition.

Chapter 4

Paleo Nutrition

· ·

In This Chapter

▶ Understanding proteins, fats, and carbohydrates

▶ Swapping out the USDA food pyramid for the Paleo pyramid

▶ Building health with surprising foods

▶ Supplementing with the "big guns"

· ·

Paleo nutrition is the cornerstone of living Paleo, and it puts real food first. Based on high-quality proteins, fats, and carbohydrates, Paleo nutrition ensures that you'll eat all the nutrients you need, so you build a better you with every bite. By following the Paleo nutrition plan, you create a new relationship with food, and eating nutritiously becomes effortless.

When your body is deficient of nutrients, everything can feel like a chore. You become tired, depressed, or anxious; weight and sleep issues damage your quality of life. In contrast, when your body is in a state of nutritional balance, you feel better than ever. You look younger and feel happier. You're energized, and your skin glows. You even get sick less often, and those nagging aches and pains disappear.

In this chapter, you discover how proteins, fats, and carbs make you healthier, and you see why the Paleo food pyramid makes more sense and feels more natural than any other nutrition "rules" ever have. In this chapter, we also explore how some surprising foods — even desserts — can contribute to healthfulness, and we identify the right supplements to further boost the power of Paleo nutrition.

The Paleo Big Three: Animal Proteins, Natural Fats, Complex Carbohydrates

The nutritional building blocks of proteins, fats, and carbohydrates are known as *macronutrients*. We like to call these macronutrients the "Paleo Big Three," and understanding them is essential to knowing how the Paleo diet works.

As historical and anthropological records show us, in the Paleolithic era (about 2.6 million years ago), hunter-gatherers of the time had many of the attributes that you're probably looking to gain. They were incredibly healthy, lean, fit, and strong. Much of this was undoubtedly attributed to what they ate. So when you eat as they did, you can expect many of the same benefits. To move forward, then, you must look backward to gather wisdom and use it as your own nutritional guideline.

The first step to forming these new nutritional guidelines is to follow the recipe for nutrition that our ancestors took by eating the macronutrients they ate. We know hunter-gatherers ate no dairy, no cereal grains, no refined sugars, and few fatty meats. Instead, they feasted on the Paleo Big Three: wild, lean animals; naturally occurring fats, especially the healthy omega-3 fats found in cold-water fish; and non-starchy, wild fruits and vegetables.

The Paleo Big Three play an essential role in fueling your body:

- ✔ **Protein** builds and repairs you, increasing lean muscle mass and reducing body fat. Adequate protein supports your physique and ensures that your appetite is satisfied.

- ✔ **Fat** is essential and not the enemy. Naturally occurring fats are vital to the health of your cells and, therefore, your entire body. When you enjoy fats from both animal and plant sources, you fight illnesses caused by inflammation and keep your body in balance. Fat also contributes to feelings of fullness so that overeating becomes a thing of the past.

- ✔ Complex **carbohydrates** supply energy. All carbohydrates are eventually turned into a form of sugar called *glucose* — and glucose is what your brain and your cells use for fuel. But just as high-quality gas serves your car's engine better, your body runs best on the carbohydrates found in vegetables and fruits, rather than processed, starchy carbs, like bread, pasta, and sugary treats.

When you're planning your meals, think about the Paleo Big Three and ask yourself, "Will my plate include lean protein, healthy fats, and complex carbs?" Also, think about whether your feast would have been welcome on a hunter-gatherer's table, too.

Paleo proteins and why animals matter

Humans are omnivores. That means that people have a meat-eating heritage and evolved to subsist on meat and plants. Anthropologists agree that our earliest ancestors were meat eaters, and scientists estimate that our genes are 99.9 percent the same as they were back then. Meat provides us with protein, essential fatty acids, and vitamins — just as it did for our hunter-gatherer ancestors.

Our ancestors ate as much as approximately 3 pounds of protein a day! The meat they ate gave them an abundance of protein, essential fatty acids, and vitamins. It allowed them to build strong muscle and to store the fuel they needed for long walks and short bursts of energy (to, say, outrun a predator or take down dinner).

For modern cave men and women, we recommend that you invest in the highest-quality protein sources you can afford. Here are a few helpful tips:

✔ **Happy animals are healthy animals.** And eating healthy animals makes you healthier. As much as possible, choose lean, grass-fed, and free-range meat. You earn bonus points for good health if it's also organic, and it should always be free of antibiotics and other fillers. Beef, buffalo, game, lamb, goat, turkey, chicken, and fish/seafood are all good sources.

✔ **Conventional can be okay, too.** If a tight budget means you need to buy store-bought, conventional meat, you can still vastly improve your health. Choose lean cuts and trim visible fat before cooking, and then drain as much of the released fat as you can after cooking.

✔ **Go fishing!** Another valuable protein source to pile on your plate is wild-caught, sustainable fish. Your best bets are fattier, cold-water fish like salmon, sardines, mackerel, cod, and herring. Tuna packed in olive oil is also a good choice. Check out the Monterey Bay Aquarium Seafood Watch (`www.montereybayaquarium.org/cr/seafoodwatch.aspx`) for more recommendations and a helpful mobile app.

✔ **Scramble up some eggs.** Eggs are a Paleo protein powerhouse. Rich in many key nutrients, especially fat-soluble vitamins A and D, egg yolk is also loaded with a B vitamin that's super brain food. Look for organic, pastured eggs with omega-3 for the best fatty acid profile. (Eggs are one food where you shouldn't settle for conventional production methods.)

✔ **Get wild!** Wild animal meat — venison, rabbit, bear, wild-caught fish, even wild boar — is an excellent choice. It's very lean and full of healthy omega-3 fats. If you're going to splurge a bit on your food bill — or really imitate hunter-gatherers and do the hunting yourself — choosing wild animal meat is a wise way to do it.

Animal proteins help you reduce excess body fat, build lean muscle, and feed your brain with the nutrients it needs for peak performance. Incorporating adequate animal protein in your Paleo approach will vastly improve your health and well-being.

Friendly fats and why they're essential

If the term *friendly fats* seems like an oxymoron, this section is for you! Our brains have been hijacked by low-fat, no-fat thinking, but we are evolved to eat naturally occurring fats (called *fatty acids*) to build our best bodies. Say it with us: "Fat is our friend."

When we talk about essential fats, we refer to fats that your body can't produce on its own. These fats, important for all systems of the body, must be obtained through the food you eat. Your skin, heart, lungs, nervous systems, brain, and all internal organs are improved and maintained by eating fatty acids. Plus, fats make food taste good and help you feel satisfied. What's friendlier than that?

The two essential fats are known as *omega-3* and *omega-6 fatty acids.* You've probably heard about omega-3 in relation to heart health, but these fatty acids are inflammation busters and also aid in other conditions, including diabetes, some cancers, skin disorders, arthritis, cholesterol, and depression.

Getting the right ratio of omega-3 and omega-6 fats

Omega-3 fatty acids are found in animal sources, such as the following:

- Cold-water fish, like salmon, sardines, herring, mackerel, and black cod
- Wild game, like venison, bear, rabbit, and boar

Omega-6 fatty acids are found in unfavorable sources, such as canola oil, corn oil, and other processed fats known as industrial oils, which are best avoided. But omega-6 fatty acids are also found *naturally* and more healthfully in the following nuts and seeds and the oils extracted from them:

- Almonds
- Brazil nuts
- Cashews
- Hazelnuts
- Macadamia nuts
- Pecans
- Pistachios
- Sesame seeds
- Sunflower seeds
- Walnuts

Before you reach for the jar of nuts, there's a catch: You need to consume these essential fats in your diet in the right ratios. The ideal fatty-acid ratio is about 1:1 omega-6 to omega-3.

Wondering what a healthy omega-6 to omega-3 ratio looks like? Our number-one pick for nuts is macadamia nuts. With a ratio of 6:3, they're definitely Paleo approved (and delicious).

Unfortunately, the ratio of omega-6 to omega-3 in the modern diet is between 15:1 and 22:1 — that means that most people are consuming far too much omega-6 fatty acid. About 15 to 20 times too much!

How did this happen? Non-Paleo-friendly fats are used to produce many processed foods found on supermarket shelves, and those types of oils are used almost exclusively in restaurants. Additionally, modern grain-fed meat supply means that the conventionally grown meat is also high in omega-6 fats. The critical balance of omega-6 to omega-3 fatty acids is teetering the wrong way.

Avoiding unhealthy fats

Here are some common fats that aren't Paleo-friendly. These refined oils have very unbalanced fatty acid ratios — corn oil is 57:1!

These fats are also sensitive to the damaging effects of heat and are often rancid on the store shelves, before you even add them to your grocery cart. Your body isn't adapted to process these oils, and they should be eliminated from your kitchen and your plate.

- Canola oil
- Corn oil
- Cottonseed oil
- Margarine
- Partially hydrogenated vegetable oil

- Safflower oil
- Soybean oil
- Sunflower oil
- Vegetable shortening

These fats can cause more inflammation in the body. Inflammation causes illness, premature aging, and weight gain. These fats are not naturally occurring, and when you eat fake fat, you get fat.

Eating healthy, natural fats

Here are some smart, healthy choices for friendly fats:

- **Monounsaturated fats:** Monounsaturated fats (MUFA) are liquid at room temperature and solidify when chilled. Good sources include green or black olives, olive oil, macadamia nuts, macadamia oil, avocado, and avocado oil. These fats aren't recommended for cooking because heat can oxidize them, turning them from friend to foe. Use MUFAs on salads or to drizzle on cooked foods.

- **Saturated fats:** Saturated fats have suffered an unfair reputation as a heart disease villain. The truth is that saturated fats have been an important and beneficial part of the human diet since our cave man ancestors gnawed on a nice, fatty chop. Saturated fat is solid at room temperature, and our favorite source is coconut. Coconut oil is ideal for cooking because it can withstand higher temperatures. Coconut flakes, coconut milk, and coconut butter are also delicious, healthful options. You should also feel free to indulge in the luscious fat found in organic, grass-fed, pastured meats and poultry, eggs, and wild-caught fish.

✔ **Polyunsaturated fats:** Polyunsaturated fats (PUFA), found primarily in nuts and seeds, are higher in omega-6 fatty acids and should be consumed in moderation. The best choices for PUFAs are almonds and almond butter, Brazil nuts, cashews and cashew butter, pistachios, and pecans.

When you enjoy Paleo-friendly fats, all your body systems function more optimally, and you fight fit, ready to ward off many modern ailments, like cancer, autoimmune diseases, neurological problems, heart disease, obesity, and a host of other issues that deficiency brings. Fake fat makes you fat — natural fats help you thrive.

Complex carbs and why they're king

To understand carbohydrates' role in your body function, you need to know a little about glucose and insulin. Carbs are your body's go-to source for quick energy. Your body transforms all carbohydrates — from whole-grain bread to broccoli florets — into glucose, and your brain and cells use glucose as a primary fuel source. Activities like reading this book, running a mile, or hugging your kids are all made possible by glucose.

Insulin is a hormone that helps your body store fat for later energy use. If you want to control the accumulation and reduction of body fat, you need to control insulin — and to do that, you need to eat the right kinds of carbohydrates. Knowing which carbs to eat is critical because the sources you choose directly dictate your insulin level. When insulin production is under control, weight loss and optimal health are the result.

The best carbohydrate sources are local, organically grown fruit and vegetables. Choose fruits and non-starchy vegetables in all the colors of the rainbow to cover the full spectrum of nutrients. Dark-colored fruits, such as blackberries and blueberries, are packed with antioxidants, and deeply colored veggies, like carrots and kale, are loaded with vitamins and minerals.

Here are some delicious examples of non-starchy vegetables:

✔ Asparagus

✔ Broccoli

✔ Brussels sprouts

✔ Cabbage

✔ Cauliflower

✔ Eggplant

✔ Onions

✔ Peppers

✔ Spaghetti squash

✔ Summer squash

✔ Tomatoes

✔ Vegetable greens: kale, collard greens, Swiss chard, mustard greens, spinach, and so on

✔ Zucchini

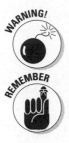

Steer clear of starch- and sugar-laden carbohydrates sources like white potatoes, rice, corn, breads (including whole grain), cereals, pasta, fruit juices, and sodas. These sugars are instantly absorbed and will affect your blood sugar insulin levels in a flash.

The Paleo approach is not a low-carb diet but a healthy-carb plan. When you drop unhealthy refined carbohydrates and replace them with vegetables and fruits, you begin to live the Paleo way.

Rethinking the Pyramid

In 1992, the Department of Agriculture created the USDA food pyramid. When it came to what to eat and how much, many families, schools, organizations, and nutritionists came to rely on this pyramid as the gold standard. This, unfortunately, was a big fat mistake. Since adopting the USDA pyramid, we've become more unhealthy, more overweight, and definitely more confused than ever. In 2010, another attempt was made to get America back on track. The pyramid was retired, and along came the USDA plate — with more confusion and misinformation. However, hope exists. It comes down to eating by design, by making your meals come from food choices that your body understands.

In the following sections, we tear down the USDA plate and retire it with the USDA food pyramid. We introduce the most effective eating guide you'll find, the Paleo pyramid. It's decisive, scientifically founded, and super easy to implement! You'll enjoy figuring out why this pyramid is the answer for modern-day cave women and men and how your concerns will be answered once and for all.

The flawed USDA food pyramid

The advice about good nutrition can be very confusing. Just browse the magazine covers at the checkout stand to see all the conflict: low-carb, no-carb, low-fat, vegetarian, vegan, no fruit. What's next — no food? No air?

We place the blame for all the confusion on the USDA food pyramid, shown in Figure 4-1.

Here are some of the biggest problems with the food pyramid:

✔ The base of the food pyramid is cereal, bread, and pasta — and a lot of it, to the tune of 6 to 11 servings. As we discuss in Chapter 2, these processed carbs are unfavorable sources of energy and, more importantly, your body does *not* require these foods to operate efficiently.

Additionally, antinutrients are found in whole grains, called *phytic acid* and *lectins*.

- Phytic acid binds to minerals, making them unavailable for you to use. This means that the more whole grains you eat, the less able your body is to take advantage of minerals like calcium, magnesium, and zinc.

- Lectins may even cause more trouble. These tricky guys bind to insulin receptors, which can lead to insulin problems, are linked to inflammatory problems, and damage your gut defenses that line your intestines. When you damage this lining, it causes you to transport food particles into the blood system and lymph system, where they don't belong. Digestion becomes compromised as well as your immune system — not very appetizing!

The USDA food pyramid identifies whole grains as a good source of fiber. Here's the real skinny: non-starchy veggies and fruits often have more than double the amount of fiber as grains.

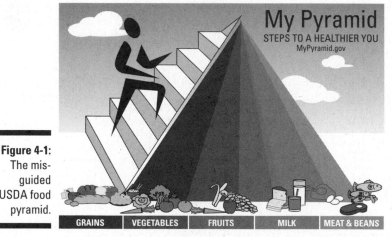

Figure 4-1:
The misguided USDA food pyramid.

Illustration © USDA

With the Paleo plan, you have no recommended daily allowance (RDA) for breads, pasta, and cereals. In fact, not only does your body not require these grains, but also your insulin management is better — so you're healthier and happier — without them.

✔ The food pyramid identifies dairy as a key component of good nutrition, but cow's milk is the number-one food allergen for humans. That's because cow's milk isn't intended for human consumption; it's the perfect food for transforming calves into very large cows. Your body just doesn't know what to do with milk — and ailments like digestive disturbance, acne, insulin resistance, and allergic reactions are the result.

Studies show that milk isn't as protective to bone tissue as once thought — and contrary to popular belief, milk does *not* reduce bone fractures! To form and maintain strong bones, your body strives to be in pH balance; the fruits and vegetables in the Paleo diet do just that.

✔ The food pyramid missteps with protein, too. Dried beans and peas can't be eaten interchangeably with animal proteins like meat, poultry, fish, and eggs. Beans and legumes have poor digestibility and don't pack the same complete protein punch as animal sources. In fact, beans, and legumes averaged about 20 to 25 percent lower than animal protein ratings in a protein quality index published by The Food and Agriculture Organization/World Health Organization.

Beans and legumes contain about three times less protein than animal sources — and the incomplete proteins found in legumes are difficult for your body to digest.

In 2010, the USDA developed the next generation of food guidelines called MyPlate, shown in Figure 4-2.

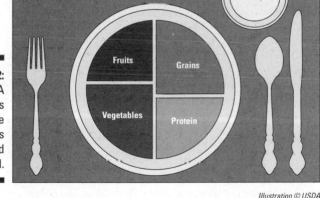

Figure 4-2: The USDA plate has the same flaws as the food pyramid.

Illustration © USDA

Although the USDA plate is more appealing to the eye than the pyramid, it suffers from the same challenges: Whole grains and dairy are still included requirements for health. The plate approach doesn't solve the old problems. Instead, our actual plates should represent what we've discovered from evolutionary science.

The Paleo pyramid

So the USDA food pyramid had major problems, and the new USDA plate didn't improve on those problems. However, the Paleo food pyramid, which you can see in Figure 4-3, is built on simple, real foods that are close to their natural state. When you create meals with the healthy building blocks of the Paleo pyramid, weight loss is effortless, and vibrant good health is a natural side effect.

The Paleo Pyramid

The Top
Paleo-friendly snacks and desserts made with nuts, dried fruit, coconut flour, and nut flours

Level Three
Naturally occurring fats and oils — nuts, seeds, coconut oil, macadamia oil, nut butters (like almond butter), grass-fed butter, and ghee

Level Two
Low-starch and low-sugar vegetables and fruits (berries, lemons, and limes)

The Base
Protein: The foundation of the Paleo Pyramid — includes meat, fish, fowl, and eggs

Figure 4-3:
The Paleo pyramid in all its glory.

Illustration by Wiley, Composition Services Graphics

Here's what good health looks like:

- ✔ **The Base:** Meat, fish, fowl, and eggs
- ✔ **Level Two:** Low-starch and low-sugar vegetables and fruits
- ✔ **Level Three:** Naturally occurring fats and oils
- ✔ **The Top:** Paleo-friendly snacks and desserts made with nuts, dried fruit, coconut flour, and nut flours

When you eat the foods that make up the Paleo pyramid, you're free from confusion — and free to eat real food. When you choose Paleo foods, you choose a plan that works with your genetics to bring out the best in everything you do. You'll soon find that the nutrient-rich foods have everything you need to become healthier and stronger and to fight aging.

The next sections go into detail about how following the Paleo pyramid gives you enough fiber, calcium, and all the vitamins and minerals your body needs for all the structures and functions of your body to flourish. The nutrients listed in these sections are ones you definitely *won't* be missing when you start living Paleo.

Yes, you'll get enough fiber

You've probably been hammered with the idea that you need to eat plenty of fiber. And, yes, fiber plays an important role in healthy nutrition. It helps stabilize blood sugar levels while lowering blood cholesterol. Fiber helps you feel more full, so food cravings are reduced, and it helps you build a stronger immune system with fewer hormonal imbalances. It also acts like a scrub brush for your colon to help keep it clean and healthy.

Based on all of that, you may be worried that if you eliminate whole grains from your diet, you'll be short on your fiber requirements. But when you enjoy appropriate quantities of vegetables and fruits, you get all the fiber you need from natural, *digestible* sources.

You may be surprised to realize that the foods you've been taught are high in fiber — whole-grain bread, whole-grain pasta, brown rice — aren't the health foods they've been advertised to be. Your best sources of fiber, in just the right amounts to keep you healthy, are fresh vegetables, fresh fruit, dried fruits, and, in moderation, nuts and seeds.

Yes, you'll get enough calcium

You probably already know that your body needs calcium to form strong bones and teeth. And like most Americans, you've been taught to believe that drinking milk is essential for getting enough calcium. But dairy can be a major source of inflammation. Instead, get your calcium from high-quality sources like plants, sardines, seafood, and some nuts.

Here are some good options for calcium that are easy for your body to absorb:

✓ **Plant sources:**
- Bok choy and cabbage
- Collard, mustard, and turnip greens
- Green beans
- Kale
- Seaweed, like kelp and dulse
- Spinach
- Watercress

  ✔ **Seafood sources:**

  - Canned mackerel

  - Salmon (with bones)

  - Sardines (with bones)

  - Shrimp

  ✔ **Fat sources:**

  - Nut and seed butters: almond, sesame, sunflower

  - Nuts: almonds, cashews, Brazil nuts, chestnuts

  - Seeds: sesame, sunflower

  ✔ **Other sources:**

  - Dried dates

  - Dried figs

  - Olives

If you eat plenty of leafy green vegetables and embellish your meals with other calcium-rich choices, you don't need dairy or calcium supplements to meet your calcium requirements.

Yes, you'll get enough vitamins and minerals

We talked about macronutrients earlier (in the section "The Paleo Big Three: Animal Proteins, Natural Fats, Complex Carbohydrates"); now it's time to address *micronutrients* — the vitamins and minerals found in the foods you eat.

Nutrients work synergistically in your body — the vitamins and minerals cooperate to keep you healthy. When you have a vitamin or mineral deficiency, merely supplementing with the one that's falling short won't correct the imbalance.

A healthy diet is the best way to supply your body with the balance of vitamins and minerals it needs. When you eat an abundance of vegetables and fruits, as well as high-quality protein and fat, the nutrients in those foods work together to keep your body functioning well.

No, you don't need whole grains and dairy

Many of us were taught that healthy meals must incorporate some whole grains, legumes, and dairy to be complete and to ensure adequate doses of vitamins and minerals. The truth is that grains and legumes include substances called *antinutrients* that are actually detrimental to your health. In the short-term, they can cause digestive distress and bloating; in the long-term, they can permanently damage your digestive system, which leads to internal inflammation.

pH and your body

Your body strives to be in a pH balance (see Chapter 2). In addition, grains, legumes, and dairy are acid-forming foods in the body. You do need some acid in your body, but a diet that's even slightly over acidic can cause bone loss, muscle loss, aging, fatigue, and illness. When you're acidic, your body starts to lose its ability to absorb minerals and other nutrients. Fruits and vegetables are very alkaline and provide you with that acid-alkaline balance — another nutritional benefit that grains, dairy, and beans can't provide.

And forget what you've heard about milk doing the body good. Once you've been weaned from your mother, you're not designed to consume milk in any of its forms. (Sorry, cheese and yogurt!) Cow's milk is evolved to nourish cows, not humans — and the pasteurization and homogenization processes further obliterate any potentially nutritious components of dairy.

The truth is that grains, dairy, and beans are more damaging than rewarding and don't add value to investments in your nutritional bank.

Real food always equals real nutrition. Your health is determined by your nutrient intake, and the Paleo pyramid supplies all the nutrients you need in delicious, natural packaging.

Beyond the Big Three

By now, you're an expert on the Paleo Big Three and micronutrients that form the framework for living Paleo. But there's more to a Paleo plate. After you're a pro at building a nutritious meal around macronutrients, you may want to spice things up or grab a meal on the go. And, yes, you may even want to have dessert.

Do you think *dessert* means cheating or doing something sinful? Think again. Living Paleo means that you can enjoy healthy choices for dessert that help you avoid the bloating, fatigue, sugar buzz, and guilt that are usually served alongside cake or ice cream.

These days, people live high-speed lives, and, sometimes, they need a meal that they can take on the go. Adding protein powders to a vegetable-and-fruit smoothie can be a fast, portable protein source when you're in a hurry — but only if you choose the right protein powder. Of course, real food should always be your first choice.

Salt, too, takes us beyond the Paleo Big Three. Both demonized and lauded for its nutritional properties, salt contains iodine and other minerals that can help keep your body at a desirable pH level. Our hunter-gatherer ancestors enjoyed the taste of salt that naturally occurs in seafood and seawater, and you can, too.

In the following sections, we show you how you can end a meal with something sweet without a sugar crash, we arm you with the info you need so you can be as healthy as possible in your busy world, and we clue you in on how you can enjoy the benefits (and flavor) of salt — in a Paleo-friendly way.

Desserts redefined

Living Paleo means redefining the foods you eat, from breakfast straight on through the day to dessert.

Your body is hardwired to desire something a little sweet from time to time. Your hunter-gatherer ancestors satisfied their sweet tooth by grabbing a handful of berries — when they were in season and when they could find them. In modern life, it's almost always berry season, so you need to temper your natural craving for sweets with moderation and sugar in its natural form: fruit and nuts.

A Paleo-friendly dessert can blast your body with vitamins, minerals, and healthy fats. Your best bets are berries and other low-sugar fruits, eaten slowly and savored for their natural sweetness. You can add natural seasonings — vanilla, coconut flakes, crushed nuts, lemon zest — that don't increase the sugar content and transform fruit into dessert. (We share some recipes in Chapter 13.)

Shakin' it up with protein shakes

Earlier in this chapter, we clue you in to all the good that protein does for your body. This macronutrient is so important that many companies have created quick sources, like protein powders, to make it easy for people to supplement their lifestyle. On the plus side: These sources can be a convenient source of lasting energy; on the minus side: Most contain unhealthy artificial sugars and flavorings. To be blunt, they're protein-ish junk in a bottle. In order to stick to our mission, which is to make sure we are 100 percent authentic in what we teach and not just espouse the popular vote, we have to assert that protein powders are not our favorite or recommended choice of protein.

Real food always trumps anything with a label. However, if protein powder can make your life easier — and make living Paleo more manageable — here are some guidelines for getting the best protein powder for your body:

✔ Look for protein sources that come from lactose-free whey isolates, egg white, or hemp. Avoid both soy and casein, which are inferior proteins that cause allergies in many people.

✔ Avoid protein powders that include multiple protein, like a mixture of whey, casein, and soy. These powders are often higher in calories and are difficult to digest.

✔ If you find yourself with a bad aftertaste, indigestion, or an allergic reaction after consuming a smoothie made with protein powder, that's a sign you're sensitive to that particular protein and shouldn't eat it again. Instead, try a hemp powder; it comes from a vegetarian source that's low-allergen and is easy for most people to digest.

Our number-one recommendation for protein powder is Primal Fuel (www.primalblueprint.com). It's completely grain-free and has the cleanest ingredients you'll find on the market. We love the added kelp — which is great for thyroid function — and it also includes some coconut for a dose of healthy fats.

Salt: Love it or leave it

Salt should be one of the seven wonders of the world! It's historically known as the *divine substance* because it provides so much pleasure by enhancing the flavor of food. More importantly, your body needs salt. Natural salt is vital to your nervous system and your adrenal glands, which are in charge of many of your body's hormones.

Here's the real deal on salt: It can make you healthier, or it can make you sick. It all depends on what kind of salt you're sprinkling on your food. Today, most table salt goes through a lot of refining. After being chemically cleaned with bleach, manufacturers add toxic anti-caking agents to ensure that the salt flows freely.

A healthy salt is loaded with trace minerals, including potassium and magnesium. These two minerals allow your cell walls to be permeable, so fluids — and nutrients — can flow in and out of your cells freely. This allows your body to re-mineralize and rehydrate easily. When your cells are permeable, your body releases what it doesn't need, eliminating the fluid retention that causes bloating and high blood pressure.

Note that natural, unrefined salts contain only trace amounts of iodine. Because adequate levels of iodine are essential for a healthy thyroid, hormones, and immune function, make sure you get iodine from these other sources:

✔ Seaweed, like kelp and dulse

✔ Protein: eggs, meat, poultry

> ✓ Vegetables: Swiss chard, asparagus, spinach
>
> ✓ Strawberries

We love the finely ground vital mineral blend of Celtic Sea Salt. It comes from one of the most pristine coastal regions of France, has zero additives, and is rich in minerals and trace elements. For more info, go to www.celticseasalt.com or call 1-800-TOP-SALT.

Paleo-Approved Supplements

Living Paleo means putting real food first. But the modern world presents some real nutritional challenges, and sometimes supplementation — for a short period of time — can be a good idea to help restore balance in your body.

Many of the foods you eat may come from depleted sources. The soils in which most vegetables and fruits grow are devoid of nutrients, and by the time you bite into that apple from the grocery store, it probably made a journey by truck then sat in a crate for weeks while its nutrients dissipated.

The standard American diet of processed food and nutrient-poor grains and dairy may have provided you with excess calories and a deficiency of nutrients. You can turn this around with Paleo nutrition, but in the beginning, you may need a boost from the right supplements. After living Paleo for some time, you'll need less supplementation because you'll get all you need from food. Until then, in the following sections, we outline the supplements with the biggest bang for your health with the reminder that you take them only when and if you really need them.

To get your supplements in the purest possible form, buy the highest quality you can afford from health professionals or a reputable natural health store. Be sure to scan labels for artificial colors, flavorings, and added sugar so you don't sabotage your good intentions.

Omega-3s

Omega fats are one of the most critical factors in nutrition today. They're vital to improving your health and slowing the aging process, but most people are severely depleted of omega-3s.

Omega-3 supplementation is important in the prevention of heart disease, cancer, diabetes, arthritis, obesity, eczema, learning problems, and many other lifestyle ailments. As omega-3 supplements reduce inflammation in the body, most people immediately feel more energy and brighter skin. They also have more comfortable bowel movements and can think more clearly.

When you buy omega-3s, purchase the cleanest source possible. Heavy metals, PCBs, pesticides, and other contaminants can be an issue when taking fish oils, so be sure to check the labels. Also, a great way to test your omega-3 oil, is to run the "freezer test": Place your supplement in the freezer; if it freezes, you may have a poor quality oil with additives. This is definitely not going to get you looking or feeling better!

We recommend Stronger Faster Healthier's super omega-3 oil (`www.stronger fasterhealthier.com`). It's available in five tasty-enough flavors, and the quality is top-notch.

Probiotics

Imagine a 25-foot long tube lined with trillions of cells. That's your intestine, and it houses 95 percent of the total number of cells in your body. That's also where almost three-quarters of your immune system is housed.

The bacteria that live within the walls of your intestinal tract are critical to your overall health. When you have an abundance of friendly bacteria, there's literally no room for the bad guys (pathogens) to attach to and damage your intestinal walls. So when you're healing your body, probiotics may be a good choice for you.

Probiotics are naturally occurring, friendly bacteria. A probiotic supplement ultimately makes your intestinal tract healthier and more resilient. Probiotics aid digestion while they protect against yeast and other bacterial overgrowth and help prevent weight gain.

Many modern ailments are the result of disturbed gut flora. Frankly, our hunter-gatherer ancestors played around in the dirt a lot more than we do. This exposure provided them with the bacteria they needed to keep their guts healthy. Our modern practices of sanitization means we don't interact with these microscopic organisms. Additionally, processed foods, antibiotics, and even stress all eliminate these helpful microorganisms.

The following questions can help you determine whether you'd benefit from a probiotics supplement:

- ✔ Have you eaten a lot of processed foods?
- ✔ Have you taken antibiotics to fight infection?
- ✔ Have you lived or worked in a sanitized environment (like a hospital)?
- ✔ Have you lived or worked in a very stressful environment?

Despite what some advertisements try to tell you, you can't get effective probiotics from yogurt or kefir. (And as we discuss in Chapter 2, yogurt can be the cause of — not the answer for — digestive issues.)

Probiotics are available in two forms: in a tablet (or capsule) or in a powdered formula. Heat can damage these fragile, friendly bacteria, so look for a dairy-free source that's stored in a refrigerator. Look for a probiotic supplement that contains multiple strains of lactobacillus and bifidobacterium — and follow the dosage recommendations on the label.

We like Primal Blueprint's Primal Flora (www.primalblueprint.com). Available in easy-to-manage capsules, each dose includes about 30 billion CFUs (colony forming units) — that's about 25 times more potent as an average serving of yogurt!

Vitamin D3

Vitamin D3 has been shown to lower the incidence of some cancers, reduce inflammation, prevent autoimmune diseases, maintain healthy bones, promote healthy moods, act as a powerful antioxidant, as well as prevent colds and flu. Pretty amazing!

Unfortunately, vitamin D3 deficiency has become an epidemic. If you spend a lot of time indoors or use sunscreen regularly, you may be low on vitamin D3. Even many windows block the UVB rays that you need to naturally produce vitamin D. Plus, the reality is that no sufficient dietary source exists.

Recently, it's been determined that the recommended daily allowance for vitamin D is too low. If you've never had your vitamin D levels checked, we urge you to request this simple blood test from your doctor. It's an essential benchmark to ensure that you're getting the correct dosage, because you can overdose on vitamin D. Be sure to ask that the lab test for the most beneficial vitamin D marker: 25-hydroxy-vitamin D. Work with your doctor or practitioner to determine the right dosage for you.

To absorb vitamin D3 naturally, you need to expose large portions of your skin to the sun for about 15 minutes daily. But be careful! More is not better. If your skin begins to turn pink or red, you've already stopped producing Vitamin D.

Melatonin

Melatonin is naturally produced in the pineal gland (which is found in the brain) when your environment starts to dim, whether it be from ambient lightning or dusk approaching. Melatonin is actually a hormone, and as levels in the blood increase, your body gets ready for sleep. Your melatonin levels start to naturally decrease at about puberty, and wane even more after age 40, which is partly the reason it becomes more difficult to get a sound night sleep as you get older.

Melatonin has been found to be safe and effective for treating sleep issues. Melatonin helps restore and regulate your brain's natural rhythms, which contributes to a good night's sleep. The double bonus is that melatonin also floods your brain with antioxidants, so it's protective as well.

Sound, restful sleep is essential to your health. No matter what else you do to improve your health, if you're not sleeping well, you're not as healthy as you can be.

Melatonin is a powerful hormone, so we don't recommend that you supplement with melatonin every night. Work with your physician to understand how long you can rely on an external source of melatonin. Ideally, your body will eventually produce adequate melatonin on its own. But during times of long periods without sleep — or stress or travel that disrupts your sleep — melatonin supplementation can help you enjoy restorative zzz's. Take one to three milligrams about one hour before bedtime to restore a normal sleep-awake rhythm.

Magnesium

Magnesium is an essential mineral in your muscle and nerve cells. In fact, more than half of the magnesium in your body is in your bones. It regulates muscle contractions. Where calcium constricts or tightens muscles, magnesium relaxes them. Magnesium calms nerve cells down, and a deficiency in magnesium interferes with nerve and muscle impulses, causing irritability and nervousness. It's also a big player in the formation of bones.

Happily, with magnesium supplementation, these ailments disappear — and the Paleo diet is packed with magnesium-rich foods so the period for supplementation can be short. Fish, meat, seafood, apples, almonds, avocados, leafy greens, and kelp are all great sources. Your levels will be back up in no time by living Paleo!

Magnesium supplementation is a great way to maintain your acid-base balance. Magnesium is very alkaline forming. Modern-day foods and lifestyles have made people very acidic, and magnesium is a great way to bring you to balance. It also moves stool through your intestines, so it's an amazing natural laxative. It relaxes you, helps you sleep, eases menstrual aches, and reduces muscle pains. Magnesium is definitely worth a try!

We recommend you take a chelated form of magnesium that's easier for your body to absorb, like magnesium citrate, glycinate, or malate. The dosing depends on your intended use. If you're taking magnesium for treatment of low magnesium levels, take as directed on your product label. If you're taking it for other reasons, consult your wellness practitioner for further consultation.

Branched-chain amino acids

Amino acids are the building blocks of protein. The term *branched chain* refers to the chemical structure of three of the amino acids that are essential to your body. *Essential*, meaning your body can't produce these amino acids, so you must get them through outside sources, such as food. These amino acids in the branched chain include L-Valine, L-Leucine, and L-Isoleucine, which are the three aminos responsible for muscle protein synthesis. In nature, we find these amino acids in red meat products, eggs, fish, and nuts (and other non-Paleo sources, such as dairy, corn, beans, rice, wheat, and lentils).

Branched-chain amino acids help your body synthesize the protein found in your own muscles to prevent that muscle from breaking down. They assist your body in slowing down the rate of muscle wasting — especially after vigorous activity — so you maintain muscle and burn fat.

Another big bonus: Branched-chain amino acids can also help reduce cravings for carbohydrates, which is very beneficial while making the transition to living Paleo. So in addition to keeping your muscles strong, they also calm your cravings.

You'll see supplemental amino acids sold in a variety of forms: multivitamin mixtures, protein mixtures, capsules, tablets, and powders. The protein in your supplement should be derived from animal or vegetable protein — and it should be labeled *free form,* which means the amino acids are in the best form for digestion.

This supplementation is great for athletes who want to improve their performance and reduce muscle breakdown. Or if you're a casual exerciser who wants to drop a few pounds or reduce carb cravings, this supplement may be a good choice for you. Dosage is 5 to 15 grams per day, depending on your activity level. Talk to your doctor or practitioner to determine your specific needs.

Avoid crystalline-free forms of branched-chain amino acids; they're made from grains. We recommend Life Extension (www.lef.org) as a Paleo-approved supplement.

Those with ALS or disorders impairing the metabolism of branched-chain amino acids should not use these supplements.

Chapter 5

Modern Challenges, Ancient Solutions

*L*iving in this modern world brings many challenges. Our inverted way of eating, moving, and living has created a pandemic of chronic illnesses, so much so that chronic illness is now killing 80 percent of the industrialized world and is the leading cause of death. By 2017, chronic illness will cost $4.3 trillion per year in the United States alone! Why all this suffering, when we're spending more money on healthcare than ever before?

The answer goes back to our ancestors. Their lifestyle patterns were so different from how we live today. Our current lifestyles have become so incongruent with our natural design that we're getting plagued with chronic illness — something that wasn't at all common with our ancestors.

The greatest factor of whether you'll be healthy and vibrant or sick and obese is your lifestyle choices. *You* are in the driver's seat. How your genes express themselves has to do with the environment you choose to live in and stay in.

In this chapter, we share the rhythm of the cave man's lifestyle so you can figure out how to make choices that express health and vitality. You discover better ways to manage stress, toxins, and electronic pollution and realize the value of sunshine, water, and sleep. We designed this chapter to walk you through some of those lifestyle patterns that are practical and important in helping you live a life that will recharge and heal you.

The Civilized Life of a Cave Man

The cave man's life appears anything but civilized. He had to deal with outside elements and had to hunt and forage for food. When he was stricken with illness and infections, he had none of our modern-day supplies and medications to heal him. Every day was a fight for survival. Somehow, though, he had a rhythm to his life. As much mayhem as there appeared to be, there was also community and a pattern that made sense.

Hunter-gatherers lived in bands of about 30 people dispersed over various land. Roles were clearly defined: The men hunted and fished while the women gathered nuts and berries and cared for the children. At night, they sat by a fire, which provided heat and light. It protected them from animals, and they used it to cook their food.

Food was scarce at times for hunter-gatherers, and hunger was sometimes a part of their reality, although they usually had enough. The food that they did have was filled with such abundant nutrition that it was ideal to maintain a very healthy existence.

Hunter-gatherers were lean and strong. Those that survived illness, trauma, and infection lived a relatively long, healthy, and fit life. They were completely untroubled by the chronic illnesses brought on by current lifestyle patterns.

Bottom line: Hunter-gatherers lived healthier lives. Regardless of what they died from, they were free from chronic illness, and they were healthy and fit and full of vitality. They didn't have diseases of modern civilization, such as heart attacks, strokes, diabetes, hypertension, and obesity. The discordance between our current lifestyle and the one we've genetically adopted is the heart of our suffering.

Should we go back in time and try to mimic everything about the Paleolithic life? Of course not. But we can learn from science and take the features from our ancestors' footprints that would most benefit us. We can choose the lifestyle patterns that will help us live a better life and leave behind those that are impractical.

In the following sections, we walk you through a day in the life of a Paleo man, including how he worked *and* relaxed — something we can definitely apply more of to our current lifestyles.

The working life of a Paleo man

The hunter-gatherers were anatomically like modern-day human beings. They had the same range in physique and biological function. They lived in a time before agriculture, so they didn't have crops or domesticated animals. Instead, people lived by hunting and gathering. They had limited shelter. They had to learn to be attuned to everything around them. They formed close relationships with all the members of their band.

Daily life included lots of activity. Children were active, and women were busy caring for children and gathering berries while meat roasted from a recent kill. The men spent their days hunting. Every moment of their day was spent on survival.

In the world of our ancestors, hunting and gathering was their only way of sustaining life. The men were the leaders in their bands. They moved with the seasons, finding game, water, and plant food. Physical activity was a central part of their day.

Hunter-gatherers were psychologically similar to modern-day man and had challenges, hopes, and pleasures just like many do today. They wouldn't hang on to anger and grievances for long periods. If aggressions formed with band members, they'd go off to live with friends or family in other bands until they decided to return. This was an understanding of conflict resolution among communities.

The people in their band were important to hunter-gatherers. They formed close relationships with these people and brought home enough kill so that their band wouldn't starve. Hunter-gatherers also planned their seasonal moves so they would always be with food and water.

Looking at the life of a Paleo man shows us how we were meant to eat, move, and live. But it also shows us that we thrive when we're around others, have a purpose, and enjoy the simple things life has to offer that can bring so much pleasure.

The relaxing life of a Paleo man

Even though daily survival was tough, our ancestors spent time during the day relaxing. Daily relaxation was a part of their life, not just every so often or when they could. Every night, they'd gather around a fire and eat, talk, play music, and sing songs, and the children played.

Our ancestors' ritual of relaxing was as important to them as anything else they did (a big contrast from modern-day lifestyles). They worked hard, but they also relaxed every day. Relaxing was a great way to combat many of the stresses of their day-to-day struggles. It was part of their daily rhythm.

Here are a few lessons we can learn from our ancestors' footprint:

- **Community:** A big factor in their ability to get through their daily stresses were that they were communal people. Knowing that they had each other kept them calm and relaxed. No matter what disappointments, hurt, or frustration they went through, they went through it together.

  They also didn't suffer from any social isolation. They experienced nurturing and love from those around them. This social safety was a form of stress relief.

- **Daily rhythms and relaxation:** They were very ritualistic people and had a rhythm to everything they did. They had regular relaxation time and connected with one another every day.

- **Purpose:** They didn't fill their life with false, needless worries or aimless patterns. They had a role in their band and knew what was expected of them. They spent their time doing meaningful, necessary tasks with people they had a close connection with. They worried about only real stresses like food, shelter, injury, infection, or trauma.

Our ancestors didn't die from diseases of stress like so many people do today. The importance of community, love, and sense of purpose allowed them to escape the harmful effects of stress that many of us experience in our modern world. Living Paleo is about creating a life that's healthy and vibrant in every area. Our hunter-gatherer ancestors valued the simple things in life, which, even today, are often the keys to relaxation and joy.

Sleep: An Essential Ingredient for Weight Loss and Health

These days, everyone is so focused on the value of doing more. However, recognizing that more important than getting stuff done is the importance of shutting your eyes can take you to the next level of health. Look at sleep as a nutrient that affects virtually every aspect of your life. Lack of sleep can make you age prematurely and make you sick and obese. It affects mood and mental health. For these reasons, you should think of sleep being as important as any other element of healthy living.

Look to our ancestors' lifestyle when it comes to sleep habits. They didn't fall prey to the diseases we have, and sleep may have been a very big part of the puzzle. When darkness fell and their nightly fire went out, so did they. They didn't have the opportunity to stay up and push to do more, and their health was better for it.

When you begin living Paleo, you *will* sleep better. When you begin to maintain good sleeping habits, it has a domino effect in your life. You'll move better, think better, and be more motivated to eat better. Sleep is your foundational piece to everything and developing living Paleo sleeping habits are key.

So sleep is one of those simple yet powerful tools that is truly a health weapon. Sleep makes you much healthier and function better, and it's an important component in weight loss.

What does sleep have to do with fat, you ask? Insufficient sleep as well as poor quality sleep provokes your body to store fat. As important as eating a nutrient-dense diet is to your waist so is adding a quality sleeping program into your regime. In fact, if your goal is weight loss, cuddle in a comfy chair and be sure to read the following sections. These are facts you'll want to know.

What happens when you're short on zzz's

Getting enough sleep was easy for our hunter-gatherer ancestors, but that's not the case for most modern people. Electricity and the widespread use of the good ol' light bulb have given us freedom. They've also given us sleep deprivation.

In 1910, the average adult slept nine to ten hours a night. Now, the average adult may get seven hours a night. That's a staggering 500 extra waking hours a year — and it's even more if you're not getting at least seven hours of sleep a night!

So many things interfere with sleep today: E-mails, TVs with 150 channels, more hobbies, social media, and smartphones have all become such a part of living in our modern world that we borrow time from sleep to do more. Because of sleep's cumulative affect, before long, we're sleep deprived, which leads us to a host of serious problems.

Sleep deprivation isn't a joke. When you lack sleep, here are some potential outcomes that may startle you:

✔ **Illness:** Going to bed too late doubles your risk of breast cancer.

    In 2004, a study in the journal *Sleep* found that women who averaged less than five hours of sleep per night had a higher death rate than those who slept seven hours.

✔ **Weight gain:** You can loose 14.3 pounds a year by getting one more hour a night of sleep. Sleep deprivation causes you to gain weight. Proper sleep helps you lose weight.

✔ **Hormonal shifts:** When you don't get enough sleep, hormones shift, causing your appetite to change. The sugars you crave shoot your insulin up, creating blood sugar problems. These hormonal shifts cause weight gain and health issues. Here are few other common hormones that can affect your weight:

   • **Leptin:** This hormone tells you when you've had enough food; when you haven't had enough sleep, it's greatly reduced. Reduced leptin tells your body that you're less full than you really are. It also makes everything you eat taste sweeter so you have constant cravings.

   • **Ghrelin:** This hormone is the green light of eating. It tells you to go ahead and eat more. When you're sleep deprived, it increases, causing your appetite to increase.

   • **Serotonin:** This hormone sends messages throughout your body that makes you feel good. When you're sleep deprived, serotonin makes you want to devour simple sugars.

   • **Growth hormone:** This is a powerful anti-aging hormone. Twenty minutes after you go to sleep, your pituitary gland begins to release high levels. Without sleep, you're deprived of this hormone.

✔ **Heart disease:** When your hormones shift, causing you to eat more sugar, you get insulin resistance (see Chapter 3). Insulin resistance causes you to gain weight. During this process, you convert all your carbohydrates into bad cholesterol and you retain water, which alters your blood pressure and paves the way to heart disease.

✔ **Pre-hibernation messaging:** When you expose yourself to unending artificial light, it registers with your brain that it's a long summer day. After long summers come the cold dark winter. So your body naturally puts on a fat base, preparing for the winter. Your body can't metabolically resist eating carbohydrates to prepare. These extra carbs cause blood sugar problems and weight gain.

✔ **Lowered immune system:** The body's immune system is weakened without sleep. The number of white cells in your body actually decreases.

✔ **Altered brain power:** Memory, concentration, and creativity are all impaired with lack of sleep.

✔ **Premature aging:** The body decreases its growth hormone needed for ongoing tissue repair, healing, cell rejuvenation, and bone function. Growth hormone can reverse the effects of aging; therefore, sleep deprivation causes aging.

✔ **Sugar handling problems:** When you're sleep deprived, the ability to metabolize sugar decreases, turning sugar into fat.

✔ **Decreased regenerative powers:** Sleep is needed to regenerate the body, especially the brain. When you don't have enough sleep, your body doesn't heal or regenerate.

✔ **Prolonged high cortisol levels:** When you're up for long periods of time with the lights on, the hormone cortisol doesn't naturally drop like it's supposed to. High cortisol occurs in nature when you need it to run fast or deal with pain from an injury. This constant high cortisol causes people to become panicky and depressive.

✔ **Cumulative effect:** Sleep deprivation is cumulative. You don't adapt to sleep deprivation; you only get more tired and, eventually, unhealthy and overweight.

Getting enough sleep and creating a natural rhythm

Sleep is closely weaved into our natural circadian rhythms inscribed in our genes by the footprint of our ancestors. This inscription allows us to live comfortably in our environment of dark and light. Because our genes are set to this dark and light pattern, sleep needs to have a required rhythm to be healthy. Just as your heart, body temperature, and metabolic process have rhythms, so do your sleep needs.

As we discuss earlier in this chapter, people are often over stimulated and ignore their bodies' signaling for sleep. When your signaling and sleep matches your outside world, your rhythms are in order. When they're not, you become out of sorts and your health is at risk. This health risk is significant enough to put your state of mind — and life — in danger.

When you constantly trick your circadian signaling by staying up too long in artificial light, your body thinks it's a long summer day. What your body naturally expects to follow is the cold, short days of winter. The concern, however, is that the expected dormant hibernation period after the long summer never comes, which makes your mind start to literally go crazy. Nature thinks you're up too long, that you've eaten more than your share of nature's goodness, and that you're likely infertile from being bathed in insulin. Your body creates a bipolar state of mind and you become depressive and manic.

Also, when the light never dims, your cortisol never drops. Chronic high cortisol and chronic high insulin put your mind in a chronic state of panic. When insulin and cortisol are constantly off, more than just moodiness occurs; you experience true manic depression and mental illness.

The National Institute of Mental Health agrees that one of the primary causes of depression and mental illness is simply being out of sync with the dark-light rhythm that your body expects. Most of the drugs for depression are aimed at putting your sleep cycles back in place.

Start looking at sleep as a nutrient! As much as we look at evolutionary eating, moving, and living as our blueprint, staying in tune with our natural sleep design is just as essential.

Sleep works together with all other areas in your life to provide you the best health; here are a few tips for getting the right amount and quality of sleep you need:

- ✔ **Go to bed at the same time every night**. If you don't give yourself a scheduled bedtime, you get distracted. Before long, your awake time will be squeezing it's way into your much-needed sleep time.

- ✔ **Go to bed by no later than 10 p.m. and wake up by no later than 7 a.m.** Set your phone, watch, or an alarm clock to remind you to close down shop for the night. Most of your body's repairing goes on before 1 a.m., and you get more growth hormone. Your circadian rhythm will also be in sync with your sleep-awake cycle.

- ✔ **Rise with the sun.** The sunlight will regulate your hormones for the day.

- ✔ **Unplug.** Make sure you're not doing anything but relaxing, journaling, or reading one to two hours before bed. This quiet time releases the hormone melatonin to get you to sleep. That means no TV, no computer, or anything stimulating. Dim the lights if you can. Doing so allows your body to start producing even more melatonin. Move away all alarm clocks or electrical devices at least 3 feet from your bed.

- ✔ **Black out your bedroom room completely.** Melatonin is produced when it's dark. Even cover the windows to prevent any light from coming in. Use blackout shades if you need to. You shouldn't be able to see even your hand in front of your face. If your room is too light when you try to sleep, hormone production slows down.

- ✔ **Keep you're room cool and well ventilated.** Keep your room at a temperature that's comfortable for you, but make sure it's on the cooler side; about 68 degrees works for most people. Some people also like an air purifier. Using one can improve the way you breathe and, ultimately, the way you sleep.

- ✔ **Limit caffeine.** Drinking caffeine prolongs the time it takes you to go to sleep and decreases the amount of deep sleep you get. The time it takes for about half of the caffeine you've had to clear out of your system is three to five hours, so plan accordingly. Caffeine limitations vary greatly from person to person, so see what works for you

- ✔ **Limit alcohol:** Alcohol may make you fall asleep quicker, but your quality of sleep is diminished. Deep sleep and REM sleep are both greatly reduced, so even if you fall asleep quicker, you'll probably wake up feeling tired.

Make sleep as essential as eating, exercising, or anything else you do that you consider important to your health (and waistline). These living Paleo sleep tips will go a long way in making you stronger, leaner, and healthier.

Sleep-inducing foods include turkey and almonds as well as seasonings like nutmeg, turmeric, and garlic. (Try herbal tea with nutmeg or turkey broth with garlic as a before-bed snack to prep for a restful night.) Calcium and magnesium are also helpful sleep aids; we give the supplement Natural Calm two thumbs up.

The Sun's Time to Shine

Hunter-gatherers woke up to the sunshine every morning. It was a normal part of their life. It was as much a part of their day as the stars were at night.

The modern-day view of sunshine has changed. We used to frolic in the sun, sunbathe (with sunscreen that was no more than moisturizer), and never had a care in the world about skin cancer. Now, we fear the sun. We've gone from enjoying the sun to feeling like we have to protect ourselves from it.

Sunshine is like sleep. It's one of those nutrients that stays under the radar, yet it's imperative to your health. Just as eating, moving, and living for health is important, so is sunshine exposure.

In this section, we discuss the evolutionary wisdom of sun safety and where sunscreens fall into the mix. We also talk about what a healthy dose of sunshine can do for you!

Sunblock and sunscreen: Making the right choice

When you went to the store to get sunscreen, you used to have only a few choices. Some people used them, some didn't. They were really just glorified moisturizers and didn't contain any sunblock. Today, you'd be hard-pressed to find anyone not lathered up in the summer. In fact, a lot of people wear sunscreen in the winter "just in case," and makeup companies and moisturizers often have sunscreen listed in their ingredients. The question is, is this a good thing or not?

Well, it certainly goes against evolutionary wisdom. Our ancestors benefited from the sun and didn't fear it. They learned to work within their ecology and understood that they weren't on the outside looking in but were very much a part of nature and their surroundings. They had an awareness to work within nature's rhythms.

Why all this fear of sun exposure? The short of it: sunburn and skin cancer. In an answer to this fear, sunscreen manufacturers tell us that their sunscreens protect against cancer.

The truth is no evidence exists that sunscreens prevent the main skin cancers, cutaneous melanoma and basal cell carcinoma. Sunscreens protect against sunburn. Sunscreens aren't an anticancer remedy. In fact, because they allow you to have prolonged exposure to the sun, you actually have a heightened risk of melanoma.

In the following sections, we dig into more detail about what exactly is harmful about sun exposure and whether sunscreen is the answer.

Steering clear of the sun's harmful rays

Is the sun dangerous? The part of the sun that causes damage is ultraviolet (UV) radiation. This UV radiation is broken into two categories, A and B:

- **UVA:** Sunscreens often don't block out UVA. Although no conclusive evidence exists as of yet, scientist are strongly postulating that UVA rays increase your risk of melanoma. These rays are strong and deeply penetrate your skin throughout the entire day.

- **UVB:** This is the portion of UV radiation that causes the burn (or redness) in your skin. For this reason, most of the sunscreen you buy blocks out these rays. These rays are low in the morning and later in the day but strong midday.

Blocking UVB rays isn't a solution but actually causes another problem. Think of UVB as your "buddy." This spectrum of light is what manufactures vitamin D production in your skin. If you block UVB, you block vitamin D from 97.5 to 99.9 percent.

Vitamin D is hands down one of the most anticancerous types of nutrients your body produces. Blocking UVB really takes away one of the best cancer- and disease-fighting shields your body has to offer.

The problem doesn't stop there. No hard evidence suggests that sunscreens protect against cancers; in fact, they contain toxic ingredients that actually cause cancers.

Using the right sunscreen/sunblock

Unfortunately, the FDA guidelines for sunscreens aren't helpful to the consumer. They fail to establish the ingredients that they find safe and effective for sunscreens. They also don't address the claim that the "higher the SPF, the higher the protection" has, in fact, negligible benefits. What the FDA does claim is that people should lather this rather toxic substance on their skin every two hours.

Sunscreen ratings

The Environmental Working Group (EWG) is a nonprofit consumer advocacy group that investigates products like sunscreen. Through its investigation, it found that many of the brand-name sunscreens contain unsafe ingredients.

The EWG offers a rating system on more than 1,700 sunscreen products on the market. Check it out at www.ewg.org/skindeep to help ensure that you purchase a safe product.

What are the solutions when it comes to sunscreens? First, you need to understand your options:

- ✔ **Sunscreens** include chemicals that your skin absorbs (going directly into the body). When your skin absorbs these chemicals, it forms a sun barrier. Although sunscreens do, in fact, prevent sunburn, no evidence suggests that they're effective in reducing skin cancer. Some statistical evidence suggests that the toxins they contain may actually increase your risk of cancer. Always avoid mists and sprays, whose ingredients have been broken down into small particles that are more dangerous internally.

- ✔ **Sunblocks** are designed so that the ingredients literally lay on top of the skin to form a barrier against the sun. They don't enter the bloodstream. If you purchase wisely, you can avoid the chemicals that some sunblocks may contain.

We recommend that you buy mineral sunblock whose active ingredient is zinc and/or titanium dioxide.

Getting a healthy boost of sunshine with slow immersion

The dangers of the sun have been exaggerated, and the benefits have been underestimated. Sunshine is a fantastic way to ward off cancers and other diseases. It also helps your body keep the hormonal rhythm of your natural light-dark cycle.

If you're sun savvy, you can use the sun as a friend and not look at it as a threat. As we explain in the previous section, many sunscreens contain toxins and may not defend you against skin cancer.

First, understand what is known to cause skin cancer. Intense infrequent exposure to the sun leading to burning, followed by little to no sun may cause melanomas and many other cancers. What you don't want, then, is to burn. That strategy is easy to implement.

Start practicing the slow immersion process by slowly immersing yourself into the sun and building a protective layer. You can build up your tolerance on a regular basis, gradually and early on in the springtime. Doing so preps your skin for the stronger sun in the summer. Try to get sun earlier in the morning where you have less chance of burning and overheating.

Try to do frequent short periods of exposure. The benefit to going in the sun without sunscreen and building a base through slow immersion is that you're welcoming the production of vitamin D. This vitamin (which is actually a hormone) helps your body ward off countless diseases. Here are just a few:

- Cancer
- Diabetes
- Heart Disease
- Hypertension
- Multiple Sclerosis
- Osteoporosis
- Psoriasis
- Rickets

How much exposure you need to get your dose of vitamin D depends on how dark your skin is and environmental factors (such as how close you live to the equator or what time of day you're sunbathing). The darker your skin, the more exposure you need. Just underscore in your mind that regular sun exposure is grossly understated as a vitally important barrier to disease.

A skin cancer secret that shouldn't be

Most people don't realize that the type of oils in your body can either increase or decrease your risk of sunburn or cancer. A study from the National Academy of Science found that low omega-6 to omega-3 ratios was the key to prevention of skin cancer. Omega-3 fats decreased cancers, while omega-6 increases risk. That's another score for the living Paleo healthy fats!

Here are some great sources of omega-3 fats to add to your health weapons:

- Brussels Sprouts
- Fish (salmon, sardines, halibut, tuna, shrimp, and scallops)
- Fish oil supplements (1 or 2 grams a day)
- Flax seeds
- Kale
- Spinach
- Walnuts

To find out more about omega-3 fats and why they're important, see Chapter 4.

The benefits of this sunshine (UVB exposure) far outweigh any adverse affects. Vitamin D is extremely protective. Have your levels checked, and if you need to supplement to "catch up," do so (see Chapter 4 for types of supplements we recommend).

Regular exposure to the sun protects against skin cancers, and intermittent exposure actually increases your odds.

Water: The Ideal Drink

Your body is made up of about 60 percent water. Just as your body needs macronutrients (such as healthy proteins, carbohydrates, and fats) to function, it also needs water. Pure, clean water is the most essential of all nutrients. You can live for weeks without consuming food, but you can't go for more than a couple of days without water.

Proper intake of water is so vital to your being that deficiency of even 1 percent can present signs of dysfunctions in your body. Slightly more dehydration, and you have exponentially more health risk.

You also need water to maintain the chemical balances in your body, such as these important functions:

- Balancing acid-base levels
- Eliminating waste from the lungs, skin, and colon
- Regulating hormones
- Transporting nutrients to the cells

Your body responds with different signals when it's dehydrated or hungry. Many times, people read the signs wrong and intervene with food, medicines, or procedures that aren't necessary. All your body really needed was some water — another one of those simple health weapons that's often overlooked because it seems so simple!

In the following sections, you discover how to decode your body's signaling in regard to hunger and thirst. Also, you find out how to make sure your body is fueling up on water that does a body good.

Recognizing your body's signs for hunger and thirst

Your brain recognizes low energy levels available for the functions of its body. Hunger or thirst fall within this signaling. Because brain signals are simultaneous, people sometimes confuse these signals and assume they need food when they actually need water. One of the main problems with this signal confusion between thirst and hunger is not understanding how much water you really need and misinterpreting the signs of dehydration. The key is to be attuned with your body and know when to drink water.

The biggest roadblock is waiting until you're thirsty to drink. Your brain center doesn't send a message until you're almost 2 percent dehydrated. By then, you've likely already encountered some problems associated with dehydration. Your kidneys receive the low signal before you do, so it responds by decreasing urine output, a big sign that you need more water.

How do you know whether you're dehydrated? The biggest tell is if you're not urinating at least six to eight times a day. Also, look at your urine; it should be fairly clear. If it's bright yellow, you need more water.

Here's how some of the signs of dehydration play out in your system:

✔ Arthritis pain

✔ Chronic hunger

✔ Depression

✔ Excess body weight

✔ Headaches

✔ High blood cholesterol

✔ High blood pressure

✔ Intestinal pain

You've probably been told that you need six to eight cups of water daily. But this amount is on the low side. You need at the *very least* six to eight cups. A great way to tell whether you're hydrated is to simply look at your urine. If it's a pale to light yellow color, you're well hydrated. If your urine is dark yellow, it's time to drink some water!

The optimal water intake should be half of your body weight in ounces. So if you weigh 100 pounds, you need 50 ounces of water daily. If you exercise, you should consume even more water. Get in the habit of drinking water before, during, and immediately after exercise.

Pre-hydrate in the morning! It's a good way to get your blood moving and transporting all the good stuff to your body!

When you get used to water as your main source of liquid, it helps a great deal. Remember your body's signaling. When you're not feeling well, feeling low energy, or feeling hungry, your first line of defense is always drink water. It's easy in this fast-paced modern world to get your tank too low!

Determining whether tap water is okay

Tap water is easy to get and low in cost. But is it healthy to drink? The Environmental Working Group (EWG) obtained almost 20 million records from state water officials. Incredibly, more than half of the chemical pollutants they found (315 total) aren't subject to any health or safety regulations, so they can show up in your water in any amount, and it's legal.

The contaminants you have to be concerned about in tap water are

- Bacteria
- Environmental chemicals
- Heavy metals
- Parasites
- Radiological pollution

Also, even public water systems, where the water is filtered, add chlorine and fluoride back into the water. You also have to think about your home's pipes. The type of pipes you have and any corrosion can cause contamination.

To make a decision about whether your water is safe, you may have to do some investigation. If you have a public water system, you have the right to ask for the results from past water tests. The Environmental Protection Agency (EPA) requires utilities to provide a consumer's confidence report. If you have well water, you'll have to have it tested yourself.

Having your water tested from a laboratory takes away all the guesswork. Your local health authority may offer free test kits. For a great resource on certified testing labs and water in your area, call the EPA's drinking water hotline (800-426-4791) or go to www.water.epa.gov/drink/hotline/index.cfm. The EWG also has an information site where you can see how your state's water ranks: www.ewg.org/tap-water/home.

Unless you know your tap water is safe, drink it only when you're desperate and look for a cleaner source. For solutions, read the next section.

Choosing clean water for wellness

One of the simplest ways you can lose weight and get healthier is to listen to your body's signal for water — clean, pure water, that is. You may not have access to pure stream or river water, but you can get close!

Water that gets into your body isn't just coming from your kitchen tap. It's also coming from all the water sources in your home (like the bath or shower).

Water bottles aren't an alternative to tap water because the plastic packaging they come in pollutes your body and the world. The chemical Bisphenol A (BPA) and phthalates contained in plastics are dangerous to your health. Even low levels of these chemicals cause disease and can create hormonal disturbances. Also, 40 percent of bottled water is simply taken from municipal tap water, so most bottled water is really nothing more than tap water in toxic bottles.

Your body needs pure, clean water without all the chorine, fluoride, and toxins. The best way to get this kind of water is through a water filtration system. Knowing what's is in your water and what needs to be filtered out is a good place to start. This is where water testing comes in (see the preceding section).

If you don't want to test your water, at the very least, make sure the filtration removes the following:

- Arsenic
- Chlorine
- Chloroform
- E. coli
- Fluoride
- Nitrites and nitrates
- Radon

You can choose from a system that filters the water in one area of your house or a whole house filtration system. The best-case scenario is to make sure all the water in your house is filtered, including bath water and cooking water. Choose a system that fits your personal needs and budget.

Stress and Belly Fat: Modern Problems for Today's Cave Man

Modern man has a challenge: to exist in a world that he wasn't designed for. We've changed our lifestyle patterns away from what our species requires to genetically express health toward what causes us to express illness. How do we sub-exist in this world and come out on the other end healthy, strong, and vibrant? The best blueprint for a healthy survival is to study the patterns of our ancestors and repeat what's practical and meaningful to our health.

You're most likely not eating meat that you or someone else caught from the wild every day. You probably don't eat berries and fruits that were picked that day year-round. You've probably even eaten boxed, canned, frozen, and refined foods. You've probably had days with not enough movement, and you may spend a lot of time with your smartphone or computer. Or maybe you don't get enough sun, sleep, or water. But don't worry: You can tweak all these things to help you live as genetically close to your blueprint as possible. For some, this may mean changing your paradigm, changing the way you used to eat, move, or live, and changing the way you look at things in your life, such as your healthcare, your food, and your lifestyle.

When you don't change your paradigm to match your blueprint, your body expresses signs of stress and, ultimately, illness. This stress can bring on cravings, which eventually gives you a belly and those not-so-lovely love handles. So you need to ask yourself, "What do I need to do to get well, be strong, and stay healthy? What do I need to do to live the most positive life I can live and have the effect I want to have in life?"

In the following sections, we talk about how modern-day stresses can affect your body, leading to belly fat, and we walk you through the changes you can make to live the healthy life you want and to relieve stress and its side effects.

Living Paleo is a lifestyle that helps the modern-day hunter-gatherer adjust to his environment in the healthiest way possible. This lifestyle programs your genes to express health and vibrancy as your body was designed to do.

Putting your body under stress

We know that, genetically, people haven't changed for thousands of years, but their lifestyles sure have. As soon as you start eating or living in a way that isn't congruent to your genetic blueprint, it's a stressor on your body. If you continue to live in a way not by design, you'll be under chronic stress.

You're not designed in any way to be under chronic stress. Your body has a built-in system called the *sympathetic nervous system,* which activates in times of stress. This system is also referred to as *fight-or-flight response.* This mechanism helps your body when you're in those moments of crisis (for example, a tiger chasing you down).

With modern-day living, people are stimulating this system constantly, which is most definitely not how your fight-or-flight system was designed to be used. This constant triggering causes problems that can lead to even bigger problems.

When you're under chronic stress, you force your body to adapt to whatever that crisis situation is. The physiological stress that this brings on your body expresses itself in many ways. Here are some of the symptoms of chronic stress adaptation:

- Anxiety
- Blood sugar problems
- Decrease in fertility
- Decreased growth hormone
- Depression
- Fatigue
- High blood pressure
- Hormonal changes
- Increased heart rate
- Memory problems
- Obesity

When you get stressed, you probably sometimes turn to medications; however, they're not the solution. Your very intelligent innate system, which you were born with, is doing exactly what it's supposed to do in response to stress. The symptoms or diseases you have occur because your body is expressing your chronic stress.

The best way to get well, stay well, and have the life you want is to remove chronic stressors from your life. Remove yourself from whatever physiological or environmental factors are causing these stressors, and put yourself in an environment (whatever that means to you) that is free of constant stress.

Living Paleo was created with that foundation in mind: to help you create a life that would reduce as many chronic stressors as possible. (For more on stress relief, see Chapter 6.)

Understanding the dangers of belly and visceral fat

Your body needs healthy fats. If you don't have healthy fat, your body can't do important functions, such as produce hormones, maintain healthy cells and nerves, insulate and protect organs, and have sufficient brain capacity. However, carrying around excess fat can be as dangerous as not having enough fat.

Knowing your body composition helps you determine whether you have healthy fat or unhealthy fat (see Chapter 3). Tracking what your body fat actually is tells you a lot about your state of health. Your body fat tells you the ratio of how much fat (including the fat just beneath the skin, within muscle tissue, and around the organs, called *visceral fat*) is in your body compared to lean mass.

Visceral fat is very dangerous. It's the hidden fat (called *skinny fat*) that even the thinnest of people can be in danger of walking around with. Because visceral fat is stored around the abdominal organs, you may even have a normal weight. That's why knowing your body fat ratio is a good idea.

Here are some of the conditions that can be associated with visceral fat:

- Cancer
- Diabetes
- Heart Disease
- High blood pressure
- High triglycerides
- Insulin resistance (precursor to diabetes)
- Strokes

You can be skinny and have visceral fat; however, an outward sign that you have hidden fat is a sizable belly, commonly identified by the "beer belly" or an apple-shaped figure. People with a wider girth are more likely to have hidden fat.

The quickest and easiest way to get answers about what type of fat you have is to measure your waist. The National Institute of Health (NIH) stated that a waist measurement above 35 inches for women and 40 inches for men — no matter how much you weigh — is an unhealthy sign of visceral fat.

Normal body fat has a variation due to factors, such as age and activity level. The normal range for women over 18 years of age is between 14 and 31 percent. The normal range for men is between 6 and 25 percent. Numbers higher than these are dangerous.

If you do have high body fat, you may already be in harm's way. Beginning a healthy lifestyle program immediately can reverse any danger. The Living Paleo 30-Day Reset (see Chapter 3) is one of the best things you can do to get your belly fat down and start moving your biology toward health. For other solutions, see the next section.

Minimizing stress and belly fat

Belly fat is resistant fat, sometimes coined *the middle-aged spread*. It's the fat that flops over your jeans. It's also dangerous fat (see the preceding section). This fat is not only unattractive but also deadly. Belly fat is definitely fat you want to minimize!

If you want to do away with stubborn belly fat, you've got to address the stressors in your life. In the earlier section "Putting your body under stress," we talk about how chronic stress manifests when you live a lifestyle that doesn't match your genetic blueprint. Your attitude, food, relationships, connection to others, environmental factors, and how physical you are contribute to stress levels.

Belly fat (dangerous midsection fat) isn't the cause of all diseases. It's your body having to adapt to the stressors that causes the belly fat. So, in the end, it's your stressors that are actually causing the diseases. Your belly fat is only a symptom.

As your stress rises, so do your stress hormones, such as cortisol. When your stress hormones rise and your feel-good hormone (serotonin) decreases, it's disastrous. The result of this combination includes the following symptoms: depression, drop in growth hormone, exhaustion, insomnia, insulin problems, and weight gain.

One of the best actions you can take to get rid of dangerous, unattractive belly fat is to remove your stressors. That means creating a lifestyle that most closely resembles your ancestors, changing the patterns in your life that are more congruent to your genetic requirements, and creating an environment that allows your body to express its fullest potential.

If we told you that we invented this miracle pill that would decrease your incidence for about every disease and make you look better, have fewer cravings, and have far less stress on your body, would you take it? Well, you already have this miracle pill. It's called exercise! One of the best ways to stimulate your brain and hormones to produce pleasure is through exercise. Exercise not only boosts metabolism, but it also changes the way your body responds to stress. Exercise is one of the most powerful things you can do to reverse stress, depression, anxiety, cravings, or negative eating patterns.

The living Paleo-approved meats, vegetables, fruits, and healthy fats are all genetically compatible foods that will help you minimize belly fat. Reducing stress is vital and is best accomplished by making sure you're in an environment that allows your body to express its fullest potential. It's important that you look at all the living Paleo patterns to maximize your results.

Combating stress and cravings

In times of stress, your body releases stress hormones, specifically cortisol. In a normal situation, cortisol regulates your blood pressure, cardiovascular function, and metabolism. When your body needs a blast of cortisol in a time of crisis, it's a great protective feedback mechanism. It's when you have that steady stream of stress (chronic stress) that causes significant damage. (For more on the affects of chronic stress, see the section "Putting your body under stress," earlier in this chapter.) Your body has a hard time adapting to this unrelenting stress, and disease and obesity are often the outcome.

Most often, stress causes a vicious cycle. This cycle is why so many people who are stressed are overweight. Your immune system decreases, so you're naturally more tired, and everything you do seems like a chore. You end up moving or exercising less.

Here's the worse part of the stress cycle: The main ingredients for stress hormones are — you guessed it — fat and sugar. That's why you crave so much junk when you're stressed. It's your body crying out for more stress hormones because it requires more! This creates a terrible cycle of craving, eating, and crashing.

This stress and cravings cycle is the reason that so many people feel like they can't control their hunger. The stress causes your hormones to change your eating patterns and brain chemistry.

The answer to this unhealthy cycle is not eating comfort foods and taking medication waiting to feel better. It's living a life that's congruent with your body's design that will naturally reduce many of your body's stressors. It's eating the foods that nourish you, moving in a way that awakens you, and living in a way that allows your body to express its best potential. Following the living Paleo plan is your road map to reduce stress, cravings, and that terrible belly fat.

You can decrease stress and cravings by increasing water consumption, vegetables, fruits, fish, and nuts, and decreasing sugar, caffeine, and alcohol.

Ridding Your Life of Toxins

If you want to live your life as closely as you can to your body's natural design, then what do you do about all the toxins that surround you 24/7?

Well, you can't live in fear or in a bubble. Your goal has to be to minimize your exposure to toxins as much as you can control — and don't let the rest create stress. (Remember that stress is a toxin that should be avoided, too!) In fact, look at this section as your living Paleo bonus. We want to be clear that by applying all the principles to cleaning up your diet, reducing stress, improving sleep, and getting some good, old-fashioned sunlight, you've come a long way! Those changes will pay off in spades! Making lifestyle changes is a transition. Your life tends to pick up a natural flow and rhythm, and your changes just start to unfold. Don't feel like you have to be perfect or do everything. Do the best you can and the rest will follow. When you start living the Paleo lifestyle, your green living will start to evolve naturally. Don't push; just lean into the change.

Living a green, or non-toxic, lifestyle doesn't require you to give up all the things you like but simply adjust your choices. You have to change your paradigm to one that understands that in order to be as healthy as possible, you have to make reducing toxins an important part of your lifestyle.

The cold hard truth is that people are exposed to thousands of chemicals daily, and scientists estimate that people carry in their bodies at least 700 contaminants no matter where they live. Some chemicals stay in your body for only a short time before you naturally detoxify them (by exhaling, sweating, and so on), but some can't be automatically removed. They leave a residue, which remains in your blood and fat tissues, muscles, bones, and organs. These are your toxic burden.

One of the goals of living Paleo is to decrease this toxic burden by introducing you to foods and lifestyle patterns that reduce your daily exposure to toxins. The following sections walk you through avoiding and eliminating some common toxins found in your skin, food, and home that may elevate your toxic burden.

Shifting your chemical culture

Many people are walking around sick and frustrated because they can't get answers to why they're chronically fatigued and unwell. With blood tests and exams revealing normal results, it can make someone feel lost. For years, this chronic, unexplained fatigue was thought to be just "all in their head," but now, we understand that many illnesses and unexplained fatigue may be the results of toxins in the system (toxic burden).

The amount of toxins that surround us are jaw dropping. Studies by the National Resource Defense council state that the use of pesticides is ten times what it was in the 1940s. In the United States alone, we use more than 1.2 billion pounds of pesticides per year. At least 70,000 chemicals are used in businesses today with 6 trillion pounds annually.

Although this information may be daunting, the marketplace is seeing more and more toxin-free foods and products every year. As awareness increases, so will the choices. It's a matter of educating yourself on where you can cut back on your daily surroundings of toxins and making different choices that fit your needs. When you shift your paradigm to wellness, you get better as you go along, and making better choices becomes fluid after you've done it for a while.

Eliminating toxins on your skin

Think about this: Your skin is your largest organ. Yes, your skin is actually an organ, and anything you put on the skin has a direct route into your bloodstream. When you put something on your skin, ask yourself, "Is this product pure enough that I could actually eat it?" If not, you probably shouldn't have it on your skin at all.

You can make toxin-free choices with these common products:

- **Makeup and moisturizers:** Makeup and moisturizers include numerous chemicals. A good way to find toxin-free options is to purchase unscented brands. They usually have no petrochemicals or their derivatives. Look for a company that makes it a priority not to use harmful ingredients. (Dr.Hauschka is one brand we recommend, which is available online and in most health food stores.)

- **Perfumes:** Perfumes can cause toxins and allergies in many people. Instead, try essential oils, which are lightly fragranced in different scents. You can even buy them in sprays or roll-ons. Most health food store and grocers carry essential oils.

✔ **Antiperspirants:** Stay away from any antiperspirants that have aluminum in them. Because you're putting these products under you arm near the tail of your breast, you need to be extra cautious. You shouldn't put anything with toxins near your breast tissue. Opt for a more natural deodorant, which doesn't contain aluminum. Tom's of Maine makes a wide variety of natural deodorants.

✔ **Nail polish:** Nail products are filled with chemicals. Actually, a nail spa can be a toxic trap if your provider uses products with chemicals. Look for holistic spas where you have a better chance of getting a more natural product (and experience all around). SpaRitual (www.sparitual.com) is a great brand that's all-natural and works well.

✔ **Toothpastes:** Toothpastes are often filled with toxins and some even contain artificial sugars. Opt for a more natural brand, like Tom's of Maine, where you don't have to worry about all the chemicals and toxins included on the label.

✔ **Shampoos:** Take a minute and read the back of your shampoo bottle. I bet you can't even say half of the ingredients! Shampoos have tons of chemicals in there. You can find alternatives pretty easily if you look. Aveda is a good option and widely available.

✔ **Dry cleaning:** This modern convenience is hard for people to break. No one wants to be scrubbing clothes and ironing all day. However, dry cleaning is one of the most toxic habits we have. Minimizing this practice as much as possible greatly reduces your toxic exposure. Dry cleaning uses the very toxic chemical *perchloroethylene,* which should be avoided.

Another great resource for many of the products you put on your skin is Environmental Working Group (EWG). Its Skin Deep website (www.ewg.org/skindeep) is chock-full of good finds.

Removing toxins from your home

Toxins in your home include any pollutants that are in your daily surroundings. Here are some common toxins and what to do about them:

✔ **Cleaning solutions:** Cleaning products can be hazardous because you inhale the chemical in the fumes that these products often give off. Drain openers, air fresheners, ammonia-based cleaners, and chlorine bleach all contain toxins. These toxins are neurotoxic chemicals, meaning that they're damaging to your nervous system. The good news is that many non-toxic cleaners are widely available, so you don't need to use neurotoxic chemicals to clean your house. Try an all-natural cleaner or use some old-fashioned ingredients, like borax, baking soda, vinegar, soap, and water.

✔ **Indoor air:** Most people spend 90 percent of their time indoors, so quality air is paramount. However, the Environmental Protection Agency (EPA) says that indoor air is two to five times more polluted than outside air because of the chemical products people use, which they come in contact with and inhale.

To reduce toxins from indoor air, you can do a couple things:

- **Get some good ol' fresh air:** Make sure you allow your home to get fresh air every day. Crack open the windows just enough to permit air flow. When it's really cold, just open them for five minutes.

- **Buy a good air purifier:** You want the purifier to filter bacteria, molds, toxic fumes, smoke, dust, dander, pollens, static electricity, and hydrocarbons (from cooking). You can find great units at most home improvements stores.

✔ **Carpets, rugs, and furniture:** Carpeting is heavily sprayed with insecticides. Toxic carpets are one of the most dangerous toxins you can have because you're exposed to them all day and all night. You can reduce toxins in carpet or rugs by airing it outside for a few days before you place it in your home. Also, instead of wall-to-wall carpets, opt for area rugs to reduce toxins. Always look for natural fibers, like wool-cotton blend, and make sure it doesn't have a latex backing.

Look for the Carpet and Rug Institute (CRI) low-emission labels before buying: www.carpet-rug.org/commercial-customers/cleaning-and-maintenance/seal-of-approval-products.

Avoiding EMFs, the invisible pollution

Wherever there's electricity, there are EMFs (electromagnetic fields). When something is plugged in but not used, it generates electrical fields, or low frequency electromagnetic waves. The EMFs generated are coined as invisible pollution called *electrosmog*. By contrast, magnetic fields are when electricity actually passes through the wires.

Much different than even 50 years ago, we now have multitudes of new inventions, all which require electricity. There are electrical poles, wires, substations, transformers, and the hidden wires in the walls of homes, businesses, schools, factories, churches, and stores. All this electricity creates a dangerous electrical environment and places new stresses on our cells. In fact, the stress placed on the cell is similar to what would be produced by heavy metals or toxic chemicals.

The BioInitiative Working Group released an extensive report in 2007, citing more than 2,000 studies that detail the toxic effects of EMFs. This report shows that chronic exposure can lead to many life threatening diseases. For a full report, go to www.bioinitiative.org/freeaccess/report/index.htm. The World Health Organization established the EMF project to assess the scientific evidence. Check out its findings at www.who.int/peh-emf/en.

To reduce EMF exposure, try the following:

- ✔ **Remove yourself:** The best way to reduce EMFs is to remove yourself as far as you can from the source. Be aware, and do the best you can to make adjustments. Try to make sure your bed is as far away from EMF sources as possible. It's best not to have a lot of wiring or electrical devices by your head for eight hours every night.

- ✔ **Eat the right food:** You can make your diet a great EMF shield, too. When your body's internal environment is expressing health, it's a great fortress against the consequences of EMF exposure. Foods like grass-fed beef, blueberries, asparagus, cinnamon, artichokes, garlic, olive oil, wild salmon, and walnuts are all superfoods for your cells.

- ✔ **Use a gauss meter:** If you want to test your house for EMF exposure, you can purchase a gauss meter for about $150 to $200. It's a small device that fits in a pocket that measures the strength of a magnetic field. You can take measurements at home or work and see whether some areas are more exposed than others. You can see how far you need to be away from the TV or other electrical devises.

- ✔ **Have an electronic-free day:** Try to go electronic-free for a day once a week. On these day, let your family and friends know that you'll be shutting down. Close the computer, shut off the cellphone, and do whatever else you can to de-wire for the day.

No matter what your view is on EMFs, our ancestors weren't exposed to all the artificial lighting and gadgetry we have today. Use common sense and try to limit your use as best you can.

Chapter 6

Incorporating Paleo Exercises into Your Life

In This Chapter

▶ Understanding how your body was designed to move

▶ Making movement a part of your everyday life

▶ Adopting a Paleo fitness program that makes your body flourish

You probably know that incorporating exercise into your daily routine makes you look better and gives you more energy. What you may not know is that when you exercise in a way that your body is designed to move, *everything* you do gets better. No matter what the activity it is, you get better at it. Whether you're a student, builder, teacher, dancer, factory worker, office worker, soccer mom, world-class athlete, or clown, when you move in a way that your body expects, you flourish in every way possible, and you're able to do everything better and with more ease.

Whether you're a newcomer to everyday physical activity or an old pro, we give you the tips and tools you need to get your body moving the way it was designed to move. We provide a workout overview and a sample program. You can either follow our sample or take tips from other workouts. We know that incorporating Paleo exercises into your life and embracing Paleo nutrition (Chapter 4) will have a profound effect on your life.

Before you start an exercise program, consult with a doctor who knows your history.

Moving the Way You Were Designed to Move

What would happen if a hunter-gatherer decided one day that he had had enough and was just going to take it easy from now on? What if he decided that he was going to spend his day sitting, sleeping in, or not walking so much? He would be without food and shelter and may even get eaten by a wild animal! He would certainly be outcast by his band members and could be left without his community.

For him, moving was a matter of survival. Foraging, walking, sprinting, crawling, and squatting were a necessary way of life. It was either move or die.

This activity was woven into our genes. Unfortunately, our human genes and our physical lifestyles have become incongruent. When our genes were selected, daily physical exertion was mandatory. Our biology, physiology, and biochemistry depend on this activity for optimal function. In fact, your body absolutely craves movement.

The following sections cover some of the ways in which your body was meant to move, including anaerobic for speed, resistance for strength, and aerobic for endurance, and we explain how much you need of each to quench your body's craving for movement.

Living Paleo resistance: Building strength and fighting age

Our ancestors needed strength — and a lot of it. They needed to climb a tree to get away from a predator, to butcher their kill, to throw the meat over their shoulder, and to carry it back to their camp. Moving their camps, building their tools, carrying children, digging, squatting, and harvesting trees and shrubs all involved intense strength.

Real fitness and strength are defined by how well you can function in your everyday life. If your muscles are big but you can't throw a water bottle over your back or carry a child, it doesn't mean much. You want to be fit and strong enough to do all the practical things in life that you need to do.

One of the main advantages of doing shorter, faster exercises is that they stimulate the production of growth hormone, which you need for strength and health. The best part, though, is growth hormone is like an anti-age shield. It not only makes you look and feel younger, but it also does the following:

✔ Boosts metabolism by about 15 percent

✔ Prevents, stops, and reverses bone loss

✔ Improves blood sugar

✔ Improves balance, coordination, and posture

✔ Elevates endorphins (chemicals your brain releases that make you feel great)

✔ Increases brain cells for improved thinking and concentration

✔ Improves cardiac fitness

✔ Reduces stress and anxiety

You're genetically wired to do resistance training at a high intensity. You need to demand more of your muscles than they're used to. Only through this process of going beyond what your muscles are used to can you improve. *High intensity* means that you're doing as much weight as you can and moving as fast as you can for a short period of time. The progression of all new activities requires a gradual progress in both the intensity and duration.

To function your best, your body has an internal blueprint for strength and power. Strength deteriorates quickly with age, so it's super important to implement strength building in your routine. We walk you through some specific exercises that you can implement for living Paleo in the section "Following the Road Map to Lean and Healthy," later in this chapter.

Living Paleo anaerobic: Building speed and power

Building speed and power is one of the greatest skills you can maintain to help you with everything you do in life. But getting these skills is one of the most poorly understood movements in fitness today. Case in point: How many people have you seen at the gym on the treadmill, elliptical, or stair stepper for what seems to be forever? Going at the same pace for long periods of time or performing movements that your body doesn't naturally do is simply not what you were designed to do. It's also not necessary to create a strong, lean, and lithe body filled with power and speed.

You're designed for all-out bursts of energy followed by conservation. When cave men hunted, or avoided being hunted, they were required to sprint. They went as fast as they could for short distances. By doing these short bursts, they naturally developed the speed they needed.

Doing short bursts of exercise followed by rest is far better than all that long, stretched-out exercise that takes forever. How often do you hear that? The exercise you need takes less time and is more effective!

Here are some of the advantages of doing short bursts of exercise, such as sprinting or performing high-intensity exercise followed by a period of rest:

- Improved endurance
- Quick results
- No cash or equipment required
- Burn more fat
- Cardiovascular health
- Spend less time working out, so much less boring

You no longer have to feel chained to all the cardio equipment to get power and speed into your physiology! Isn't living Paleo liberating? For specifics on a sample program and implementation, see the later section "Following the Road Map to Lean and Healthy."

Living Paleo aerobic: Doing what you love to build endurance

Hunter-gatherers had to be concerned with food preparation, they had to carry firewood and water back to the camp, and they had to build nightly fires where they also sang and danced. They sprinted, lifted, and walked an average of nine miles per day. Their rhythm was to move a lot and rest every day. As a result, we need to have certain energy expenditures daily.

Here's the good part: To meet this need, all you have to do is incorporate movement into your daily routine, or do what you already love, at a lower intensity pace. For example, if you like to hike, go for a hike. If you like to walk, bike, or swim, do those things; just enjoy what you do while moving. Playing with the kids counts, carrying groceries count, walking up and down the stairs counts. You just have to be conscious that your body needs this movement and be sure to get it every day.

While doing what you like to satisfy your living Paleo cardio requirements, your heart rate should be at about 55 to 70 percent of your maximum. You can figure out your heart rate by simply listening to your body. You shouldn't be huffing and puffing. If you are, you're doing too much. For more methods to find your ideal heart rate range, see the next section.

Determining how much movement you need and how often

Our goal is always to mimic the physical patterns of our ancestors and make the exercises as practical as possible. In the following sections, we break down the types of exercise you need into daily and weekly chunks that fulfill the movement requirement for a healthy, Paleo lifestyle.

Note: These movements are guidelines, and you may have to modify them to meet your fitness level or schedule. Just remember that whenever you start a program and just start moving, you improve your body and your life.

Your body has different systems for using the energy it needs. Anaerobic (weight lifting, sprinting) is done in short spurts, and your body relies less on oxygen. Aerobic (running, dancing) increases your heart's pumping over an extended period of time, and your body depends more on oxygen.

Resistance: Building strength and fighting age

Do resistance exercises about two to three times per week (for most people, two days is enough) for no more than 30 minutes. If you don't feel like that's enough for you, check your intensity level; it should always be as much as you can tolerate.

You have to push the muscle outside of its comfort zone to improve. Always think, "I'm going to go as hard and as fast as I can." Tell yourself the workout won't last long, so give it your all. That's how you get results.

Recovering between workouts is extremely important, so two days provides ample recovery time between resistance training and endurance. But depending on your previous conditioning, three days a week may be fine for you. You must have a break in between workouts, no less than 48 hours is optimal. If you do three days, make sure you stagger your workouts between 10 and 30 minutes and take a day off when your body tells you to. Slowly progress into the intensity and duration. Going too hard, too heavy, or too quickly is a pitfall you want to avoid.

Anaerobic: Building speed and power

To gain power and speed as you're designed, add one to two days of endurance conditioning to your weekly workout regimen.

The most effective way to build speed and power is through sprinting. You can choose from a number of activities — running sprints, hill sprints, stair sprints, bike sprints, or body sprints, like squat jumps or running in the sand. Or if you're just starting out, have bad knees, are injured, or have a health condition that prohibits you from this type of exercise, you can do low-impact sprinting options, like the pool, bike, rowing, or elliptical.

Sprinting exercises also improve your aerobic capacity because you're affecting all the muscle fibers. So these exercises help you in your power, speed, and endurance.

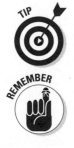

Give this exercise your all-out effort, but be sure to listen to your body and sprint only on the days you feel maximum energy and are well rested.

Aerobic: Doing what you love to build endurance

To fulfill your aerobic requirements, you must move your body for one hour *every day.* Although some of you may think that one hour of aerobic movement every day is a lot, just remember that your body was designed to move. So you need to incorporate movement into your daily life to keep your body healthy.

You can check this hour off by doing what you love to do: Walking, taking stairs, chasing after the kids, doing hobbies, or taking a hike. You can even break up the hour into 10-, 20-, or 30-minute increments — whatever works in your life and schedule — just make sure you move for a minimum of one hour a day at a slower pace. For a higher fitness levels, move a little more.

If you want to track how much you're walking, try using a pedometer, which shows you how many steps you take. The average person walks about 700 steps in an hour (that's 3.5 miles).

Stop counting how many calories you're burning. Think about aerobic movement as a daily requirement because it's what your body is programmed to do. Just because you're moving at a slower pace doesn't mean it's not effective. This slower paced movement helps with daily stress, weight maintenance, blood sugar control, muscle tone, joints, improved fat metabolism, stronger immune system, and increased energy. If you're doing your resistance and sprinting exercises, slower movements during the rest of the week are plenty. And on the days you sprint, you get double bonus because sprinting also improves your endurance!

When doing your slower-paced movements, keep track of your heart rate; you shouldn't be huffing and puffing. You should be at 55 to 70 percent of your maximum heart rate. Figuring out where your heart rate should be in this range depends on your fitness level. This calculation is personal, and you have to adjust according to your needs and history. If you're an elite athlete, higher than 70 percent may be appropriate. The important thing to keep in mind is to go at a slower, more moderate pace.

To help you incorporate this daily movement into your life, pick a time of day that you ask yourself, "Did I get my hour of movement in today?" It's as important as anything you can do for your health and longevity.

The Road Map to Lean and Healthy

We know that our ancestors' day was filled with physical exertion that was like modern-day cross-training. Their daily regimen involved several components, including strength, endurance, and power, which gave them incredible body composition, core strength, and overall health.

Our goal in this section is to provide you with a road map that emulates this cross-training pattern so you can gain the physical and metabolic effects. We provide tips for warming up and stretching, give you some specific exercises to follow, and show you how to just chill out.

Warming up and stretching yourself

We recommend three ways of stretching: dynamic motions, low-intensity exercise, and static stretches. Here's the difference:

- **Dynamic motions:** These movements prepare your muscles and nervous system for your workout. They include low-intensity functional movements where you swing your arms or legs in a controlled fashion.

- **Low-intensity exercise:** Low-intensity exercise works as a warm-up before your regular exercise. For example, if it's a sprint day, you can build up to your sprint with a light jog; if you're doing resistance, warm up with a couple of light weights. These low-intensity movements get your blood circulating and warm up your muscles.

- **Static stretches:** These stretches involve a stretch-and-hold pattern, such as touching your toes and holding, and should be done after a workout. They're designed to stretch a muscle while at rest. The stretch comes from tension, which leaves your limbs loose or relaxed.

Make sure you don't engage in any static stretches before a workout; they can have a negative impact on any high-intensity, short workout because they leave your limbs relaxed and flaccid. Static stretches should be done after exercise or on an off day, when you're not doing resistance training or sprinting, to avoid tearing fibers.

The following sections provide step-by-step instructions for dynamic motions and static stretches.

Dynamic motions (pre-workout)

Arm swings prepare your upper body for exercise. They warm up your arm and shoulder muscles and get them ready for action. Warming up your shoulder muscles is important to safeguard against injury.

1. **Stand with your feet under your hips.**

2. **Swing one arm to an overhead position, then down, and backward as far as you comfortably can.**

3. **Do about 10 repetitions, and then repeat.**

When you're going for a run, sprint, or doing any kind of movement that involves the lower body, first do some **leg swings.** Legs swings open up your hips and get them ready for movement and get the blood moving through your biggest muscle, your gluteus. Be sure to give those hamstrings in the back of your leg a nice warm up because they can be easily strained.

1. **Place both feet under the hips and hold on to something sturdy, like a wall or a chair.**

2. **Swing one leg forward and backward while the other is planted firmly on the ground.**

   Gradually increase your range of motion until the leg swings as high as it can go.

3. **Repeat on the other side.**

Knee hugs are a nice way to stretch out your quads in the front of your leg that you use in so many functions of movement and exercise.

1. **As you take a step forward, grab your leg and hug your knee to your chest.**

2. **Step and repeat on the alternating leg.**

Butt kicks are hamstring heaven. They get those muscles in the back of your legs ready for some hard work, and they give the muscles in the front of your leg a nice stretch as well. They're a very effective lower body stretch.

The steps for butt kicks are super simple: Kick your heels up toward your butt, keeping a nice pace in between kicks. Make sure your body is upright and aligned.

Static stretches (post-workout)

Squatting is one of the best exercises you can do because it's a natural motion. It's definitely one of our favorite stretches! And the **deep squat** is just an all-around good stretch that does the trick for both the upper and lower body. It's a great way to end your exercise. Doing this stretch may be a little challenging at first or even difficult to stay steady once you're in the squat, but keep trying to progress at this stretch because it's just so good.

1. **Place your feet shoulder-width apart.**

2. **Bend your knees and lower your torso all the way down, almost to the ground.**

3. **Extend your arms in front of you.**

   Be careful that your knees stay behind your toes.

4. **Hold for 15 seconds.**

   Build up to more time as you progress.

You're going to just love the **hang** stretch. Our guess is that it'll become a favorite. The hang stretch emulates our ancestors who often hung from trees. It's so relaxing and feels so good yet is effective at giving your body that post-workout stretch it needs. Hanging is fantastic for your spine and nervous system. Because most people sit all day, this stretch is a great way to relieve your spine of all the impact (spinal decompression).

The hang stretch involves simply hanging from a branch or a bar, or anything you can find to hang from.

Gathering the equipment for strength training

To do the exercises we outline in this chapter, you need some of the following basic equipment:

✔ **Range of dumbbells, comfortable to very heavy in weight:** For women, pick a range in weights from 10, 15, to 20 pounds, and for men, 20, 25, to 30 pounds. You can purchase these weights at any sporting goods store or even Wal-Mart.

✔ **Standard medicine ball:** Purchase a 10-pound and a 14-pound medicine ball. Dynamax is a good brand (www.medicineballs.com/product/).

✔ **Jump rope:** Using a jump rope makes interval training fun and builds up fitness levels quick. And jump ropes are easy to travel with.

These simple pieces of equipment are easy to store and are a great investment. With them, you can do a highly intense workout any time you please!

If you have the room and a little extra cash to spend, you may want to consider purchasing the following equipment:

✔ **Pull-up bar:** Any door frame pull-up bar will work, which you can find at a number of manufacturers and sporting goods stores. Prices range from $20 to $60. If you want to get a more professional model, for about $140, you can get a Stud Bar pull-up bar (www.studbarpullup.com).

✔ **Fitness bands:** Until you gain strength, you can use these bands to assist you with pull-ups. Simply strap the band around the pull-up bar and loop the ends together, and then step onto the band as you pull your body upward. You may have to start with a heavy resistance and work your way up to a light resistance.

Check out some quality fitness bands at www.rubberbanditz.com/store/fitness-bands. Before long, you won't need a band, and you'll be able pull yourself up on your own.

✔ **Kettlebell:** Kettlebells are basically weights with handles. They're easy to use and great for building strength. You can get a great workout from a kettlebell alone! Choose a weight in your midrange (about 15 pounds for women and 25 pounds for men). Be extra careful of form so you don't get a back injury!

Performing Paleo strength exercises

Your goal is to exercise for about 10 to 30 minutes two times per week. The strength exercises in this section involve major muscles groups, which help burn fat and release growth hormones. Be as explosive as you can while keeping form. Remember to progress appropriately. Building strength takes time, and trying to progress too quickly isn't worth the risk of injuring yourself, which can really set you back.

Starter strength exercises include pull-ups with a band, push-ups done on your knees, lunges and squats without the weights, and dumbbell presses or rows with a light weight. The deadlift is one of the most effective exercises to build strength, but it isn't a beginner movement, so take your time to work up to it.

Many of the exercises we list in this section involve doing a squat. Here's a quick and dirty rundown of some of the basic principles of all squat movements to keep in mind:

1. Before you squat, brace your abdominal muscles to create spinal stability. To do this, pretend someone is about to punch you in your stomach.

2. To initiate any squat, push your hips backward first (as opposed to leading with the knees).

3. Keep the lower back in its natural arch; don't round your back!

4. Keep your weight in your heels throughout the entire movement.

5. Never, ever let your knees cave in toward one another. Keep them tracking over your toes.

6. Keep your eyes trained on a spot 30 to 45 degrees above normal eye level.

    Your squat depth depends on your joint mobility and muscle flexibility. Squat only as low as you can without your form breaking down in any capacity.

For all the dumbbell exercises in this section, choose a weight that you can do for full repetitions. You may have to experiment to find a proper weight. You want to *progress* and focus on *form first*. When you nail down form, you're ready to increase weight and volume. The idea with strength exercises is to focus on *intensity,* not time.

Wall balls

Wall balls are a favorite to many. Because they strengthen many muscles, wall balls are considered a full-body workout. When you build up your intensity, you can get a cardio workout in there as well!

To do wall balls, you need a medicine ball. Typically, men use about a 20-pound ball and women about 14 pounds. You may need to vary this weight depending on your strength and conditioning. Starting out at 8 pounds is perfectly okay. You can progress as your fitness improves.

Refer to these steps and Figure 6-1 for one repetition of wall balls:

1. **Choose a spot on the wall to focus on, approximately 8 to 10 feet from the floor.**

    If you're just starting out, 8 feet may be more comfortable; you can progress to 10 feet (or higher). This spot is your target.

2. **Start in a standing position, about 15 to 24 inches away from the wall, feet shoulder-width apart, toes turned out slightly if that's more comfortable for you in the bottom position, and your weight on your heels. Hold the ball with your hands and elbows underneath the ball at chin level.**

3. **Keeping the ball at chin level, descend into the bottom position of a squat (or close to it).**

4. **Quickly reverse the motion, explosively extending your hips and knees. You may come up onto your toes as you transfer the momentum of your body into your arms and launch the medicine ball at the target.**

   This movement should end with your body fully extended, fingers pointed toward the target.

5. **As the ball bounces off the wall, catch it in a position near your chin, and let the weight of the ball push you back into a front squat to seamlessly begin your next rep.**

Note: The key to this exercise is to get an even tempo, where each rep flows into the next in a quick, controlled manner. Ideally, no pausing should occur between steps.

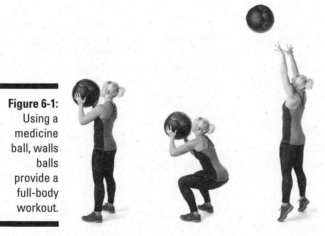

Figure 6-1:
Using a medicine ball, walls balls provide a full-body workout.

Photos by Bob McNamara

Dumbbell Romanian deadlift

The dumbbell Romanian deadlift (Figure 6-2) is another effective workout because, with this one movement, you're strengthening both your upper and lower body. To avoid back injury, it's imperative to follow good form.

1. **To get in starting position, follow these steps:**

   a. With the dumbbells on the floor, stand with your feet slightly wider than shoulder-width apart.

   b. Squat down to grasp the dumbbells.

   c. Keeping your spine neutral, come to a full standing position with the dumbbells resting against the fronts of your thighs, elbows straight. Keep your shoulder blades pulled down and pinched together.

2. **To initiate the lift:**

   a. Shift your hips backward and bend forward, almost as if you're bowing.

   b. Keeping the dumbbells close to your body, lower them only as far as you can while maintaining the natural arch of your back — shoot for just below the knees (the precise bottom point varies by individual).

3. **Return to standing and repeat.**

Figure 6-2:
The dumbbell Romanian deadlift works both the upper and lower body.

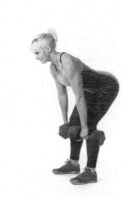

Photos by Bob McNamara

Dumbbell squat

Squats are one of the most functional movements you can do. You squat in different ways every day, such as picking something up or reaching down to tie a shoe. The dumbbell squat (Figure 6-3) works your entire lower body.

1. **Stand, holding a dumbbell in each hand at your sides, palms facing your legs. Position your feet about shoulder-width apart.**

2. **Keeping the weights hanging down at your sides, slowly lower your torso by pushing your hips backward and bending your knees.**

   Maintaining the natural arch of your back, descend as low as you're able to with perfect form.

3. **Return to the starting position by driving through your heels.**

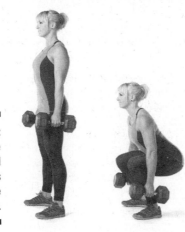

Figure 6-3: The dumbbell squat is great for the lower body.

Photos by Bob McNamara

Note: An alternate version to this exercise, the dumbbell front squat, allows you to increase the intensity by placing the dumbbells on your shoulders, as shown in Figure 6-4. You may find that you can squat more deeply with this variation (thus engaging more of your glutes!) because of where you're holding the weights.

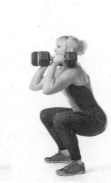

Figure 6-4: Increase the intensity with a dumbbell front squat.

Photos by Bob McNamara

Dumbbell lunge

To perform the dumbbell lunge exercise, follow these steps and refer to Figure 6-5:

1. **To get in the starting position, stand, holding a dumbbell in each hand at your sides, palms facing your legs. Your feet should be about shoulder-width apart.**

2. **Take a large step forward with one leg, simultaneously bending both legs until they're at 90 degrees. (The top of your front thigh will be parallel to the ground.)**

   Keep your chest up and head in a neutral position, looking ahead.

3. **Pushing through the heel of your front foot, step back into your starting position.**

   Either repeat the movement on the same side or alternate sides.

Note: You can increase the intensity of this exercise by performing walking lunges: String the lunges together, moving forward and alternating legs with each step.

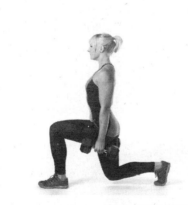

Figure 6-5:
The dumb-
bell lunge
strengthens
the lower
body.

Photos by Bob McNamara

Push-ups

Traditional push-ups stick around the exercise circuit because they're a fantastic way to strengthen the upper body and build core strength. If you're traveling or are somewhere where you just can't get to any equipment, the push-up is a great standby, on-the-go exercise.

To perform a standard push-up, follow these steps and check out Figure 6-6:

1. **To get in starting position, place your feet and hands on the floor, with hands slightly more than shoulder-width apart and feet hip-width apart.**

2. **Lower yourself to the floor, stopping when your chest is a few inches from the ground.**

3. **Press away from the floor, straightening your arms.**

   The rest of your body should remain stiff as a board, maintaining the straight line from head to toe.

4. **Pause at the top and repeat.**

If you're new to push-ups, try this modified version (shown in Figure 6-7) and progress slowly until shoulder and chest strength develops:

1. **To get in starting position, place your hands and knees on the floor, with hands slightly more than shoulder-width apart and knees hip-width apart; cross your legs at the ankles.**

   Make sure your arms are straight and your body forms a perfectly straight line from head to knees.

2. **Lower yourself to the floor, stopping when your chest is a few inches from the ground.**

3. **Press away from the floor, straightening your arms.**

   The rest of your body should remain stiff as a board, maintaining the straight line from head to knees.

4. **Pause at the top and repeat.**

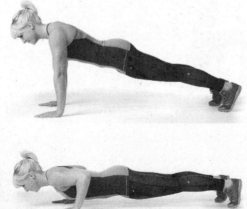

Figure 6-6:
The traditional push-up, with hands and feet on the floor.

Photos by Bob McNamara

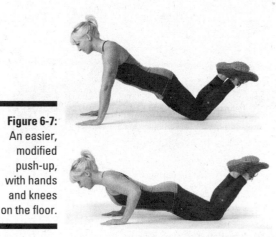

Figure 6-7:
An easier,
modified
push-up,
with hands
and knees
on the floor.

Photos by Bob McNamara

Dumbbell press

The dumbbell press builds your upper body, working your chest, shoulders, and triceps. Your back and your biceps assist you in the movement, so dumbbell presses are a great all-around exercise to build strength.

The following steps walk you through the dumbbell press, using a bench (see Figure 6-8):

1. **To get in starting position, follow these steps:**

    a. Sit on the bench with the dumbbells resting on your lower thighs. Use your thighs to help bump the weights up to your shoulders one at a time and lie back.

    b. Rotate your wrists forward so that the palms of your hands are facing away from you.

    c. Lower the weights to chest level with a bent arm under each dumbbell, creating a 90-degree angle.

2. **Press the dumbbells upward until your arms are extended and parallel.**

    Your dumbbells should touch ends at the top position.

3. **Lower the weights in a smooth controlled fashion to the starting position. Repeat.**

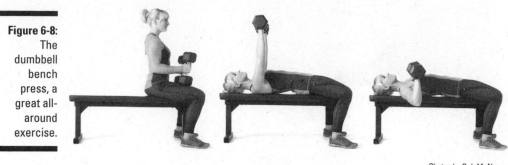

Figure 6-8:
The dumbbell bench press, a great all-around exercise.

Photos by Bob McNamara

To sit back upright, use these steps to protect your back:

1. **Lift your legs from the floor, bending at the knees.**

2. **Rotate your wrists so that the palms of your hands are facing each other and place the dumbbells at the top of your thighs.**

3. **Tighten your abdominals and roll up while pressing the dumbbells on your thighs. Slightly kick forward to give yourself the momentum to sit up.**

If you don't have a bench available, try the dumbbell press on the floor, as shown in Figure 6-9:

1. **To get in starting position,**

    a. Sit on the floor with the dumbbells resting on your lower thighs. Bringing the weights with you in front of your chest, lie back, knees bent.

    b. Maneuver the weights so that your forearms are vertical and your elbows and upper arms are flush with the ground.

    c. Rotate your wrists forward so that your palms are facing away from you.

2. **Press the dumbbells upward until your arms are extended and parallel.**

    Your dumbbells should touch ends at the top position.

3. **Slowly lower the dumbbells down until your upper arms are resting on the floor again. Repeat.**

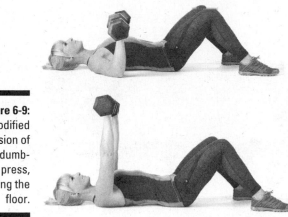

Photos by Bob McNamara

Dumbbell row

Your back is so important for the stabilization and strength of your entire body. That's why dumbbell rows (Figure 6-10) are such a great addition to your workout regimen. They develop and strengthen many of your back muscles (both upper and lower) and also work your shoulders, arms, and core.

1. **To get in starting position, follow these steps:**

   a. Stand near a stable bench, table, or chair. Hold the dumbbell in the hand farthest from the bench.

   b. Take a large step forward with your foot closest to the bench and place the same-side hand on top of the bench to brace yourself.

   c. Lean forward so that your back is almost parallel to the floor.

      The dumbbell should be hanging down toward the floor, with your knees slightly bent and your eyes focusing on a spot on the ground somewhere in front of you.

2. **Pull your shoulder back and row the dumbbell up to your ribs, pulling your elbow to the ceiling as far as you can without forcing it.**

   Your forearm should be nearly vertical from start to finish.

3. **Lower in a smooth and controlled manner and repeat.**

4. **To change sides, switch the direction you're facing and follow the same procedure.**

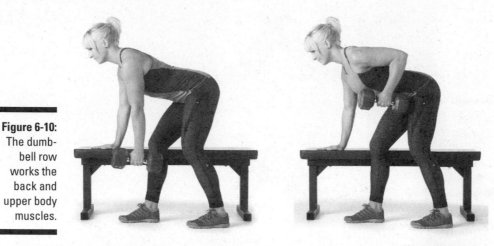

Figure 6-10:
The dumb-
bell row
works the
back and
upper body
muscles.

Photos by Bob McNamara

Dumbbell swings

The dumbbell swing is one of the best exercises you can do for full-body strength and power. Dumbbell swings work all your major muscles, and, when using a lighter weight, you can do a lot of repitions for a great cardiovascular workout.

Check out the following steps and Figure 6-11 for the dumbbell swing. (You can also use a kettlebell for this movement, as shown in Figure 6-12.)

Note: Keep your chest up and your back in its natural arch at all times, and keep your gaze focused forward throughout.

1. **To get in starting position,**

   a. Place the dumbbell between your legs, with your feet slightly wider than shoulder-width apart and your toes pointing slightly outward.

   b. Squat down and grab the handle of the dumbbell with both hands interlocking your fingers around the handle.

2. **Hike the dumbbell back between your legs to build momentum. Then, keeping your arms straight, immediately stand upright and snap your hips forward, swinging the dumbbell upward until it's at about shoulder height.**

   The power should come from your hips and glutes — don't raise it with your arms.

3. **As the dumbbell arcs downward again, fold forward at the hips to about 45 degrees, bending your knees slightly, and guide the dumbbell between your legs.**

   This step completes one repetition.

4. **Continue from that point, forcefully straightening your hips and legs so that the dumbbell again reaches shoulder height.**

   You may need to start out with swings that only reach belly button height until you get comfortable with the movement.

Note: The lower back has little to do with this exercise. Maintaining a neutral back with no rounding or bending over is important. Progress slowly to avoid injury.

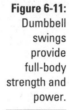
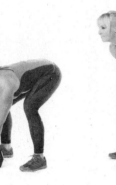
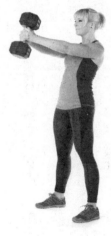

Figure 6-11: Dumbbell swings provide full-body strength and power.

Photos by Bob McNamara

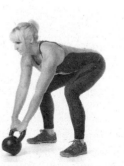
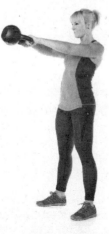

Figure 6-12: Dumbbell swing, using a kettlebell instead.

Photos by Bob McNamara

Pull-ups

Pull-ups are a great exercise to develop upper body strength. They work your back, chest, and arms. Pull-ups are a more challenging exercise for many, but you just have to dig in and start somewhere.

Using a pull-up bar is the best-case scenario for this exercise. If you have to improvise, find a smooth fence or a piece of playground equipment.

1. **Grab the pull-up bar with your hands placed about shoulder-width apart and your palms facing away from you, arms fully extended (see Figure 6-13).**

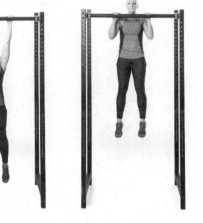

Figure 6-13: Traditional pull-ups with a pull-up bar.

Photos by Bob McNamara

2. **Pull your body up until your chin is over the bar.**

   Concentrate on keeping your shoulder blades down and pinched together as you reach the top (which will keep you from chicken-necking over the bar).

3. **Slowly lower yourself down to the hanging position and repeat.**

If you need assistance doing pull-ups until you build strength, try exercise bands with different levels of assistance (see Figure 6-14). The thicker the band, the more support you get.

1. **Choke the band around the pull-up bar, looping one end through the other and pulling it tight over the bar. Place one foot in the exercise band, and cross the other foot in front to keep the band in place.**

2. **Grab the pull-up bar with your hands placed about shoulder-width apart, your palms facing away from you.**

3. **Pull yourself upward until your chin is over the bar, and keep tension on the band by keeping your leg straight and knee locked out.**

4. **Slowly lower yourself down to the hanging position and repeat.**

Note: You can use bands as you work toward progression. They'll help you either achieve a pull-up or increase the number of repetitions.

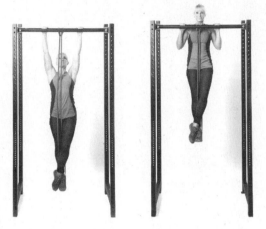

Figure 6-14: Assisted pull-ups with pull-up bar and exercise bands.

Photos by Bob McNamara

Push press

Every time you lift up your arms, your shoulder muscles are working. That's why it's so important to keep your shoulders strong and conditioned. The push press targets all your shoulder muscles and even works your legs a bit. It's a great all-around shoulder exercise that you'll want to add into your exercise rotation, but be sure to start slowly to avoid injury.

Here are the steps to the push press exercise (also see Figure 6-15):

1. **Start with your feet hip-width apart, and rest the dumbbells on the fronts of your shoulders.**

   Make sure you have a firm grasp on the handles.

2. **Take a small breath and dip slightly by bending your knees, keeping your torso upright and your head up.**

3. **Immediately reverse the movement, using your legs to drive the dumbbells off of your shoulders. Use this momentum to press the dumbbells overhead.**

   This should be done explosively but under control.

4. **Pause for a moment in the top position, and then lower the dumbbells back to your shoulders. Repeat.**

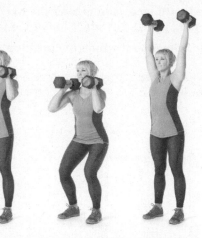

Figure 6-15:
The push press keeps shoulders strong.

Photos by Bob McNamara

Progressing through sprinting and recovery exercises

If you're just beginning, then sprinting one or two days a week is a great start. You'll know you're ready for more advanced sprinting when the activity becomes easier and your breathing isn't so labored after you've completed a sprint. Running as fast as possible can be a liberating and even fun experience, especially if you haven't done it since you were a kid. Enjoy yourself.

For purpose of these exercises, we assume that you're sprinting on a track.

Beginner's track

If you're just starting out, progression is the key to sustainability in exercise. This intensity is for those who are hitting the pavement for the first time or have been away for a while:

1. **Do some dynamic motions (see earlier section "Warming up and stretching yourself") and a light jog around the track to warm up.**

2. **Go as fast as you can for 6 to 30 seconds.**

3. **Rest for 3½ to 4 minutes by walking or jogging very lightly.**

4. **Repeat Steps 1 through 3 as many times as you can, working up to six bursts.**

5. **Cool down by walking or jogging lightly around the track.**

Progress slowly as you need to and work up to six bursts. Just moving makes a difference in your overall fitness and health.

Advanced track

When the beginner's sprinting routine starts to get easy, it's time to try some advanced sprinting.

1. **Do some dynamic motions (see earlier section "Warming up and stretching yourself") and a light jog around the track to warm up.**

2. **Go as fast as you can for 6 to 60 seconds.**

3. **Rest for 1½ minutes by walking or jogging very lightly.**

4. **Repeat Steps 1 through 3 as many times as you can, working up to eight bursts.**

5. **Cool down by walking or jogging lightly around the track.**

Be sure to get proper recovery in between workouts and eat carb-dense food, like a sweet potato, afterward. Also, drink plenty of water.

Chilling out with yoga

Okay, we know that yoga doesn't have all functional movements. We also know that the kind of stretching involved for some people may be counterproductive for others. But we also can't dismiss the many who have benefited from the mental relaxation and the wellness that yoga bestows. As long as you're careful of any discomfort and adapt your movements as needed, we give yoga a thumbs-up. We believe the benefits far outweigh any potential risk. Yoga may be something you want to do on your "do what you love" days (see the section "Living Paleo aerobic: Doing what you love to build endurance," earlier in this chapter).

The healing benefits of yoga are so great, and most people feel better after just one session. One of the main reasons for this high success in yoga healing is that yoga relaxes and de-stresses you on a deep level. In Chapter 5, we discuss the stress cycle and the impact on your body. It can make you sick, depressed, anxious, and fat. Finding ways to calm your body and eliminate stress is priceless. Yoga does that for your body and does it well. The difference in energy you feel and the difference in stress levels make this practice worth the effort to buy a DVD that you can do in the comfort of your home or to join a local class.

Yoga sometimes ends with guided relaxation/meditation. In guided relaxation, your teacher (guide) speaks to the class or reads something that helps you go into a deep state of relaxation or inner stillness — one of the most powerful ways to de-stress and bring about positive changes in your life. Now you can also find many smartphone apps and CDs that have guided meditations for you to follow in the comfort of your own home.

Designing Your Personal Paleo Exercise Program

This program is all about you. It's about giving you the tools you need to express health and to become lean, strong, and energized.

Through the anaerobic program of sprinting, you build power and speed. Through resistance training, you build incredible strength and look younger. Through the aerobic program of doing what you love, you build endurance.

When you begin to cross-train in these short but powerful bursts and find time to move by doing what you love, you make physical activity a part of your life as your ancestors did. Soon your body will reach its potential and flourish.

Some of you may need a little help building your personal program. In this section, we provide three sample weeks of exercise, from beginner to advanced workouts. Pick the program that fits your fitness level now, and work toward the next level. You'll know you're ready to progress on to the next level when the exercises become effortless and less challenging to you. When you have the form down solid and you feel ready for a little more zest, you're ready to move on.

In these exercises, a *burst* is the actual sprint, where you go as hard and as fast as you can for 6 to 60 seconds. When doing the metabolic conditioning (met-con) exercises for time, you do the suggested number of rounds as quickly as possible with good form, keeping track of the time it takes to complete the exercise so you can track improvements.

Beginner sample week

It's hard not to hit the ground running when you're excited about starting something new and important to you. However, try to keep the end in mind, which is to build a strong, healthy, lean body by working out on a *consistent* basis. If you get injured or over-exhausted because of doing more than you should, you'll be forced to interrupt your program. Starting slow can sometimes be frustrating, but maintaining a pace that works for you and your fitness level is the smartest strategy. Table 6-1 provides a sample workout week for the beginner level.

Table 6-1	Beginner Workout Week Sample	
Day	**Exercise**	**Time**
Day 1	*Walking sprint	2 bursts in 15-minute walk
Day 2	**Do what you love	1 hour
Day 3	Met-con: 12 push-ups, 9 dumb-bell squats, 6 pull-ups (use fitness band until you build strength to do without)	3 rounds for time
Day 4	***Do what you love (slow, play pace)	1 hour
Day 5	Met-con: As many wall balls as you can do in 12 minutes	12 minutes
Day 6	Walking sprint	2 bursts in a 15-minute walk
Day 7	Do what you love	1 hour

*You always have the option to sprint by doing track, hill, bike, or treadmill. We start you with walking because it's a beginning exercise and a great way to build a foundation for sprinting.
**Do what you love (walk, swim, hike, stairs, yoga, chase after your kids, or anything that gets you moving).
***Do what you love (slow, play pace): This is your day to take it easy. Your one hour of movement should be simple, non-strenuous, slow movements, like walking from one place to another.

You may wonder why you don't see those three words common to most exercise programs: *Day of rest*. We don't include a day of rest because your body is designed to move a minimum of one hour every day. You don't have to push your body or force anything. The hour of *doing what you love* can be walking around in the grocery store, or even chasing the kids around — it all counts. You just need to carry the mental framework that you gotta move!

Intermediate sample week

The sample exercise program in Table 6-2 is for people who are beginning to progress past the newcomer's stage and are starting to develop the rhythm and flow that works best for them.

In this stage, you've started to build your cardiovascular base as your body becomes more efficient, and you feel the first blush of increased strength and energy throughout your day. At this point, you may even begin to notice the physical affects of your commitment to move, as your body becomes leaner.

Table 6-2	Intermediate Workout Week Sample	
Day	**Exercise**	**Time**
Day 1	*Running sprint	3 bursts in a 20-minute run
Day 2	**Do what you love	1 hour
Day 3	Met-con: 15 dumbbell lunges, 12 dumbbell rows, 9 push-ups, 6 kettlebell swings	3 rounds for time
Day 4	***Do what you love (slow, play pace)	1 hour
Day 5	Met-con: 15 wall balls, 12 kettlebell swings, 9 pull-ups, as many rounds as you can do in 20 minutes	20 minutes
Day 6	Running sprint	3 bursts in a 20-minute run
Day 7	Do what you love	1 hour

*You always have the option to sprint by doing track, hill, bike, or treadmill. We have running for this week because it's a good intermediate exercise.
**Do what you love (walk, swim, hike, stairs, yoga, chase after your kids, or anything that gets you moving).
***Do what you love (slow, play pace): This is your day to take it easy. Your one hour of movement should be simple, non-strenuous, slow movements, like walking from one place to another.

Advanced sample week

When you progress in your resistance training to go harder and faster in a shorter period of time and your sprinting leaves you feeling like you could do more, you're ready for advanced training. At this stage, your hard work and commitment will be noticeable to you — and those around you. You'll feel leaner, stronger, and more energetic. Table 6-3 provides a sample workout week for the advanced level.

Be careful not to *over*train. Overtraining does exactly the opposite of what you're trying to achieve. It leaves you chronically tired, prone to injury, and wide open for illness. If you're starting to feel like your workouts are exhausting you more than giving you energy, it's probably time to pull back and take a rest. In the long run, a rest will help you, not set you back.

Table 6-3	Advanced Workout Week Sample	
Day	Exercise	Time
Day 1	*Track, hill, bike, or treadmill sprint	4 bursts in a 25-minute workout
Day 2	Met-con: 12 pull-ups, 9 dumbbell presses, 6 dumbbell deadlifts, 12 push-ups	3 rounds for time
Day 3	Met-con: 15 kettlebell swings, 9 dumbbell lunges, 6 dumbbell presses, as many rounds as you can do in 12 minutes	12 minutes
Day 4	**Do what you love (slow, play pace)	1 hour
Day 5	Track, hill, bike, or treadmill sprint	4 bursts in a 25-minute workout
Day 6	Met-con: 150 wall balls	150 wall balls for time
Day 7	***Do what you love	1 hour

*For advanced sprinting, doing a track, hill, bike, or treadmill sprint are all consistent with this level of conditioning.
**Do what you love (slow, play pace): This is your day to take it easy. Your one hour of movement should be simple, non-strenuous, slow movements like walking from one place to another.
***Do what you love (walk, swim, hike, stairs, yoga, chase after your kids, or anything that gets you moving).

Chapter 7

Stocking a Paleo-Friendly Kitchen

. . . .

In This Chapter

▶ Clearing your kitchen of non-Paleo foods

▶ Restocking your kitchen for Paleo success

▶ Identifying essential Paleo cooking tools and methods

▶ Finding your way through the grocery store

▶ Foraging for food in new ways

. . . .

*Y*our commitment to living Paleo begins with changing your eating habits, so it's time to create your base of operations for success: the Paleo kitchen.

In this chapter, you say goodbye to the pasta and processed foods in your cabinets and replace them with palate-pleasing Paleo staples. You see how to stock your refrigerator with fresh meats, vegetables, and fruits that keep you and your family energized throughout the day.

Whether you're an experienced cook or just finding your way around the kitchen, we show you how to equip your kitchen with the tools you need and the best Paleo-friendly cooking methods to keep you and your family well fed. Thanks to modern conveniences, you don't need to actually track and hunt your dinner, but instead we show you a new way to prowl the aisles of the grocery store for just what you need — and provide tips for foraging in new locations to make the most of farmers' markets, health food stores, and online retailers.

With a little bit of prep work in the kitchen and a few new shopping habits, living Paleo will soon be second nature.

Cleaning Out Your Kitchen

This task may hurt a little, but it must be done. Think of it as ripping off a Band-Aid. Your first step in setting up your Paleo kitchen is removing all the non-Paleo foods from the house, which serves two important purposes:

- ✔ It signifies the beginning of your commitment to your new lifestyle. A fresh start can be very motivating.

- ✔ It removes temptation from your immediate vicinity and helps you keep your new commitment. If the wrong foods aren't in the house, you can't accidentally eat them in a flurry of cravings or wavering commitment.

So roll up your sleeves, grab a trash bag for castoffs and a cardboard box for food to donate, and then take a deep breath and start your new lifestyle by cleaning up your kitchen. We walk you through each area of your kitchen in the following sections.

As you rid your kitchen of non-Paleo foods, dump all open packages and jars directly into the trash bag. Place *unopened* packages in the box to donate to a local food bank or shelter. Although you're choosing not to eat these foods because they don't provide optimal health, the calories can be helpful to other people who are hungry and striving to feed themselves.

If you live with family members or friends who aren't making the switch to living Paleo, you may be forced to share your Paleo kitchen with non-Paleo foods. Although doing so is undoubtedly a challenge, you can prevail! Talk to your housemates and explain your commitment to living Paleo, and then designate a shelf of the refrigerator, a cabinet, and an area of the freezer where they can store their non-Paleo foods. Avoid coming in contact with these designated areas as much as possible to minimize your discomfort and possibility for temptation. And maybe, eventually, your new Paleo habits will rub off on your companions, and the whole kitchen will become Paleo.

The cabinets and pantry

Start with the cabinets and pantry, and remove all non-Paleo foods, such as the following. Read labels carefully to see whether anything can be salvaged, but in all likelihood, most of it will need to go.

- Agave syrup
- Breakfast cereal, granola, and oatmeal
- Candy
- Canned chili, soup, stew, and so on
- Canned tuna that contains soy
- Commercial sauces and condiments that contain any non-Paleo ingredients
- Cornstarch
- Crackers and chips
- Flour

- Fruit and vegetable juice
- Fruits packed in syrup or containing sweeteners
- Jam and jelly
- Microwave meals
- Pasta
- Rice
- Salad dressing
- Soy sauce
- Vegetable oils (canola, corn, peanut, safflower, and so on)
- White and brown sugar

Less-processed, natural sweeteners like raw honey and pure maple syrup can stay but shouldn't be eaten during your 30-Day Reset (see Chapter 8).

The refrigerator

Next up is the refrigerator. You may be tempted to hold on to open jars and containers to finish before switching to Paleo. Resist that temptation and toss non-Paleo items into the trash bag. The food is only wasted if you eat it because it only does you harm, so instead of being concerned about wasting food, try to view this purge as your first step toward good health.

- Bacon that contains nitrates and/or sweeteners
- Butter
- Cheese
- Commercial sauces and condiments that contain any non-Paleo ingredients
- Cream
- Deli meats that contain nitrates and/or sweeteners
- Fruit and vegetable juice
- Half-and-half

- Jam and jelly
- Leftovers that contain non-Paleo ingredients
- Margarine
- Milk
- Salad dressing
- Sausage that contains nitrates and/or sweeteners
- Soy sauce
- Tofu and vegetarian "meats"
- Yogurt

The freezer

The freezer is the last stop on the kitchen cleanup tour. Old favorites like ice cream and frozen meals may be hard to banish to the garbage bin, but again, resist the temptation to hang on to these foods that conflict with the new lifestyle you're creating.

- Frozen meals and pizzas
- Frozen yogurt
- Homemade foods that contain non-Paleo ingredients
- Ice cream
- Popsicles and frozen fruit bars that contain sweeteners

Restocking Your New, Paleo-Friendly Kitchen

The hard part is over! You've bid farewell to those old foods, and your kitchen is ready to be provisioned for living Paleo. Now the fun part begins: restocking your larder with delicious, nutritious Paleo-approved foods. We show you just what your new and improved kitchen needs in the following sections.

Paleo protein

Animal protein is going to be the basis of your Paleo meals, and you want to buy the highest-quality meat, poultry, eggs, and fish you can afford. If your budget can support it, the optimal choice for animal protein is meat from organic, grass-fed, pastured, or free-range animals. Factory farming is damaging to the environment and produces animals that are less healthy than their humanely raised counterparts. (See more on why grass-fed meat is important in Chapter 4.)

- **Beef:** Your best bets are all cuts of grass-fed beef, preferably organic and definitely free of antibiotics. Consider organ meats, too, for an extra dose of nutrition.

✔ **Pork:** Look for pastured pork or wild boar to avoid the hazards of the omega-6 fatty acids found in factory-farmed pork. If you must eat conventionally grown pork, remove all visible fat and don't eat sausage or bacon from factory-farmed pigs. Pastured, sugar-free bacon is *technically* Paleo, but it's a food you should eat in moderation because of its high proportion of fat to protein.

✔ **Lamb:** All cuts of pastured lamb are a healthful choice, and, again, organ meats are delicious and nutritious.

✔ **Poultry:** Look for organic, pastured chicken that's also free of antibiotics. All cuts, including the tasty chicken livers, are good choices.

✔ **Game meats:** Game meats, like elk and bison, are naturally low in fat and high in protein. Look for pastured, organic, antibiotic-free brands.

✔ **Eggs:** The labels on eggs are particularly confusing. Your healthiest choice for eggs is organic and pastured. You know the chickens were humanely and healthily raised if the carton says *Certified Humane* or *Food Alliance Certified* — but avoid *United Egg Producers Certified,* which permits factory farm practices. Also beware squishy terms like *vegetarian fed* and *natural,* which have no bearing on the quality of the eggs.

✔ **Fish and seafood:** Wild-caught fish, seafood, and shellfish are healthier than farm-raised varieties and better for the planet, too. Avoid all farmed fish and seafood to ensure that the fish you're eating has consumed a healthy, natural diet itself. For specifics about the wisest choices both for the environment and your health, visit the Monterey Bay Aquarium Seafood Watch at `www.montereybayaquarium.org/cr/seafoodwatch.aspx`.

If your grocery budget doesn't allow you to invest in this higher-quality protein right now, that's okay. You can still improve your health by eliminating processed foods and focusing on animal protein, vegetables, fruits, and high-quality fats. If you must buy conventionally raised meat, these tips can help improve its healthfulness:

✔ Buy the leanest cuts of red meat and pork you can find.

✔ Remove excess fat from red meat and pork, and the skin from poultry, before cooking.

✔ Drain excess fat after cooking.

✔ Chill soups and stews after cooking, and then remove and discard congealed fat from the surface before eating.

Paleo produce

Eating too many vegetables is practically impossible, so let yourself loose when you hit the produce department, and choose a wide variety of vegetables in a rainbow of colors. Buying organic isn't always necessary (see the later section "Choosing whether to buy organic"), so vegetables are an economical way to satisfy hunger and improve your health.

Fruit, in moderation, is also an excellent source of nutrient-dense calories — and who doesn't like something a little sweet now and then?

For both fruits and vegetables, choose what's in season for the freshest, most nutritious options. And if your favorite isn't available fresh, frozen fruits and vegetables — because they're flash frozen just after picking — are a solid, nutritious alternative to fresh.

Here are some ideas to get you started, but let your senses be your guide in the produce department and farmers' market (and see the later section "Creating your Paleo-approved grocery list" for more options):

- ✔ **Leafy greens:** High in fiber, vitamins, and minerals, leafy greens are some of the best veggies to put on your plate. Try beet tops, bok choy, collard greens, kale, mustard greens, Napa cabbage, spinach, Swiss chard, and turnip greens.

- ✔ **Hearty vegetables:** Roasted, sautéed, grilled, or steamed, these veggies serve up plenty of flavor and nutrition. Dig into artichokes, asparagus, beets, broccoli, Brussels sprouts, cabbage, cauliflower, carrots, eggplant, fennel, onion, parsnips, spaghetti squash, summer squash, turnips, and zucchini.

- ✔ **Salad vegetables:** Fresh, crisp, and filling, a salad can be a meal in itself or a tantalizing side. Toss in alfalfa sprouts, arugula, bell peppers, celery, cucumber, jicama, lettuce, mushrooms, radicchio, radishes, red cabbage, sunflower sprouts, tomatoes, and watercress.

- ✔ **Carb-dense vegetables:** These starchy and carbohydrate-dense vegetables play an important role in helping you recover from exercise and stress. Roast a batch of acorn squash, butternut squash, sweet potatoes, and yams.

- ✔ **Paleo-approved legumes:** Although these vegetables are technically legumes, they include more pod than bean — and they're green! Snap into green beans, string beans, snap peas, snow peas, and wax beans.

- ✔ **Fresh herbs:** Leafy herbs like basil, cilantro, dill, garlic, ginger, mint, oregano, parsley, rosemary, and thyme add a big dose of flavor to any meal.

- ✔ **Fruits:** Eaten whole or in salads, raw or cooked, colorful fruits are a good source of vitamins and taste oh-so-sweet. Savor every bite, from apples to UGLI fruit.

Paleo fats

High-quality fats, such as the following, are essential for optimal health and weight loss, and they not only make your food taste good but also provide a satisfying mouthfeel.

- ✔ **Coconut fats:** Coconuts are an excellent source of saturated fat and produce so many delicious varieties of Paleo-approved fats, including coconut oil (best for cooking), coconut butter, coconut flakes, and coconut milk.

- ✔ **Olives and avocados:** Both olives and avocados are favored sources of monounsaturated fats. Use olive oil and avocado oil for drizzling on salads, and nibble on both olives and avocados in salads or as snacks for healthy fat intake.

- ✔ **Animal fats:** Animal fats are an excellent choice for cooking but only if the fats come from organic, grass-fed, pastured animals. If you can find a good source, then fats like lard, tallow, and ghee (clarified butter) are healthful, delicious options.

- ✔ **Nuts, nut oils, and nut butters:** In moderation, nuts and nut butters (excluding peanuts and peanut butter) are tasty options to add fat to meals, snacks, and desserts. Nut oils are a nice way to add unexpected flavors to salads but shouldn't be used for cooking.

Cooking at high heat can damage some oils, causing oxidation that makes otherwise healthy oils likely to cause inflammation. Avoid cooking with extra-virgin olive oil and nut oils; instead, use those oils to toss on salads or drizzle over cooked food. For high-heat cooking — on the stovetop or grill or in the oven — use saturated fats from animals or coconut.

Paleo pantry staples and spices

Now that you've rid your cabinets of grains, legumes, and processed foods, you need to fill those empty spaces with the flavor enhancers that help ensure that your meals are as good to eat as they are nutritious. In the following sections, we share our ideas for pantry items and spices that every Paleo kitchen should have.

Pantry palate pleasers

A well-stocked pantry can mean the difference between enjoying an appetizing Paleo meal and a desperate phone call to the local pizza delivery shop. Here's a list of staples to keep enticing meals flying out of your Paleo kitchen:

- ✔ **Arrowroot powder:** Substitute for flour and cornstarch to thicken soups, stews, and sauces.

✔ **Coconut aminos:** Substitute for soy sauce in Asian food.

✔ **Coconut oil:** Choose unrefined coconut oil, and use it for sautéing, roasting, and baking in place of vegetable oils and shortening.

✔ **Unsweetened coconut:** Enjoy flakes as a snack, and use shredded coconut to add fat and sweetness to curries, salads, and desserts.

✔ **Coconut milk:** Avoid the coconut milk in the carton and use the variety in cans. You can substitute coconut milk for yogurt and cream in recipes — or splash it into coffee instead of half-and-half. Most brands of coconut milk include some kind of stabilizer; the only Paleo-approved stabilizer is guar gum.

✔ **Extra-virgin olive oil:** Use on salads or drizzle over cooked vegetables and meats.

✔ **Dried fruit:** Eat in moderation; add to stews, sautés, and vegetables to add texture and a hint of sweetness.

✔ **Olives:** Look for packaged olives that contain only water, olives, and salt; avoid chemical additives and stabilizers. Toss them into salads and cooked foods to add healthy fat.

✔ **Nuts:** Raw or dry roasted are your best bet. Eat them in moderation; add to cooked foods for crunch, or enjoy a few as a snack.

✔ **Pickles:** Examine labels for chemical, non-Paleo ingredients, and then enjoy pickles whenever you want a tart bite.

✔ **Broth/stock:** Review labels for non-Paleo ingredients, especially soy and hidden sugars; use in place of water or wine in sauces, soups, stews, and sautés.

✔ **Nut butters:** Examine the label for added sugar. Enjoy nut butters in moderation; they're great for snacks, sauces, and desserts.

✔ **Tomato paste:** Use to add depth of flavor to sauces, soups, and stews.

✔ **Canned tomatoes:** Make your own quick marinara sauce or add to soups and stews for a savory touch and extra veggies.

✔ **Canned fish:** Examine labels for non-Paleo ingredients, especially soy. Tuna, salmon, sardines, and kipper snacks are all good choices.

✔ **Curry paste:** Examine labels for non-Paleo ingredients, especially soy and added sugar. These pastes are great to have on hand to make a quick meal with coconut milk, protein, and veggies.

✔ **Canned chiles:** Examine labels for non-Paleo preservatives. Mild green, jalapeño, or chipotle chile peppers add zing to everyday ingredients.

✔ **Jarred salsas**: Examine labels for non-Paleo ingredients, like chemical preservatives, sugar, corn, and wheat.

Sweet, savory, sensational spices

Spices are an easy, Paleo-approved way to turn boring into *booyah!* If you're not accustomed to cooking with spices, you may be intimidated by this list, but don't feel like you need to stock up all at once. Think of your spice cabinet as a collection that grows over time as you expand your palate and recipe adventures. A new spice can open up a whole new world of flavor, and you just may find some new favorites.

- **Bay leaf:** Use in soups, stews, and braises, especially in Mediterranean cuisine.

- **Cardamom:** Essential in Indian curries.

- **Cayenne pepper:** Add a kick of heat to just about anything.

- **Chives:** Use in French and Swedish cooking; they add a light oniony flavor.

- **Cinnamon:** A kitchen essential for both sweet and savory foods.

- **Cloves:** Use in Indian, Vietnamese, Mexican, and Dutch cooking for sweets and savory dishes.

- **Cocoa:** Use Unsweetened cocoa to add richness and depth to tomato-based dishes and sweets.

- **Coriander:** Use in Middle Eastern, Asian, Mediterranean, Indian, Mexican, Latin American, African, and Scandinavian foods.

- **Cumin:** Earthy flavor great for North African, Middle Eastern, Mexican, and some Chinese dishes.

- **Garlic powder:** A good substitute for fresh garlic when you're in a hurry.

- **Ginger:** Essential for Indian curries and Asian dishes.

- **Ground mustard:** Use in homemade mayonnaise, salad dressings, and spice blends.

- **Mint:** A key ingredient in Middle Eastern and Mediterranean cooking.

- **Oregano:** Use in Italian, Greek, and Mexican foods.

- **Paprika:** Bring a peppery bite and pleasing color to Moroccan, Middle Eastern, and Eastern European recipes.

- **Pepper:** A cooking staple.

- **Salt:** Highlight the flavor of food. Look for iodized sea salt.

- **Thyme:** Use in Middle Eastern, Indian, Italian, French, Spanish, Greek, Caribbean, and Turkish cuisines.

Spice blends: Delicious shortcuts

Many spice vendors offer their own spice blends, in addition to freshly ground individual spices. From more familiar names, like chili powder, Italian herb blend, or curry powder, to more exotic options, like Chinese five-spice powder or Middle Eastern Za'atar, these spice blends instantly add international flair to humble vegetables and protein. Be sure to read the ingredients list because some blends include sugar. Online spice retailers like Penzeys (www.penzeys.com) and Savory Spice Shop (www.savoryspiceshop.com) also provide recipes that show you how to make the most of these exciting additions to your kitchen.

Gathering Essential Paleo Cooking Tools

Among the many advantages of not *actually* being a cave man or woman is that you have access to cooking tools that are easier and safer to use than an open fire with a spit. The following sections highlight the kitchen appliances, gadgets, and cookware that make cooking Paleo a cinch.

Appliances

You can ditch your toaster, rice cooker, and Easy-Bake Oven, but these kitchen workhorses are essential tools for transforming Paleo ingredients into culinary masterpieces.

- **Food processor or blender:** You can get by with one or the other, but to cover all your bases, you may want both. A food processor or blender is irreplaceable for whipping up sauces (like the Homemade Mayonnaise recipe in Chapter 14) and puréed soups. A food processor makes quick work of grating and slicing vegetables, and you can use it to grind meat, too.

- **Standing or hand mixer:** If you have a solid food processor, you may not need a mixer, but this appliance can handle more volume and is useful for turning coconut milk into Whipped Coconut Cream (Chapter 12).

- **Slow cooker:** The slow cooker is the ultimate hands-off cooking tool because it does the work while you sleep or play or work. It's perfect for preparing large batches of soups or stew and is also handy for roasting meats. (See ideas for slow cooker recipes in Chapter 11.)

- **Grill:** Any season of the year, grilled meats and vegetables taste great. A gas or charcoal grill is a good weapon to have in your arsenal because you can cook large quantities in a short amount of time so you have handy leftovers in the fridge.

Gadgets and cookware

These tools help you prep meals with a minimum of fuss and aggravation. With the following gadgets and cookware at your fingertips, you'll be ready to make just about any Paleo recipe your taste buds desire:

- **Chef's knife:** If you have only one good knife in your kitchen, make it an 8-inch chef's knife — and keep it sharp for maximum safety and effectiveness.

- **Large cutting board:** Just about everything worth eating begins with something that needs to be chopped.

- **Chili/soup pot:** Invest in a pot that's larger than you think you need and choose a nonstick surface for easy cleanup.

- **Large sauté pan:** A 12-inch, nonstick skillet is the perfect size for omelets, sautés, and stir-fry.

- **Large baking sheets:** Two large baking sheets with rims are ideal for roasting vegetables, baking meatballs, and catching drips when placed under other pans in the oven.

- **Durable mixing bowls:** A set of bowls in graduated sizes comes in handy for prep work, mixing, marinating, and tossing.

- **Wire sieve/colander:** You're not draining pasta anymore, but a sieve is helpful for washing produce, sweating raw vegetables (like Zucchini Noodles; find recipe in Chapter 12), and draining fatty meats or steamed vegetables.

- **13-x-9-inch baking pan:** A large, deep baking pan is great for casseroles, roasted vegetables, and baked desserts.

- **Measuring cups and spoons:** A collection that includes dry measuring cups, ranging in size from ¼ cup to 1 cup — plus measuring spoons from ¼ teaspoon to 1 tablespoon — will have you covered for every recipe. A 2-cup liquid measuring cup is also a good addition.

- **Storage containers:** A cornerstone of living Paleo is cooking in advance and taking advantage of leftovers. Invest in a set of BPA-free storage containers in a wide variety of sizes.

- **Julienne peeler:** This specialized tool is worth the $10 investment because it turns zucchini, summer squash, cucumber, and eggplant into noodles in a flash.

- **Citrus zester:** The zest of a lemon, lime, or orange adds zip to savory and sweet foods, and a citrus zester ensures that the zest is a snap to make.

Trying Paleo-Approved Cooking Methods

No reason to be afraid of fat, but living Paleo does mean a commitment to eating the right kinds of fat in quantities that support your weight goals and good health. And that means that some traditional cooking methods — like breading and deep frying — are banished from the kitchen. Happily, you can pick from plenty of other ways, such as the following, to cook meats and vegetables that preserve their nutrition and infuse them with good taste:

- **Grilling:** A hot grill not only cooks your food but also adds a slightly smoky quality that enhances the flavor and requires little to no added fat for cooking — so you can get your fats from the meat itself or from a drizzle of a luscious sauce. The possibilities for flavorful grilled steaks, chops, kebabs, and chicken parts are endless, but barbecuing is also a great way to cook vegetables. The large surface means you can cook a lot of food at once for leftovers you can rely on all week. Marinate both meats and vegetables before grilling to infuse them with flavor.

- **Braising:** When meats are braised, they're first browned on high heat to caramelize the outside then slowly cooked in flavored liquid to tenderize the meat and steep it in seasonings. Braising can be done in a covered pan in the oven or on the stovetop in a heavy pot with a tight-fitting lid. The meat can be simmered in water or stock spiked with herbs, spices, and vegetables. This method works well with inexpensive, tougher cuts of meat, coaxing them into tenderness.

- **Sautéing and stir-frying:** A nonstick skillet means you can take advantage of the taste bud–pleasing flavors of sautéing, without needing to add excess fat. When you pan-cook thinly sliced, uniformly sized meat and vegetables in a little fat, the ingredients are lightly browned, which means the sugars caramelize, adding pleasing depth to the natural flavors. You can add a variety of seasonings to change the taste of the dish; for example, go Asian with Classic Stir-Fry Sauce (see recipe in Chapter 14) or simply add a crushed garlic clove, a little olive oil, and a handful of fresh herbs just before the end of cooking.

- **Roasting:** It doesn't get much easier than placing a chicken or beef roast in a pan, surrounding it with hearty vegetables, and tucking it into the oven for a few hours. The meat cooks in its natural juices, and you can turn the drippings in the bottom of the pan into a sauce (after simmering and straining). Simple, healthy, and easy.

- **Slow cooking:** The magic of the slow cooker is that it does all the work while you do other things like exercising, working, grocery shopping, or even taking a nap! Meats and vegetables cook on low temperatures over longer periods of time than other cooking methods, so the meat gets tender and the flavors meld. You can make everything from roasted meats to curries and soups in a slow cooker with minimal fuss.

✔ **Steaming:** This method may be the best way to optimize the nutrition and flavor of vegetables. The steam locks the nutrients into the vegetables, brightening their color and making them tender to the bite. Steamed vegetables store well in the refrigerator and can be reheated and seasoned with your favorite fats and spices — or eaten cold and tossed with your favorite salad dressing.

✔ **Poaching:** Chicken breasts and fish fillets are ideal for poaching, either to be eaten on their own or used in salads. Simmering these cuts in liquid — water, stock, or broth enhanced with herbs — gently cooks them, retaining their natural, tender texture without drying them out.

Navigating the Grocery Store

The grocery store can either be a wonderland of enticing things to eat or a nightmare landscape of temptation — and it all depends on how prepared you are to tackle the store and which path you take through the aisles.

You may have heard this advice before, but it's never been more true than when you're adapting to living Paleo: Shop the perimeter of the store. You can find most of what you need on the edges of the store — the produce department, the butcher and meat department, and the dairy section for eggs only (!) with a side trip into key inside aisles for a few pantry staples. The sample grocery list we provide in this section will help you on your quest to avoid non-Paleo booby traps while you shop.

In this section, we also help you navigate the seemingly endless options at the grocery store, including how and what to look for on food labels.

Going grocery shopping when you're hungry is never a good idea. Be sure to eat a Paleo-approved snack before foraging for food, and take a bottle of water with you to sip on while you shop

Creating your Paleo-approved grocery list

A big part of Paleo success is preparation. You don't need to plan every meal and when you'll eat it, but having a pantry and refrigerator stocked with the Paleo Big Three will help you stay on track. To make sure you don't stray from your path, you need to hit the grocery store with a shopping list in hand.

Adapting to your new grocery needs may take a few weeks as you find the foods you love to replace the non-Paleo foods that got the heave-ho. You may discover that you're eating more protein and produce than you were before, so you may have to make supplemental grocery runs during the week. Don't be discouraged! You'll figure out how to estimate what you need — and how much of it you need — to keep you and your family fed and happy. Here are a few tips to get you started:

- ✔ **Load up on stand-bys:** The basis of your Paleo diet is the Paleo Big Three, so you can make your grocery management easier by identifying the foods you want to buy every week. Maybe your favorite vegetable is broccoli, so you buy some every trip — or you know you always want to have boneless, skinless chicken breasts in the house for emergency meals. After you make your list of must-haves, you can check your inventory before each shopping trip and start your grocery list with the replacements you need.

- ✔ **Pick out a few recipes:** New recipes are a great way to avoid the boredom of food burnout — and the ingredients list of a recipe can go straight onto your shopping list.

- ✔ **Try a new vegetable:** When you're making your grocery list, think about a vegetable that you've never tried or that's in season, and add it to your list. Maybe you'll find a new favorite, and eating what's in season is a great way to amp up your nutrition.

- ✔ **Stick to the perimeter:** You've heard this already, but it bears repeating: Follow your list like a treasure map and avoid the pitfalls of the inner aisles of the grocery store. The bright, shiny packages can be very alluring, so make it easy on yourself and avoid them.

To aid you when you go shopping at the grocery store, we've organized the sample shopping lists in the following sections around the departments in the grocery store. Any item in the following lists is okay to buy.

Produce department

You should be spending a lot of your shopping time in the produce department. You can tell from the long list of recommended items that the bulk of your diet should be coming from this part of the grocery store.

Some vegetables found in the produce department aren't Paleo approved. For example, although corn is bright in color, it's a grain, so it's on the "no" list, along with white potatoes because they're nutrient-poor and cause an unfavorable insulin reaction. Following are the vegetables on the "yes" list that can go right onto your grocery list and into your cart.

- Acorn squash
- Artichokes
- Arugula
- Asparagus
- Beets
- Bell peppers: Green, orange, red, and yellow
- Bok choy
- Broccoli
- Broccoli rabe
- Brussels sprouts
- Butternut squash
- Cauliflower
- Chile peppers
- Chinese cabbage
- Carrots
- Celery
- Celery root
- Cucumber
- Eggplant
- Garlic
- Green beans
- Green cabbage
- Greens: Beet, collard, mustard, and turnip
- Jalapeños

- Jicama
- Kale
- Leeks
- Lettuce: Boston, butter, iceberg, leaf, and romaine
- Mushrooms
- Onions
- Parsnips
- Plantains
- Raddichio
- Radishes
- Red cabbage
- Snap peas
- Snow peas
- Spaghetti squash
- Spinach
- Sprouts
- Summer squash
- Sweet potatoes and yams
- Swiss chard
- Tomatoes
- Turnips
- Watercress
- Yucca
- Zucchini

REMEMBER

Although no fruits are off limits, if you're trying to lose weight, limit fruit to one or two servings per day. Your healthiest options for everyday fruits are those low in fructose, so choose berries and cherries most often. But for some variety, the following are good choices to include on your list:

- ✔ Apples
- ✔ Apricots
- ✔ Avocados
- ✔ Bananas
- ✔ Blackberries
- ✔ Blueberries
- ✔ Cantaloupe
- ✔ Cherries
- ✔ Dates
- ✔ Figs
- ✔ Grapefruits
- ✔ Grapes
- ✔ Guava
- ✔ Honeydew melons
- ✔ Kiwi fruits
- ✔ Lemons
- ✔ Limes
- ✔ Mandarines
- ✔ Mangoes
- ✔ Nectarines
- ✔ Oranges
- ✔ Papayas
- ✔ Peaches
- ✔ Pears
- ✔ Pineapples
- ✔ Plums
- ✔ Pomegranates
- ✔ Raspberries
- ✔ Rhubarb
- ✔ Strawberries
- ✔ Tangerines
- ✔ UGLI fruit
- ✔ Watermelons

Meat and seafood department

In many grocery stores, the meat department is being invaded by pre-made, processed entrees and other meat-like foods. Needless to say, avoid them. Stick to the raw stuff that you can prepare at home.

- ✔ Beef
- ✔ Bison
- ✔ Chicken
- ✔ Clams
- ✔ Duck
- ✔ Elk
- ✔ Fish
- ✔ Goat
- ✔ Lamb
- ✔ Mussels
- ✔ Ostrich
- ✔ Oysters
- ✔ Pheasant
- ✔ Pork
- ✔ Quail
- ✔ Scallops
- ✔ Shrimp
- ✔ Turkey
- ✔ Venison
- ✔ Wild boar

Deli meats, bacon, jerky, and sausages can also be eaten in moderation as long as they don't include any non-Paleo ingredients.

If you can't get grass-fed, organic, pastured meat from a local source, here are a few excellent online resources that deliver high-quality meat:

- ✓ Gourmet Grassfed: www.gourmetgrassfedmeat.com
- ✓ U.S. Wellness Meats: www.grasslandbeef.com
- ✓ Rocky Mountain Organic Meats: www.rockymtncuts.com
- ✓ Lava Lake Lamb: www.lavalakelamb.com

Middle aisles

The middle aisles at the grocery store contain a lot of junk. Avoid temptation and stick to this list:

- ✓ Arrowroot powder
- ✓ Avocado oil
- ✓ Broth/stock: Beef, chicken, and vegetable
- ✓ Butter (clarified, organic, grass-fed only)
- ✓ Canned chiles
- ✓ Canned sardines
- ✓ Canned tomatoes
- ✓ Canned fish: Kipper snacks, salmon, sardines, and tuna
- ✓ Coconut aminos
- ✓ Coconut butter
- ✓ Coconut flakes (unsweetened)
- ✓ Coconut flour
- ✓ Coconut milk (in a can)
- ✓ Coconut oil (unrefined)
- ✓ Curry paste
- ✓ Dried fruit
- ✓ Eggs
- ✓ Extra-virgin olive oil
- ✓ Olives
- ✓ Pickles
- ✓ Nuts
- ✓ Nut butters
- ✓ Nut meal
- ✓ Salsa
- ✓ Spices
- ✓ Tomato paste

After your 30-Day Reset, you may choose to enjoy honey and maple syrup in small quantities.

Reading and understanding labels

As we discuss in the earlier section "Paleo pantry staples and spices," even though a few processed foods — olives, canned fish, coconut milk, and curry paste, for example — are included on the Paleo-approved list, generally, you want to avoid any factory-produced food.

Here's a bit of advice to carry you through your Paleo grocery shopping experience: If you don't recognize the ingredient as food, you shouldn't eat it. That's an oversimplification, of course, but you really can't go wrong following that advice.

Even seemingly innocuous products, such as herbal tea, "all natural" salsas, and instant coffee, can include hidden varieties of wheat, corn, soy, and sugar, so you must be diligent in reading labels even on foods that seem safe. When reading ingredient labels, you want to look for scientific names and variations on problematic ingredients, like wheat, soy, sugar, and corn, as we describe in detail in the following sections. You should also be on the lookout for any ingredients to which you have an allergy — and beware of any ingredients that you can't pronounce, even if they don't appear on the lists in the following sections.

The terms *artificial flavorings* and *natural flavorings* are used as a catchall for flavor enhancers, and manufacturers are *not* required to disclose exactly what they are. Both of those labels can indicate wheat, gluten, corn, and soy, so even if everything else in the product is Paleo approved, steer clear of foods that include those ingredients on their labels.

Sneaky names for wheat and gluten

If the following ingredients appear on a label, it contains wheat and/or gluten:

- Artificial flavoring
- Bleached flour
- Caramel color
- Dextrin
- Flavorings
- Hydrolyzed plant protein (HPP)
- Hydrolyzed vegetable protein (HVP)
- Hydrolyzed wheat protein
- Hydrolyzed wheat starch
- Malt

- Maltodextrin
- Modified food starch
- Natural flavoring
- Seasonings
- Vegetable protein
- Vegetable starch
- Wheat germ oil
- Wheat grass
- Wheat protein
- Wheat starch

Sneaky names for soy

If the following ingredients appear on a label, it may contain soy:

- Artificial flavoring
- Hydrolyzed plant protein (HPP)
- Hydrolyzed soy protein
- Hydrolyzed vegetable protein (HVP)
- Miso
- Natural flavoring
- Soy albumin
- Soy fiber
- Soy flour
- Soy lecithin
- Soy protein

- Soy sauce
- Stabilizer
- Tamari
- Tempeh
- Textured soy flour (TSF)
- Textured soy protein (TSP)
- Textured vegetable protein (TVP)
- Tofu
- Vegetable broth
- Vegetable gum
- Vegetable starch

Sneaky names for sugar

If the following ingredients appear on a label, it contains added sugars:

- Agave nectar
- Barley malt syrup
- Cane crystals
- Corn sweetener
- Corn syrup
- Crystalline fructose
- Dehydrated cane juice
- Dextrin
- Dextrose
- Disaccharide
- Evaporated cane juice
- Fructose
- Fruit juice concentrate
- Galactose
- Glucose
- High-fructose corn syrup

- Invert sugar
- Lactose
- Maltodextrin
- Malt syrup
- Maltose
- Monosaccharide
- Polysaccharide
- Ribose
- Rice syrup
- Saccharose
- Sorghum or sorghum syrup
- Sucrose
- Treacle
- Turbinado sugar
- Xylose

Artificial sweeteners: Worse than sugar?

Artificial sweeteners not only add zero calories to food, they add zero nutrition and may actually cause damage. When you taste something sweet, your body expects to have calories associated with that flavor — and that sets off a whole slew of reactions in your body to deal with those calories. The chemical manipulation of artificial sweeteners is harmful and can lead to insulin resistance. Avoid these artificial sweeteners on their own and in processed foods:

- Aspartame
- Equal

- NutraSweet
- Saccharin
- Splenda
- Stevia
- Sucralose
- SweetLeaf
- Sweet'N Low
- Truvia

Sugar in the form of fruit juice concentrate often appears in high-quality sausages, and some nut butters include dehydrated cane juice. These are minimal amounts of sugar, so after your 30-Day Reset, it's up to you how much of these acceptable sugars you allow in your everyday diet.

Sneaky names for corn

If the following ingredients appear on a label, it contains corn derivatives:

- Artificial flavoring
- Corn alcohol
- Corn flour
- Corn meal
- Corn oil
- Corn starch
- Corn sweetener
- Corn syrup solids
- Dextrin
- Dextrose
- Food starch
- High-fructose corn syrup

- Maltodextrin
- Mazena
- Modified gum starch
- Sorbitol
- MSG
- Natural flavorings
- Vegetable gum
- Vegetable protein
- Vegetable starch
- Xantham gum
- Xylitol

Living Paleo on a Budget

Throughout this chapter, we explain what foods you need to stock your Paleo kitchen, but you may be wondering about the cost of all this high-quality food. The truth is that meat, vegetables, fruits, and healthy fats are more economical in the long run than packaged food that's devoid of nutrition.

If you decide to invest in grass-fed, pastured meats and organic produce, you may see an increase in your grocery tab at first, but that extra expense will be offset by the long-term health benefits — plus fewer meals at restaurants — of living Paleo. In the following sections, you see how, with a little creativity and exploration, you can find reasonable prices on high-quality foods that are as good for your wallet as they are for your body.

Choosing whether to buy organic

Eating local produce that's in season is the best option, both for the health of your body and your bank account. But not all your produce needs to be organic. Every year, the Environmental Working Group (EWG) identifies the dirty dozen of produce: fruits and vegetables with higher levels of pesticides. If you can afford it, buy organic versions of the produce on that list, but if your budget can't support it, buy local, conventionally grown produce and wash it well under running water before eating. We list the produce you should strive to buy organic and also the ones that are okay to buy from conventional growing methods in the following sections.

The dirty dozen

Buy organic versions of these fruits and vegetables whenever possible:

- Apples
- Bell peppers
- Blueberries
- Celery
- Cucumbers
- Grapes
- Lettuce
- Nectarines
- Peaches
- Potatoes
- Spinach
- Strawberries

The clean 15

When you can't find or afford to buy organic, buying conventionally grown versions of these fruits and vegetables is okay; just be sure to wash them thoroughly under running water:

- Asparagus
- Avocado
- Cabbage
- Cantaloupe
- Eggplant
- Grapefruit
- Kiwi

- Mango
- Mushrooms
- Onions
- Pineapple
- Sweet peas
- Sweet potatoes
- Watermelons

Assessing your meat options: Grass-fed and pastured or factory-farmed

Grass-fed, pastured meat is better for you and better for the environment than factory-farmed animals. This high-quality meat is more expensive than conventional, grocery store meat, but the payoff for your health and the planet is worth the investment, if you can afford it.

Grass-fed pastured animals live as they should, in humane, natural conditions that don't require that they're fed antibiotics. Healthier animals mean healthier, more nutritious meat for you. Grass-fed, pastured meats have healthier fat, too. They're up to four times higher in vitamin E than feedlot beef. The meat is lower in overall fat, too, and it's higher in health-friendly omega-3 fatty acids.

If your budget can't support buying pastured meat on a regular basis, treat yourself when you can, and the rest of the time, the following cuts are a good second choice:

- Skinless chicken or turkey breast
- Eye of round roast or steak
- Sirloin tip side steak
- Top round roast and steak
- Bottom round roast and steak
- Top sirloin steak
- Low-fat ground beef

Chapter 8

Paleo Jump Start: The 30-Day Reset

In This Chapter

▶ Reviewing the guidelines for the 30-Day Reset

▶ Understanding the value of journaling

▶ Knowing what to expect during each week of the 30-Day Reset

*T*he 30-Day Reset is an important step in living the Paleo lifestyle. In just 30 days of intentional, healthy, Paleo eating, you can break lifelong habits that contribute to poor health and well-being. Your body detoxes so you have more energy, your skin glows, and your sleep quality improves. Throughout the 30 days, you also start setting new patterns that will carry you through the rest of your life.

In this chapter, we provide the guidelines for the 30-Day Reset so you have all the information you need for success. Strictly following the guidelines is essential to experience all the benefits of the 30-Day Reset.

Although living Paleo doesn't require many of the trappings of a traditional "diet," like measuring and weighing food or keeping a food journal, we encourage you to keep a journal during the 30-Day Reset; we tell you how and why in this chapter. We also give you a glimpse of what to expect during each week of the 30 days so you understand what you may feel physically, mentally, and emotionally as you remove toxins from your body, slay the sugar demon, and nourish your cells with high-quality, Paleo foods. In addition, we provide tips on what to do if you feel like this whole Paleo thing just isn't working the way you expected.

At first, 30 days may seem like an eternity, but you'll quickly start to feel the effects of powerfully healthy foods that nourish your body and your spirit. And at the end of the 30 days, you'll be ready to begin your Paleo lifestyle full time.

The Rules for Your First 30 Days

We discuss the reasons for committing to the 30-Day Reset in Chapter 3. To reap the rewards of living Paleo, you don't need to be perfect. In fact, if you follow the Paleo guidelines 80 to 90 percent of the time, you'll enjoy the majority of the benefits and vastly improve your health. However, during the 30-Day Reset, you need to follow the Paleo guidelines stringently. To put it in plain language: There's no cheating during the 30-Day Reset. To really detox and heal your body, you need to grit your teeth and get through the 30 days with no slip-ups, no compromises, no excuses, and no gray areas. Doing so isn't always easy, but you're tougher than any loaf of bread or bowl of pasta. You can outsmart a doughnut, and you can absolutely triumph over happy hour.

Ready to jump in? Here are the guidelines for your 30-day immersion into living Paleo; see Chapter 3 for more details:

✓ **Omit the foods on the "no" list.** The purpose of the 30-Day Reset is to remove inflammatory foods from your plate, which means you need to avoid consuming processed foods, all grains, vegetable and seed oils, soy, legumes, added sugars, dairy, and alcohol.

✓ **Embrace the foods on the "yes" list.** The good news is that you can eat until you're satisfied from these food groups: all animal proteins, vegetables, fruits, and naturally occurring fats.

✓ **Stay hydrated.** Your body needs water to help you detox, and drinking plenty of water can also help you manage your appetite. Get yourself a BPA-free water bottle and commit to drinking fresh water throughout the day. You'll feel more energetic, your skin will look refreshed, and you'll quickly figure out how to distinguish between thirst and hunger.

✓ **Get moving!** In Chapter 6, we show you how much fun — and how easy — it can be to move your body. The 30-Day Reset is an excellent time to add movement to your routine. Even 30 minutes of walking every day can make a remarkable difference in your metabolism, your stress level, and your mood.

✓ **Practice eyeballing portions.** Chapter 2 shows you how to eyeball your food to ensure that you eat enough to support your body's energy needs without overeating. The 30-Day Reset is a great time to practice your portion skills. It may take a few weeks to understand your body's hunger and satisfaction signals, but as you break the sugar cycle and the toxins leave your body, your hormonal systems begin to function correctly, and eating "right" becomes effortless.

✓ **Record your "before" you.** Chapter 3 explains a variety of ways you can document your personal "before," so you can celebrate your Paleo improvements. Try any or all the recommendations in that chapter, and then get ready to make note of the changes at the end of the 30 days.

Although you may be tempted to weigh yourself during your 30-Day Reset, we don't recommend doing that. Instead, take your measurements or weigh yourself before starting the 30 days, and then forget about *results* and keep your focus on how you *feel* along the way. The 30-Day Reset is a liberating experience that helps you create healthy new habits and may very well change your relationship with the food you eat. Banish the scale for a month and free yourself to learn and grow.

Dear Diary: Guidelines for 30 Days of Journaling

Keeping a journal during the 30-Day Reset can be a valuable tool to help you learn from the experience and identify challenges or issues specific to you and your body so that you can make corrections. Your journal is all about you, so you can treat it like a diary to capture your entire emotional experience during your 30-Day Reset, or you can view it as more of a scientific document in which you simply record data from your day. Here are some suggestions for the kind of information to include so your review at the end of the 30-Day Reset is helpful and informative.

- ✔ **Foods you eat:** Document everything you put into your mouth — especially if you find yourself eating between meals. Doing so helps you identify triggers that may spark your appetite and compel you to eat when you're not hungry. Making note of the quantities you eat, at least in the beginning, can also be helpful. Knowing how much you eat helps you see the connections between your intake and your hunger.

- ✔ **Where and when you eat:** Focusing on and savoring your food go a long way toward appetite control and satisfaction. Do you feel differently when you eat on the run versus when you eat at the dining table? Do you eat more or less when dining with others? That kind of information can help you create positive new habits.

- ✔ **Cravings:** Especially during the first week or two of the 30-Day Reset, you may experience cravings for specific foods. Your journal can be an effective tool in helping you overcome those cravings. It's essential to your long-term success that you not surrender to the cravings during the 30-Day Reset. Make note of the craving in your journal, and do something to distract yourself from the craving, such as drink a glass of water, go for a walk, or call a friend. If you're truly hungry, a small snack of fat and protein can help curb cravings, particularly if the craving is for sugar.

- ✔ **Amount and quality of sleep:** Sleep is vital to your health and can be impacted by the foods you eat. Keep track of when you go to sleep, when you wake up, and the overall quality of your sleep. You may find that certain foods or other behaviors influence your sleep patterns.

- ✔ **Activity:** Tracking your activity — both formal exercise, like a walk or run, a fitness class, strength training, or playing a sport, and casual activity, like gardening or playing with a pet — can provide valuable insight into your energy levels and caloric needs.

- ✔ **Mood:** Food is a powerful mood adjuster, and, especially during the 30-Day Reset, you'll feel the difference when you make the switch from the standard high-carb diet to a Paleo lifestyle. Just make note of when you feel upbeat and energetic or cranky, stressed, or moody. Later, you may be able to draw conclusions from these notes that can help you adjust your eating, exercise, and sleep habits.

- ✔ **Other goals:** Although you don't want to take on too much at once, the 30-Day Reset can be an excellent time to add in other good habits. Have you always wanted to start a meditation practice? The 30-Day Reset is a fine time to add that into your routine, and you can track your progress in your journal. Other good goals may be watching less TV, drinking a specific number of glasses of water per day, cutting out caffeine, going to bed 30 minutes earlier than usual, and so on. Use the 30 days to dial in your healthiest habits, and use the journal to keep track of your new behaviors and how they make you feel.

Week 1: Cleaning Up and Jumping In

The first week of your 30-Day Reset can be an exciting, optimistic time. You're fired up and ready to banish old habits and sprint right into your new Paleo lifestyle. You've written your new goals on sticky notes attached to your bathroom mirror, and you've stocked your kitchen with Paleo-approved foods. There's no stopping you now! Or is there?

Maybe you're on the other end of the spectrum. Your brain has bought into the concepts of Paleo, and you know it's the healthy choice for you, but you're apprehensive about the 30-Day Reset. Thinking about an entire month of new eating habits is intimidating — and you're not sure whether you can commit to giving up your morning bagel and latte.

Both of these reactions — or an alternating pattern between the two — is completely normal. You're taking on a significant challenge, and change is always somewhat uncomfortable, even when it's a change you want to make.

This section is packed with tips and advice to help you get through the first week of living Paleo. We show you how to get organized, how to reward yourself for a first week of success, and how to cope if your first few days of detox don't feel too great.

What's happening?

Welcome to your sugar and junk food detox! If you've been eating a relatively "healthy" diet, you may not feel too much difference during the first few days of your new eating habits. If you typically indulge in a fair amount of restaurant food, fast food, and junk food, you may feel the effects of their absence somewhat quickly. And even if you eat "healthy," if your diet has typically been based on high consumption of grains, legumes, and low-fat packaged food, you may feel the effects of the sudden withdrawal of that sugar.

Your body doesn't really differentiate between the sugar found in a candy bar and the sugar in a bowl of whole-wheat pasta or brown rice. After you chew the food and it makes its way into your digestive system, your body identifies it as sugar. So even if you eat "healthy," you're probably consuming more sugar than you need, and your body will react when that source of sugar is removed.

By turning off the sugar faucet, you're depriving your body of the quick source of energy to which it's become accustomed, and it may not respond positively at first. Here are some of the physical symptoms you may feel as you replace grains, legumes, and sugary treats with vegetables and fruits.

- ✔ **Low energy:** You may feel a bit low on energy during this first week, and that's completely normal. You need to challenge yourself to be patient during this time; try not to rely on caffeine or fruit to help you through the afternoon slumps. Ease off the intensity of your workouts if you need to, take a nap if you can, and try to get to bed an hour earlier this week so your body can rest and adapt. Your body is beginning its transition from using sugar as fuel to burning fat. Ultimately, using fat for energy is far more effective — who doesn't want to burn more fat? — but the *transition* can be uncomfortable.

- ✔ **"Carb flu":** Feeling like you're getting a cold during the first week of the 30-Day Reset isn't uncommon, especially if you've typically eaten a diet high in processed carbohydrates and fast food. These symptoms are more evidence of your body making the transition from sugar to fat, so don't be alarmed if you feel sniffly, tired, and foggy-headed. These symptoms will pass in a few days They're a sign that the 30-Day Reset is working just the way it's supposed to.

- ✔ **Crankiness:** Feeling short-tempered and moody, like you want to smash things for no reason? There is a reason: Your brain is throwing a hissy fit because it misses the foods you're not giving it — your evening glass of wine, cheese, cookies. But again, be patient. This symptom will pass in a few days, and if you give in to your cravings and your unpleasant mood, you'll never make it past your reliance on these non-Paleo foods. The moodiness is related to blood sugar regulation, and eating quality, Paleo foods eventually regulates your blood sugar and has you smiling again.

✔ **Detox pox:** While you're making this transition, you may experience other odd symptoms brought on by your body adapting to the new diet and healing from the effects of the old one. Digestive distress, allergies, and acne/blemishes may pop up. And, unfortunately, they may get a little worse before they get better. But they will get better, usually by the second week of the 30-Day Reset. Remember that this is your body healing — it's just throwing a small temper tantrum while it does.

Tasks and assignments

Your first week is all about setting up your environment for success. You need to create your Paleo kitchen, spend time thinking about the habits you want to focus on during your 30-Day Reset, and plan non-food rewards to acknowledge the positive changes you're making in your life. The following tips can help:

✔ **Clean out your kitchen.** At the start of your 30-Day Reset, check out Chapter 7 for the list of foods you need to banish from your kitchen. If you have family members or roommates who aren't joining you in your strict 30 days, move their non-Paleo foods to a place that's out of your eye line. Make it easier on yourself by removing as much temptation as possible from your immediate environment.

✔ **Stock up on the Paleo Big Three.** Use the sample grocery list in Chapter 7 to restock your kitchen with nourishing, Paleo-approved foods. Make it fun by buying a vegetable you've never tried before or buying a perfect, grass-fed ribeye steak to treat yourself.

✔ **Equip your kitchen.** Living Paleo means cooking most of your meals at home, so you may want to invest in some new tools. You don't have to spend a lot of money, but some basics — a large sauté pan, a sharp knife, a blender or food processor — ensures that you can cook delicious foods that help you stay committed to your goals.

✔ **Set up your journal.** If you decide to make journaling part of your 30-Day Reset, set up your journal so you're ready to go on your first day. Spend time thinking about the aspects of your experience that you want to document and be sure to think about when you'll make time each day to fill out your journal. Will you do it throughout the day before or after each meal? At night before bed? In the morning before you start your day? Now is the ideal time to set up this new habit.

✔ **Minimize your schedule.** The first week of the 30-Day Reset can be unsettling to your normal energy patterns. You may feel supercharged — or you may feel sleepy, cranky, or blue. This isn't the time to take on other big challenges in your personal life or at work. As much as you can, remove stressful or important events from your schedule for the week. The goal is to minimize your commitments and your stress level so you can focus on the changes you're making to your diet and lifestyle.

✔ **Plan a special meal.** Keep your first week of meals simple so you're not overwhelmed by the need to buy special ingredients or tackle a bunch of new recipes. Build most of your meals around a nicely grilled pork chop or chicken with fresh veggies and a big salad. But if you enjoy cooking, you may want to plan one special meal for the week. Pick out a new recipe, invite family or friends to join you, put flowers on the table, maybe even light a few candles — make it an event and realize that the new Paleo habits don't actually mean giving up all the pleasures associated with eating.

✔ **Plan a social event.** If you're giving up happy hour with friends or a standing date to have a big brunch every Sunday morning with your favorite people, you may feel like Paleo is ruining your social life. Instead of abandoning these opportunities, replace them with something else. Invite your brunch friends to a Sunday movie matinee instead, or plan a group hike, a night out dancing (with club soda instead of cocktails), or a shared yoga class. You never know: These new social events may turn out to be even more popular than your food-focused fun.

Troubleshooting challenges

In the earlier "What's happening?" section for Week 1, we list some of the things you may experience while you're adapting to your new diet. In the following sections, we give you more concrete advice to help you weather those potentially uncomfortable physical symptoms.

Sugar cravings

The worst thing you can do to alleviate a sugar craving is to give in and eat sugar. Your brain may be crying out for a cookie, and it may try to trick you by giving you a craving for an apple or a dried fruit and nut bar. But feeding the sugar demon with sugar is no way to defeat it. Instead, drink a large glass of water and, if you're still hungry or distracted by thoughts of food, a small amount of healthy fat — a few nuts or olives, a few spoonfuls of avocado, or a handful of coconut flakes. These fatty foods will appease your appetite without giving fuel to the sugar demon.

Low energy

The great promise of the Paleo diet is that after you go through this transition, your energy levels skyrocket. But that's a small consolation when all you want to do is lie down. During your first week of the 30-Day Reset, you may need to get more sleep than usual, so if you can manage it, take a 20- to 30-minute nap in the early afternoon to help recharge your batteries. In addition, if you have a history of following traditional diets, you may want to check in with yourself to make sure you're not treating Paleo like a "diet." Are you eating portions that are too small for your energy needs? Review the guidelines for how much to eat in Chapter 2 and make sure you're taking in enough fuel. Even if weight loss is your goal, now is not the time to deprive yourself. Instead, eat plenty of vegetables with adequate protein and fat, especially during this transition.

Constant hunger

Read the guidelines in Chapter 2 to determine how much you should be eating and make sure you haven't put yourself on a "diet" — and, if necessary, consider adding more vegetables and a bit more protein and fat to your meals. Eating more at breakfast can actually help you manage your appetite, especially if you feel like snacking after dinner. You may also be dehydrated — your body often confuses thirst with hunger — so try drinking more water throughout the day.

Week 2: Creating New Habits and Being Strong

The second week of the 30-Day Reset may feel less exciting than the first seven days. You're on the cusp between new behavior and entrenched habit, so it's a crucial but potentially less exciting time. After a week or ten days, the Paleo way of eating begins to feel more comfortable, but it hasn't quite reached the stage where you can safely call it a habit. There's still more work to be done to make living Paleo feel like second nature.

The good news is that many of the benefits of the Paleo lifestyle — consistent energy levels, quality sleep, clear skin, energized workouts, and a positive outlook — begin to appear. These are all signs that the healing process in your body has started. And that positive trend will continue as long as you continue to fuel your body with quality, Paleo foods and restore it with adequate rest.

What's happening?

After more than a week of Paleo foods, your body is continuing to adapt from burning sugar for energy to using your fat stores for fuel. This is a good thing, and you want to do everything you can to support that process. That means sticking to your no-sugar guns and eating plenty of high-quality fats and vegetables.

You may be surprised to find that cravings make an unwelcome reappearance sometime during your second week, and they may be for foods you didn't even realize you missed. This is your body trying to trick you into giving it the familiar foods you don't need — kind of a last-ditch effort to test your resolve. But you're so close to experiencing the full effects of the Paleo lifestyle, so don't give in to those false signals from your brain.

Right around the ten-day mark, you should start to feel some of these celebration-worthy effects:

- **Renewed energy:** You'll probably find that you wake up feeling bright and energized — and that energy remains pretty consistent throughout the day. Your workouts begin to feel turbo-charged, and you bounce back from them faster than before.

- **Buoyant mood:** You just may find yourself feeling inexplicably happy. This is the result of stable blood sugar and quality fuel. You manage daily bumps in the road effortlessly and probably feel less stressed by the things that previously troubled you. You also find that concentrating is easier, and, like your energy, your moods have become more consistent.

- **Detox pox:** The odd symptoms — like digestive distress, allergies, and acne/blemishes — brought on by your body adapting to the Paleo diet begin to disappear. If you have longstanding health issues, you should notice them starting to alleviate. The changes may not be dramatic at this point, but you should feel your body beginning to heal and grow stronger.

- **Looser-fitting clothes:** At this point, you may start to notice that your clothes are fitting a little differently, maybe your pants are a little loose around the waist, or you have to move your belt a notch. This is a direct result of decreasing the inflammation in your body, reducing bloating, and beginning to lose excess body fat.

At this point, you may be feeling so good that you're tempted to step on the scale to see whether you've lost weight. This is a terrible idea! Instead, keep the scale in the closet, and keep your mind on the goal: To complete the 30-Day Reset with no cheats, no treats, no slip-ups, and no deviation from the plan.

Tasks and assignments

Your second week is all about staying on track, settling into your new habits, and continuing to focus on self-care. You want to create a support system for yourself in case you hit a snag, try some new foods to help fight boredom, move your body, and plan how you'll celebrate your halfway point.

✔ **Recruit an ally.** Forcing family or friends to join you in the 30-Day Reset is a bad idea; people need to decide for themselves when they're ready to take on the challenge. But asking people to support *you* in your mission is 100 percent appropriate — and as you move through the 30-Day Reset, it's vital to have people you can rely on if your resolve begins to waiver.

You may want to identify two people to be on your 30-Day Reset team — someone to help you during the day when you're at home or at work and someone to be your rock during the evening to make sure you don't run into trouble between dinner and bedtime. Simply ask them whether you can reach out — on the phone, via e-mail, or in a text message — if you need a word of encouragement. If you feel uncomfortable sharing with people you know, take advantage of online communities. The support you can get from others trying to make the same lifestyle changes is invaluable.

✔ **Try a new recipe.** If you kept your meals simple during your first week, you may be ready for something more enticing this week. Choose a recipe from Part III of this book or search for Paleo recipes online to add a new flavor sensation to your routine. (Just be sure to double-check the ingredients list to make sure they're compliant with the 30-Day Reset.) Something as simple as a new recipe can help renew your enthusiasm if it starts to flag at your midway point.

✔ **Have some fun.** Get outside and play; it's the easiest way to lighten your mood and help take the focus away from food, without losing sight of your Paleo goals. Go for a hike, take advantage of the swings at the playground, toss a Frisbee, or simply take an extended stroll around your neighborhood. The act of getting outside taps into something primal within us and helps us reconnect to our natural selves. You don't have to actually live like a cave man, but enjoying fresh air and natural light goes a long way toward contributing to a more balanced lifestyle.

✔ **Plan your celebration.** At the end of your second week, you'll be halfway through the 30-Day Reset. How will you celebrate? To reinforce your success and acknowledge the changes you're making, marking the occasion is important. Choose an activity or reward that's not associated with food, and make a fuss! Buy yourself the shoes you've had your eye on — or set aside an afternoon to read a book you've been wanting to dig into or to watch your favorite movie with your feet up. Maybe indulge in a full-body massage or take in an art exhibit. Just choose the reward that helps you celebrate the special commitment you've made to yourself over the last two weeks — and one that will help you stay motivated through the final two weeks of the 30-Day Reset.

✔ **Review your journal.** If you make journaling part of your 30-Day Reset, review it from time to time to see the evolution of your experience. How has your sleeping pattern changed? What's happening with your cravings? How have your workouts been affected? Seeing patterns emerge can be enlightening, and by reading your journal, you can see how far you've come in a very short time.

Troubleshooting challenges

In the earlier "What's happening?" section for Week 2, we share some of the positive things you may experience in the second week of the 30-Day Reset. But what if you're still having some struggles? Here are more tips to help you manage potential pitfalls.

Cravings

The sugar demon is probably in hibernation by now, but that doesn't mean that you're immune to cravings. Your brain and body may be trying to convince you that you "deserve a treat," or you may find yourself in a situation — a work event, a party, an unexpected trip to a restaurant — that puts you directly in the path of some former food favorites. You don't need to give in to those cravings; you're stronger than that. To help combat cravings, review your journal and remind yourself of all the hard work you've put in so far. This is where your mental toughness needs to kick in. Decide that you will absolutely not give in to signals to eat foods you don't *really* want. Be stubborn, ride out those feelings, drink a glass of water, take a walk around the block — whatever it takes to not give in. If you're truly hungry, give yourself permission to eat a Paleo snack — but fight the temptation to eat non-Paleo foods.

Weird dreams

Some people report odd and even food-related dreams during their second week of the 30-Day Reset. To alleviate sleep-related discomfort, you may try eating a small snack of protein and fat before bed — a hard-boiled egg and a few olives or a small piece of chicken with Homemade Mayonnaise (see recipe in Chapter 14) — and do some intentional relaxation. The relaxation exercise in Chapter 6 can help you ease your way into restful sleep.

Even just three minutes of conscious breathing can improve your sleep or help you manage a sudden temptation. Sit comfortably, close your eyes, and breathe deeply, inhaling for a count of four and exhaling for a count of six. This mini break helps you stop the chatter in your brain and regain control of your intentions.

Week 3: Feeling Great and Sharing Your Success

Three weeks into the 30-Day Reset, you should really be feeling like a champ. For the most part, your cravings have been kicked to the curb, the sugar demon has been banished to an unknown location, and rather than thinking about the foods you miss, you're thinking about the goals you want to tackle when your 30-Day Reset is complete. In short, you're well on your way to creating your new Paleo lifestyle.

But your transition isn't complete yet; that's why you need to hunker down for the full 30 days. Some people may be unsettled by the return of a craving or two during the third week. Try not to be disappointed or frustrated if you do feel some unwelcome cravings. Their appearance is totally natural and not unusual. And by now, you have the mental tools to overcome those temptations.

This week is key because during these seven days is when your new behaviors that you've been honing since the beginning of the 30-Day Reset really start to become concrete habits.

If your eating habits before the 30-Day Reset involved a lot of fast food, processed and packaged foods, sugary treats, and/or alcohol, you may not feel the "magic" of Week 3 the way others do. Don't despair! Your easier time is coming; it just may take a little bit longer for your body to rid itself of unwanted compounds and to heal. Stay the course, and be patient with the plan and yourself.

What's happening?

Your body is still adapting, but the finish line of transitioning from a sugar-burner to a fat-burner is in sight. If you've traditionally eaten a diet high in processed foods and sugar, your inflammation is easing off and your body is healing. Inside, your systems and tissues are beginning to be at peace, no longer inflamed by antinutrients and blood sugar spikes. You're well on your way to living Paleo.

- **Fat burning for energy:** Since the beginning of the 30-Day Reset, you've been feeding your body smart carbohydrates — in the form of vegetables and fruits — and high-quality fats. These foods allow your body to access your stored body fat for energy, and during this third week, that transition really kicks into high gear. Your insulin response to the food you eat is moderate and appropriate, so you don't get mood swings or sugar highs (and the associated crash), and your energy is stable throughout the day.

- **Consistent mood:** Because your blood sugar is no longer swinging to extremes like Tarzan, your moods are more predictable and appropriate to the situation. You feel light-hearted and optimistic.

- **No more detox pox:** The symptoms of digestive distress, allergies, and acne/blemishes brought on by your body adapting to the Paleo diet are usually cleared up, and other long-term ailments are drastically alleviated and continue to improve.

- **Less hunger:** You may find that you no longer need to snack, and you certainly don't need to eat every three hours the way you may have following a "healthy," high-carb diet. Your appetite may fluctuate during this week, and you may find that you simply have no desire to eat as much as you used to. As long as your energy and mood don't suffer, pay attention to your body's signals and eat less. You can make all your meals smaller, or simply skip a meal if you're not hungry. Just be sure to take note if cravings reappear or if your energy or sleep suffers. You may find that simply eating less at lunch or dinner resolves your appetite issues, without impacting other facets of your lifestyle.

Tasks and assignments

Your third week is all about feeling empowered by your new behaviors and success. Now is the time to share your experience with others and try out some new restaurant-related skills to help you make the transition from the rules of the 30-Day Reset to a real-world, Paleo lifestyle.

✔ **Tell a friend.** By now, the people around you may be noticing your sunny outlook and your slimmer silhouette. This is the ideal time to share what you've been doing and to lead by example instead of trying to blatantly recruit them to the Paleo lifestyle. Use your journal to jot down the key points that you think make living Paleo the right choice, and when a family member, friend, co-worker, or even your doctor comments on your vibrant health, you'll be ready to share your short list of ways living Paleo has improved your health and well-being.

✔ **Eat in a restaurant.** During your 30-Day Reset, you've probably been eating your meals at home or packing food with you when you venture out into the world. It's time to be brave and face the challenge of a restaurant menu. Chapter 16 is packed with tips for how to eat according to your Paleo principles in restaurants. Choose a restaurant where you know you can enjoy a quality piece of protein — like grilled steak, roast chicken, or broiled salmon — with a side of fresh vegetables, and a salad with olive oil and vinegar. A meal in a restaurant is a welcome treat, and it gives you the confidence to know you can take your new habits with you everywhere you go.

✔ **Plan your celebration.** In just one more week, your 30-Day Reset will come to an end. You owe it to yourself to mark the occasion with a non-food reward. Avoid the temptation to fantasize about "celebrating" the end of your strict 30 days with a forbidden food. Instead, plan an event that commemorates the mental and physical strength you gain during 30 days of Paleo eating.

Troubleshooting challenges

In the earlier "What's happening?" section for Week 3, you discover that by the third week, the positive effects of clean eating are making a regular appearance. But for some people, it may take a little more time.

Bodies are wonderful, unique entities, and although most people begin to experience significant improvements by the third week of the 30-Day Reset, in some situations, the adaption and healing process take longer. If you have a medical issue — for example, hypothyroidism, IBS, or diabetes — the transition may take more time. If you have a history of obesity or yo-yo dieting, you, too, may need a bit longer for the magic to happen. And if you consumed fast food, packaged and processed food, sugary treats, and alcohol for an extended period of time before beginning your 30-Day Reset, it may take more than three weeks to reverse the damage. But the damage can be reversed!

No matter what the cause, if you're in the third week of the 30-Day Reset and aren't enjoying positive changes to the degree you'd like, your best option for success is to consider extending your 30-Day Reset beyond 30 days. That is probably unwelcome news, but the only way to rid your body of inflammation and transition from sugar-burning to fat-burning is to continue to let your body rest by providing it with high-quality nourishment — and to completely avoid stressing your body with the problematic qualities of grains, dairy, legumes, sugar, and alcohol.

Week 4: Celebrating Success and Preparing for What's Next

You're almost finished with 30 days that can reset the pattern for the rest of your life. Congratulations!

Now that you've most likely slain the sugar demon and created new, healthy habits, it's time to start planning the rest of your Paleo life, without the rules — and the safety net — of the 30-Day Reset.

You're probably feeling pretty excited about finishing the 30-Day Reset, and you may experience some anxiety, too. During these 30 days, the rules were fairly concrete, and although it may not always be easy to follow them, they gave you a well-defined path to follow. Now, it's up to you to decide how closely you want to follow the Paleo rules. Your body is healed and your habits are reset, so you have an opportunity to decide how often you'll stray from "perfect Paleo," what your treats will be, and how you'll move forward with eating, exercise, and rest to create your optimal lifestyle.

That should be both exhilarating and, possibly, a little daunting, but you're up to it. After 30 days of clean eating, you're ready for just about anything.

What's happening?

Your body is probably feeling great right now. Insulin is rising and falling properly to manage your blood sugar, and your sleep is sound and restful, which adds up to consistent energy and mood throughout the day. Now that you're comfortable eating Paleo foods, you're probably enjoying your meals more than ever. And you're probably also increasing your muscle mass, shedding body fat, and noticing that your clothes fit better than before.

You're on the threshold of your new Paleo lifestyle, and you can look forward to the benefits of the 30-Day Reset stretching far beyond this month, as long as you continue to treat yourself well. You can expect your high, consistent energy levels to continue, along with your upbeat, optimistic attitude. Sleep will continue to be restful and restorative, and the glow of your skin, eyes, teeth, hair, and nails will make you look like a pampered celebrity.

After the 30-Day Reset, revisit the health markers outlined in Chapter 3, and retake your measurements to see the progress you've made. At this point, it's even okay to hop on the scale if you're curious about weight loss, but remember that the scale doesn't indicate increased muscle or decreased body fat, so its numbers can be misleading. It's far better to judge your success against factors like how good you feel and how your clothing fits.

Tasks and assignments

The final week of the 30-Day Reset is all about preparing for what's next: your on-going Paleo lifestyle. Revisit your allies to make sure they're ready to act as your support system, expand your collection of Paleo recipes, and decide on your personal philosophy for the when-why-how-what of Paleo treats.

- ✔ **Gather your troops.** During Week 2, you recruited allies to help you if you were tempted to stray from your Paleo path. Now is a great time to recharge your support system and remind them that you're about to make another tricky transition from the 30-Day Reset to living Paleo. Knowing you have people to turn to just to talk through the everyday challenges of making these new habits stick can be comforting.

- ✔ **Make a meal plan.** Now that you're free of the rules of the 30-Day Reset, you may be tempted to eat out more often or loosen up the "no non-Paleo foods in the house" rule. A meal plan for the week can help you avoid overdoing it on indulgences and help you make the behaviors of the last 30 days become lifelong habits. Plan which meals you'll eat in restaurants and when you may enjoy an occasional treat — write them on the calendar or in your journal — and stick to your plan. Review the guidelines for eating out in Chapter 16 so dining in a restaurant is enjoyable *and* healthy.

✔ **Define your treats philosophy.** In Chapter 9, we help you recognize the difference between a "cheat" and a "treat." In Chapter 17, we tell you how to indulge in treats so you feel good, mentally and physically. Review the guidelines in Chapter 17 carefully before the end of your 30-Day Reset so you're prepared to fully enjoy a non-Paleo treat, if that's what you most desire.

✔ **Review your journal.** If you keep a journal during your 30-Day Reset, you have a valuable weapon in your arsenal against backsliding into old habits. Go back to Week 1 and remember how lousy you felt at the start of the transition from sugar-burning to fat-burning. Relive the triumph of Weeks 2 and 3, when you started to feel energized and more motivated than ever. Nothing is a more powerful motivator than your own experience and recollections of your 30-Day Reset.

Troubleshooting challenges

When you've eaten strict Paleo for four full weeks, the transition to fat burning and Paleo living is almost complete, and you're probably telling yourself and others that you'll never go back to your old ways. But sometimes life throws curveballs, and good intentions are overwhelmed by everyday stresses and surprises. Here are a few tips to help you if you start to lose your way.

Not feeling the "magic"

A month of strict Paleo may not be enough for you to revamp lifelong eating patterns or heal systemic inflammation. That doesn't mean you've failed. Instead, it means you just need to dig in a little deeper and give your body — and your mind — more time to adapt to new Paleo habits. Consider extending your 30-Day Reset for an additional two weeks. Keep a journal and make it your mission to understand how your body works and how you can use the Paleo framework to reach your optimal health and well-being.

Too many treats

If you reach the end of your 30-Day Reset and "fall off the wagon," rest assured that you're not the first or only person to get free of the rules and go a little bit wild. The good news is that you can quickly, easily recover from indulging in too many treats; simply follow the rules of the 30-Day Reset for three to seven days. How long you need to do the mini reset depends on how you feel. You want to follow the strict Paleo rules — with no treats — until you feel healthy and balanced again. How do you know when you've had too many treats? Your body tells you, loud and clear! Digestive distress, blemishes, interrupted sleep, moodiness, and lethargy are all common symptoms when you overindulge in gluten, sugar, grains, dairy, and alcohol. The effects of eating too many non-Paleo foods are similar to a hangover and just as unpleasant. The fastest remedy? High-quality Paleo food, water, and rest.

Part III
Paleo Recipes for Success

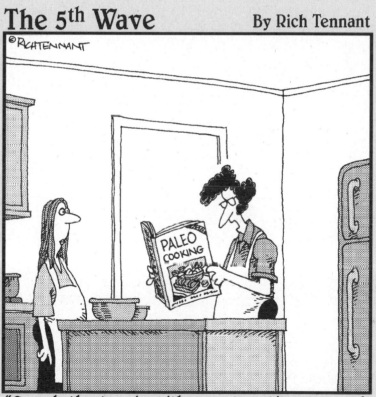

The 5th Wave   By Rich Tennant

"Smash the turnip with a rock until pulpy and then heat in the nearest volcano."

In this part . . .

It's time to get cooking! These recipes will keep you satisfied and energized throughout the day. We look at how you can really connect with your food to improve satisfaction and curb cravings, and we provide recipes that make the most of simple Paleo ingredients. With family-pleasing entrees, easy one-pot meals, enticing vegetables dishes, sauces and seasonings, and even a few treats, you can mix and match dozens of great meals.

Chapter 9

Slow Down, Savor, and Keep It Simple

*L*iving Paleo is about more than just what you eat — and eating Paleo is about much more than the food that ends up on your plate. In a healthy, balanced, Paleo life, food is an essential part of celebrations, everyday dinners, quick work lunches, and leisurely weekend meals.

But *how* you eat can be just as important as *what* you eat. Before getting to Paleo recipes, this chapter explains some of the important ways you can connect with your food — and yourself, your friends, and your family — by adopting new eating habits.

Living Paleo means you'll probably eat more home-cooked meals and eat in restaurants less often, but that doesn't mean dining out can't be fun. In this chapter, you discover how to re-create some of that restaurant experience at your own table, and you pick up tips for packing lunches and snacks so your good habits translate into your workplace or your kids' school cafeteria.

You also come to understand the difference between a *cheat* and a *treat* and how to create a set of mental tools to help you decide when it's the right time to indulge in a treat, Paleo or otherwise.

Connecting with and Enjoying Your Food

For centuries, people have come together over food. Whether they're celebrating or mourning, closing a business deal, or catching up with old friends or loved ones, food is often involved. One of the joys of the Paleo diet is that unlike traditional diets that may stress food as merely fuel or as something to be strictly measured and managed, living Paleo acknowledges that, in addition to food being nutritious, it can be fun — and delicious.

But modern lifestyles have made people disconnect from food and from eating together. Mindless eating has become the norm for too many people. Zoning out in front of the TV with takeout or hitting the drive-thru for fast food can lead to overeating and a damaging lack of awareness of exactly *what* and *how much* they're consuming.

In earlier chapters, we discuss why knowing where your food comes from and investing in the highest-quality protein, vegetables, fruits, and fats you can afford is important. How and where you eat your Paleo food is just as important as its origin — food is nourishment for both your body and your mind.

The demands of modern life don't always allow for a leisurely meal with your whole family seated around the table with napkins on their laps and polite conversation. But you'll enjoy your food more, physically and emotionally, if you make it a habit — as often as possible — to slow down, savor your food, and mindfully relish each bite.

In the following sections, we explore ways you can truly enjoy and connect with your food by being mindful of what and where you eat, by preparing meals and snacks ahead of time, and by changing things up a bit in the kitchen and around the table.

Eating at the table

One of the most important steps you can take in managing your health and weight with food is to approach your meals with mindfulness. That means serving your food on a plate and sitting down at the table. You don't need a formal dining room or fine china, but the act of slowing down to eat in a space *dedicated to eating* puts you in the right mindset to pay attention to what you're taking in. Send the message to your brain that says, "I'm eating now," so that all your senses are involved in the act of nourishing your body. Here are a few tips to do just that:

✔ **Turn off the TV:** Studies show that people eat much more when they're distracted by the television or computer while eating. The same is true for movie theaters, too. The entertainment on screen doesn't allow you to turn your attention to the food you're eating, and you mindlessly consume extra calories that leave you feeling unsatisfied because your brain hasn't registered the satiety that should be attached to the food.

✔ **Use a plate, bowl, and utensils:** When dining alone, eating right out of the skillet or while standing up may seem more convenient, but again, doing so disconnects you from the act of eating. You feel more satisfied — and are more successful in achieving your health and weight loss goals — if you place appropriate servings of protein and vegetables on your plate. And the smaller the plate, the better. Normal portions served on small plates trick your brain into thinking you're eating more, and you, therefore, can feel more satisfied when you've cleaned your plate.

✔ **Eat slowly; chew well:** Place your fork on the rim of your plate between bites to ensure that you don't shovel it in too quickly, and chew each bite of food between 30 and 50 times. Research shows that digestion and satiation improve when food is well chewed before being swallowed.

✔ **Wait 20 minutes:** Before hitting the kitchen for seconds, wait 20 minutes after finishing your food, which is how long it takes for the "I'm full" message to reach your brain. If after 20 minutes you still feel unsatisfied, add another serving of vegetables to your plate and dig in.

Creating the restaurant experience at home

As your palate adapts to the bright, fresh flavors of Paleo foods, you may find that restaurant food doesn't taste as delicious as you remember. But restaurants bring more to the table than just food — eating at a restaurant is an *experience*. With a few of the following tricks, you can re-create some of that experience at home so home-cooked meals satisfy your eyes and imagination, as well as your tummy:

✔ **Go for garnish:** As an old saying goes, we eat first with our eyes; and there's no reason you can't make a beautiful restaurant-quality presentation with your food at home. In just a few seconds, you can transform a boring plate of food into a feast for the eyes. Rather than throwing all the ingredients for a salad in a giant serving bowl, try making a pretty arrangement of the elements on a plate and drizzling them with dressing. Instead of putting a pile of vegetables next to grilled meat, why not place the meat in the center of the plate and surround it with a ring of vegetables. Edible garnishes, like freshly chopped herbs, wedges of citrus, or just a few roasted nuts, make the plate not only look pretty but also taste great.

✔ **Set the table:** Pick up a few inexpensive plates and bowls that tickle your fancy. A package of chopsticks or a pretty sushi plate can make eating Asian food at home just as engaging as eating in a restaurant. Go thrift shopping at flea markets for vintage plates, or find the perfect deep bowls for homemade chili, stews, and soups. These aesthetic touches make your table feel special, even for a weeknight dinner.

✔ **Keep the drinks flowing:** Keep a pitcher of water on the table so you can refill your glass, just like a waiter would. And make it special by placing a slice of lime or lemon on the rim — or drop a mint leaf or a few cucumber slices into the water for a fresh zing.

✔ **Eat in courses:** At a restaurant, you probably linger over an appetizer and move on to a salad before digging into your entree. Why not re-create that experience at home? Physically, taking a five-minute break between courses means your brain and digestive system have time to get in sync. Mentally, that pause between courses forces you to slow down, savor your food, and relax.

Packing lunches and snacks

If you work outside your home, packing your lunch becomes an essential part of living Paleo. You can absolutely eat at restaurants while following the Paleo diet (see Chapter 16), but for optimal control over what you're putting into your body, you'll want to pack your lunch most of the time.

And the same rules apply for kids. A lunch packed at home — consisting of quality protein, fat, and lots of vegetables and fruits — is a healthier, better-tasting alternative to the sugar- and grain-laden lunches served in schools. A packed Paleo lunch is a wonderful way to grow a healthy kid.

Try these tips to make your co-workers envious of your luscious lunches and to ensure that your kids don't trade what's in their lunchbox for their friends' junk food:

✔ **Invest in BPA-free containers:** A collection of containers in various sizes makes packing entrees, sauces, small servings of nuts, giant salads, and go-alongs easy. Be sure to get BPA-free containers with tight-fitting lids.

✔ **Make a schedule:** One way to take the stress out of packing lunches is to set up an easy weekly schedule. Designate each day of the week with a theme and repeat each week. For example, tuna salad day, tossed salad day, stir-fry day — the possibilities are endless, but the peace of mind makes eating Paleo a breeze.

- ✔ **Put salad dressing on the bottom:** If you're packing a green salad with protein, try this trick to minimize containers but maximize freshness: Place the salad dressing in the bottom of the container and top it with protein. Then add vegetables on top in layers, starting with sturdy ones like cucumbers or bell pepper strips and ending with lettuce on top. When it's time to eat, dump it into a large bowl to toss or make sure the lid is on tightly and give it a good shake, and you have a ready-to-eat salad with no fuss!

- ✔ **Welcome the leftovers:** Try doubling some of your favorite recipes so you can enjoy leftovers for lunch. Anyone eating a cold sandwich will certainly eye your hot meal with envy.

- ✔ **Eat at the table:** If your workspace provides a break room for lunch, take advantage of it! The same guidelines apply to eating at the office as they do at home: Sit at the table, use a real plate, chew slowly, and savor your food.

Redefining your meal options

One challenge of living Paleo is redefining your ideas about which foods are right for breakfast, lunch, and dinner. A "traditional" breakfast of cereal or eggs and toast isn't going to cut it — and the go-to lunch of a sandwich and a bag of chips is out, too.

Instead of trying to retrofit your old meal ideas into the new Paleo format, try eating whatever combination of protein, vegetables, and fat sounds appealing at the time. Hungry for steak and sweet potatoes at breakfast time? Fire up the cast-iron skillet. Craving a comforting omelet for dinner? Get scrambling.

Work lunch in a flash

Don't have time to pack a healthy lunch for work? You can't use that excuse anymore with these instructions at your disposal:

Place two servings of frozen vegetables in a portable container then drizzle with olive oil and a generous sprinkle of garlic powder, salt, and ground black pepper. Add a serving of protein on top — grilled chicken, frozen cooked shrimp, browned ground beef, or whatever you have on hand — and place the lid on the container. In a separate container, pack a small amount of salad dressing or other sauce to drizzle on your lunch later.

When it's time to eat, simply microwave the container of veggies and protein for a few minutes. When it's heated through, transfer to a plate and drizzle with the sauce. It's nutritious, fast, and tasty, and no real cooking is required.

Breakfast is the most challenging meal for people new to living Paleo, and getting used to the idea of chowing down on veggies for breakfast may take a while. But that's what other cultures do all over the world. Here are some tips for unusual but satisfying breakfasts to get you started:

- ✔ **Keep the veggies mellow:** Vegetables like broccoli, spinach, zucchini, and asparagus all pair well with eggs. A quick scramble or omelet is a tasty way to start your day with a healthy dose of veggies.

- ✔ **Sip on soup:** Especially nice in colder months, a mug of soup can be a gentle, delicious way to start the day. Try creamy butternut squash soup or simple beef or chicken broth poured over vegetables, cooked protein, and a hard-boiled egg.

- ✔ **Try a fry-up:** The traditional British fry-up includes grilled tomatoes and mushrooms with eggs and breakfast meats. It's a hearty way to start the day and comes with built-in vegetables.

- ✔ **Keep it cool:** Arrange a plate with cold smoked salmon, a few hard-boiled eggs, a cucumber cut into thin slices, and a handful of grapes or berries. It hits the Paleo Big Three in a deliciously big way.

- ✔ **Dig into leftovers:** No one says you can't eat leftover lasagna or chili for breakfast. Think of it as brunch served a little early. And just about any casserole or curry feels like breakfast when you top it with a fried or poached egg.

Distinguishing Between Your Emotional Appetite and True Hunger

Unlike other animals, humans eat for all kinds of reasons not associated with hunger: happiness, sadness, boredom, excitement, stress, and exhaustion, to name a few. Some people, like athletes, are very focused on eating fuel for their workouts. Others may just enjoy the pleasurable taste of their favorite foods.

Eating something tasty may provide a momentary distraction and momentary pleasure, but whatever emotion you're facing will continue to exist after you've eaten. In many cases, depending on *what* and *how much* you eat, you can actually worsen your emotional state. Remember that food itself can't be a balm for your feelings.

The exception to this rule, of course, is if you're eating because of true hunger. The key to success with food is to listen to your body's true hunger signals and to feed your emotional appetite with something other than food so you can properly deal with your emotions.

This kind of mindful eating can be challenging at first. The trick is to be as present as possible and to be honest with yourself. Here are a few tips to help you manage emotional eating and true hunger:

- ✔ **Ban all non-Paleo foods from your kitchen.** The benefit of doing this comes into play when your emotions trigger a bout of overeating; you'll have only Paleo-friendly foods on hand to consume.

- ✔ **Drink a glass of water.** This simple action helps you slow down and think about what you're doing. A short breather can help you determine whether you *need* to eat because you're truly hungry or if you just *want* to eat.

- ✔ **Be stubborn.** Remember that you've deliberately decided to make your physical and mental health a priority. Be relentless in that commitment.

- ✔ **Set a 20-minute timer.** Challenge yourself not to eat anything until the timer goes off. In that 20 minutes, examine your physical and mental state. If you're truly hungry at the end of the 20 minutes, eat a Paleo meal or snack.

- ✔ **Set kitchen hours and stick to them.** You can outwit your emotional appetite by declaring the kitchen closed.

- ✔ **Enlist an ally.** Make a deal with a family member, neighbor, online friend, or someone else you can call on to commiserate and to help you analyze whether you're hungry or trying to feed an emotion.

Setting a Time For (Occasional) Treats

When you're able to discern between the different types of appetite (see the preceding section), you can introduce foods that exist purely to satisfy your taste buds for pleasure: treats.

Eating Paleo-approved foods 80 to 90 percent of the time helps you feel your best, but sometimes you're going to decide to eat foods that fall outside of the boundaries of the Paleo Big Three. The trick is to incorporate non-Paleo foods (and even Paleo treats) into your habits with intention and to eat them occasionally and mindfully. We show you how to do that in the following sections.

Choosing treats, not cheats

If you've ever followed a traditional diet, you're probably familiar with the idea of cheating. A diet is defined by its food rules and any time you stray away from those requirements, you're cheating. With most diets, a very clear division exists between "good" and "bad," both in foods and behavior. But nourishing your body shouldn't involve judgment.

Although the Paleo diet does outline "yes" and "no" foods, it's a flexible framework that allows you to customize your approach based on your needs. In addition to giving you lots of latitude to eat the foods you like and avoid the ones you don't, this framework also allows you to remove the guilt associated with cheating on a traditional diet. When you're living Paleo, you don't have to cheat. Instead, occasionally, you may decide to enjoy a treat.

Treats can be divided into three broad categories:

- **Non-Paleo foods:** Once in a while, you may mindfully choose to enjoy foods and drinks that aren't on the Paleo-approved list, such as a favorite holiday cookie, champagne to celebrate a special occasion, or even a middle-of-the-week fiesta with corn chips and salsa.

- **Technically Paleo treats:** Baked goods made with almond or coconut flour, nut butters, and dried fruit are healthier choices than conventional baked goods. These Paleo versions, made without grains and refined sugar, are still treats, but they deliver the taste sensation of traditional goodies without the problems of gluten and refined sugar.

- **Larger quantities:** In Chapter 2, we help you assess how much food you need at each meal. Sometimes, you may decide to eat more than you need — maybe a double serving of sugar-free bacon at breakfast or an extra lamb chop. Consuming a little extra Paleo-approved food in this way can also be an occasional treat.

Punishing yourself with guilty feelings or self-recrimination after enjoying a treat is counterproductive to your success. Plan in advance when you'll enjoy a treat so the decision is intentional and celebratory, and banish the word *cheat* from your vocabulary.

Deciding when a treat is okay

Deciding when it's time for a treat is a personal decision based on how you're feeling physically, mentally, and emotionally. So how do you decide when it's the right time for a treat, and how do you determine what that treat should be?

The most important factor in enjoying a treat is *making the decision* to eat it. Mindlessly grazing at work parties or family celebrations and eating sweets or snack foods that don't even really taste very good are easy traps to fall in to. In restaurants, the bread or chip basket can suddenly empty out and into your body before you even realize it.

Eating in these kinds of social situations can be a mindless habit and are the worst use of a treat because, in reality, you often don't enjoy that food. It's a rote action: Reach for food, shove in mouth, chew, and swallow; repeat.

Be sure to mindfully choose when you'll enjoy a treat. Make the decision to eat outside the Paleo guidelines and take the time to think about why that food or that occasion is worth straying outside the framework of the Paleo Big Three.

You may decide that you're going to limit yourself to a certain number of treats per week or per month. Track them on your calendar and when you've used up all your "treat credits," eat only from the Paleo-approved foods list until it's time for a new batch of credits.

After you've enjoyed your treat, jump right back into eating Paleo-approved foods at your very next meal. One meal "off track" won't do too much damage to your body or your mindset.

If you have a diagnosed illness, like celiac disease, or a known allergy or sensitivity to certain foods, choose your treats wisely. For many people, gluten is never a good idea, and even treats must remain gluten free.

Savoring your food

You deserve the best, so when you choose to eat a treat, make sure you pick the very best version of that treat you can find. If it's a cookie you crave, go for freshly baked from your oven or your favorite bakery, instead of grabbing a packaged cookie in the work break room. If you must have pizza, bypass the processed, frozen stuff in the grocery aisle and treat yourself to the best pie in town.

When it's time to dig in, follow the guidelines for connecting with your food (as we discuss earlier in this chapter). Eat slowly. Use all your senses. Mindfully enjoy every bite.

A Note About the Recipes in This Book

All the recipes include nutritional information, but one of the best attributes of the Paleo diet is that if you eat a wide range of protein, vegetables, fruits, and fats, you don't need to worry about the details. You can just eat.

If you eat real food in amounts that are satisfying and follow the guidelines outlined in Chapter 2, you don't need to worry about calories or what percentage of them came from fat or carbohydrates.

Here are a few things to keep in mind about the recipes in this book:

- ✔ **Serving sizes:** The number of servings in a recipe is a guide for planning, based on an average serving. For most people, a serving of protein is about 4 ounces and a serving of vegetables is about 1 cup. Keep these serving sizes in mind if you're cooking for well-muscled athletes or small children and adjust accordingly.

- ✔ **Cooking fats:** For higher temperature cooking, like sautéing and baking, use coconut oil or clarified, organic, butter. All fats in recipes can be swapped with each other in a 1:1 ratio. Don't use olive oil for cooking; high heat causes olive oil to oxidize, which has some health ramifications. Reserve olive oil for drizzling on already-cooked foods and salads and for making Homemade Mayonnaise (Chapter 14).

- ✔ **Cooking temperatures:** If you're cooking grass-fed meats, use medium-high heat. High temperatures can make this leaner, high-quality meat taste tough.

- ✔ **Omitting ingredients:** Many of these recipes include optional ingredients, and all spices and seasonings are always optional. Adjust amounts and ingredients according to your personal preferences.

- ✔ **Nuts and dried fruit:** All nuts, seeds, and dried fruit included in these recipes are optional. If you're trying to minimize your omega-6 fatty acids or fruit or sugar intake, you can omit the nuts and fruit without damaging the recipe.

- ✔ **Salt:** Taste food throughout the cooking process to adjust seasonings.

All the recipes can be modified according to personal tastes and food sensitivities. The more you can make the recipes your own, the deeper connection you'll feel with your food.

Chapter 10

Everyday Entrees

. . . .

In This Chapter

▶ Revamping family favorites with Paleo-approved ingredients

▶ Creating main dish salads packed with flavor

. . . .

L iving Paleo doesn't mean you have to give up all your favorite comfort foods. With some ingredient substitution and lots of vegetables, translating old favorites into your new Paleo lifestyle is easy. And when you prepare satisfying foods in advance, you stock your refrigerator with healthy options so you never feel deprived.

In this chapter, you find recipes that make transitioning from old family favorites to Paleo-approved meals a painless process. From diner classics, like meatloaf, chicken fingers, and club sandwiches, to elegant, easy-to-make salads, these recipes are stick-to-your ribs good and Paleo approved.

Making Family Favorites Fit in Your Paleo Lifestyle

The first seven recipes in this chapter are designed to leave you with leftovers that you can turn into meals and snacks throughout the week. You can easily double many of the recipes, so you can freeze a batch for future meals to get dinner on the table in record time.

 Casseroles, soups, and stews all freeze well. Place individual servings of your favorites in small containers and freeze. They're easy to transport to work or school for lunch and can be quickly defrosted or reheated in the microwave for a meal at home.

Tossing Together Main Dish Salads for Paleo-Approved Meals

Sometimes you just want a really big salad! The last three recipes in this chapter combine protein, veggies, and fruit in unexpectedly delicious ways. And when you have already-cooked protein on hand, you can throw together a salad in no time.

Here are a couple salad-related tips:

- ✓ **Toss for two.** The secret to great-tasting salad is making sure you don't skimp on the toss. These recipes include just the right amount of dressing to supply you with energy-enriched fats and plenty of flavor. To optimize flavor, be sure to toss for at least two minutes to coat each element of the salad with dressing.

- ✓ **Make it to go.** Salads work great in packed lunches; just be sure to pack the dressing separately from the salad ingredients — or place the dressing in the bottom of a large container and top with protein, followed by the vegetables. Keep the tender veggies separate from the dressing until it's time to eat.

A little history on salads

The first cookbook that recommended people eat salads was published about 300 years ago in London, called *Acetaria: A Discourse of Sallets*. It explained that salads should be made from only the freshest greens plucked straight from the garden, sprinkled with water, and dried well. It went on to recommend that salads be dressed with young olive oil, quality vinegar, and sea salt. It also emphasized the addition of dark greens, such as spinach, endive, and arugula, and suggested that cooks could spice things up with fennel, celery, and radish for flavor. Sound familiar? Add in some Paleo protein, and the book described a thoroughly modern, healthy meal.

All-American Meatloaf

Prep time: 30 min • **Cook time:** 80 min • **Yield:** 8 servings

Ingredients	*Directions*
½ cup **Cave Man Ketchup** (see recipe in Chapter 14)	*1* Preheat the oven to 350 degrees. In a small bowl, mix the Cave Man Ketchup with the vinegar and honey (if desired); set aside.
½ **tablespoon cider vinegar**	
1 **tablespoon honey (optional)**	
½ **head cauliflower**	*2* Break the cauliflower into florets, removing the stems, and then place in a food processor and pulse until the cauliflower is the texture of fine breadcrumbs, about ten to fifteen 1-second pulses. Place in a large mixing bowl.
2 **teaspoons coconut oil**	
1 **medium onion, diced**	
2 **cloves garlic, minced**	*3* Heat coconut oil in a medium skillet over medium-high heat. Add the onion and garlic and sauté until soft, about 5 minutes. Set aside to cool.
2 **large eggs**	
½ **teaspoon dried thyme**	
1 **teaspoon salt**	*4* To the cauliflower, add the eggs, thyme, salt, pepper, mustard, coconut aminos, hot pepper sauce, coconut milk, and parsley. Mix with a wooden spoon until combined, and then add the cooked onions and garlic and ground beef; mix well.
½ **teaspoon ground black pepper**	
2 **teaspoons Dijon mustard**	
2 **teaspoons coconut aminos**	
¼ **teaspoon hot pepper sauce**	*5* Pat into a meatloaf pan with a perforated bottom, or pat into a loaf shape with your hands and place on a roasting rack set on a baking sheet to catch drippings. Brush the loaf with half of the ketchup glaze; bake for 45 minutes.
½ **cup coconut milk**	
1 **cup fresh parsley leaves, minced (about ⅓ cup)**	
2 **pounds ground beef**	*6* Brush with the remaining half of the glaze and continue to bake another 20 minutes. Remove from the oven and allow to rest for 15 minutes before serving.

Per serving: Calories 342 (From Fat 178); Fat 20g (Saturated 10g); Cholesterol 144mg; Sodium 446mg; Carbohydrate 11g; Dietary Fiber 2g; Protein 29g.

Tip: Serve with Mashed Cauliflower (Chapter 12) for a classic comfort food dinner.

Vary It! Try a combination of ground meats by substituting veal, pork, or ground turkey for beef.

Spaghetti Squash and Meatballs

Prep time: 10 min • **Cook time:** 40 min • **Yield:** 4 servings

Ingredients	Directions
1 large spaghetti squash	**1** Preheat the oven to 375 degrees. Cover two large baking sheets with parchment paper.
3 tablespoons water	
¾ pound ground beef	**2** Cut the squash in half lengthwise, and scoop out the seeds with a large spoon. Place squash cut side down on the baking sheet. Sprinkle the water onto the paper around the squash. Set aside.
¼ pound ground pork	
½ cup fresh parsley leaves, minced	
1 large egg	**3** In a large bowl, mix the meat, parsley, egg, 1 clove garlic, salt, and black pepper with a fork until combined. Measure a tablespoon of meat and roll into a ball between your palms. Line up the meatballs on the prepared baking sheet, about ½ inch apart.
1 clove plus 2 cloves garlic, minced	
1 teaspoon salt	
½ teaspoon ground black pepper	**4** Place both baking sheets in the oven and set timer for 25 to 30 minutes.
1 tablespoon coconut oil	
One 28-ounce can diced fire-roasted tomatoes	**5** While the meatballs and squash are roasting, place the coconut oil and 2 cloves garlic in a saucepan over medium-high heat. Cook until the garlic is fragrant, about 30 seconds, and then add the tomatoes and basil. Stir to combine, increase heat, and bring to a boil.
8 large basil leaves, slivered	
Salt and ground black pepper to taste	
	6 Reduce heat to low and simmer, uncovered, until slightly thickened, about 10 minutes. Season with salt and pepper to taste. Cover and reduce heat so sauce is just kept warm.

7 When the meatballs are golden brown and cooked through (about 25 to 30 minutes), add them to the tomato sauce to keep them warm. Leave the spaghetti squash in the oven to bake for an additional 10 minutes.

8 Remove the squash from the oven and, using a hot pad to hold it, scrape the inside with a fork to shred the squash into spaghetti-like strands. To serve, mound spaghetti squash on individual plates and top with sauce and meatballs.

Per serving: *Calories 373 (From Fat 183); Fat 20g (Saturated 9g); Cholesterol 124mg; Sodium 695mg; Carbohydrate 22g; Dietary Fiber 4g; Protein 26g.*

Meals in minutes

The following list provides some quick meal ideas that require no recipe, so you can whip them up in no time. With protein, vegetables, and fat, all these dishes are complete meals that you can make with minimal ingredients and fuss.

✔ **Bunless Burgers:** You'll never miss the bun! Thick, juicy burgers made from beef, turkey, pork, lamb, bison, or a combination taste great when you top them with all the traditional fixings and serve them alongside a big tossed salad or your favorite cooked vegetables.

✔ **Antipasto Plate:** Line a plate with lettuce leaves and then top with tuna, a hard-boiled egg, green pepper strips, cucumber slices, diced tomato, artichoke hearts, and a few olives. Drizzle with extra-virgin olive oil and red wine vinegar.

✔ **Rotisserie Chicken:** Take advantage of pre-made foods at the grocery store. Build a dinner plate with a serving of rotisserie roasted chicken alongside salad made from pre-washed greens and broccoli slaw. Drizzle with extra-virgin olive oil and balsamic vinegar.

✔ **Stuffed Avocado:** Cut an avocado in half and fill the well with tuna, shrimp, crab, or shredded chicken that's been mixed with lime juice, salt, pepper, cumin, and chili powder. Serve carrot sticks, red pepper strips, and cucumber slices on the side.

✔ **Stuffed Baked Sweet Potato:** Brown ground beef or lamb with salt, pepper, garlic powder, and a pinch each of cinnamon and chili powder. Spoon the meat into a baked sweet potato and top with chopped fresh herbs.

✔ **Sardines and Crudité:** Line a plate with lettuce leaves. Use a fork to remove boneless, skinless sardines (packed in olive oil) from the can and arrange on the plate with cucumber slices, jicama matchsticks, red pepper strips, and white mushrooms. Drizzle the vegetables with the olive oil from the can and sprinkle with chopped parsley.

Leafy Tacos

Prep time: 2 min • **Cook time:** 20 min • **Yield:** 4 servings

Ingredients	Directions
2 teaspoons coconut oil	*1* Heat coconut oil in skillet over medium heat until hot, about 2 minutes; add onion and cook until softened, about 4 minutes.
1 small onion, minced	
3 cloves garlic, minced	
2 tablespoons chili powder	*2* Add the garlic, chili powder, cumin, coriander, oregano, cayenne, and salt. Stir until fragrant, about 30 seconds.
1 teaspoon ground cumin	
1 teaspoon ground coriander	
½ teaspoon dried oregano leaves	*3* Add the ground beef to the pan and cook, breaking up the meat with a wooden spoon until no longer pink, about 5 minutes.
¼ teaspoon ground cayenne pepper	
½ teaspoon salt	*4* Add tomato paste, chicken broth, and vinegar. Stir to combine and bring to a simmer. Reduce heat to medium-low and cook uncovered for 10 minutes, until the liquid has reduced and thickened. Taste and adjust seasonings with salt and pepper.
1 pound ground beef	
2 tablespoons tomato paste	
½ cup chicken broth	
2 teaspoons cider vinegar	*5* Spoon taco meat into individual lettuce leaves and top with garnishes.
1 large head lettuce (butter, romaine, or leaf)	
Garnishes: diced avocado, onion, tomato, jalapeño; minced cilantro	

Per serving: Calories 304 (From Fat 159); Fat 18g (Saturated 8g); Cholesterol 80mg; Sodium 548mg; Carbohydrate 10g; Dietary Fiber 5g; Protein 27g.

Note: Commercial taco seasonings often contain hidden sugars, grains, and soy. Why eat processed seasonings when making your own is so easy — and flavorful? You can also top your tacos with your favorite tomato salsa; just be sure to check the label for non-Paleo ingredients.

Tip: This recipe is easy to double. Use leftovers tossed in a taco salad, spooned into a baked sweet potato, or scrambled into eggs.

Chicken Fingers

Prep time: 10 min • **Cook time:** 20 min • **Yield:** 4 servings

Ingredients	Directions
⅔ **cup almond meal**	**1** Preheat the oven to 425 degrees. Line a large baking sheet with parchment paper and place a wire baking rack on top.
1 teaspoon paprika	
1 teaspoon coarse (granulated) garlic powder	**2** In a shallow bowl or plate, combine the almond meal, paprika, garlic powder, salt, pepper, thyme, and allspice. Mix with a fork to combine. In another shallow bowl, beat the egg white until frothy.
1 teaspoon salt	
½ **teaspoon ground black pepper**	
½ **teaspoon dried thyme**	**3** Pat chicken dry with paper towels and then dip into egg white, shaking to remove excess. Roll in almond meal and place on the prepared baking sheet. The chicken tenders should not touch. Repeat until all pieces are coated.
¼ **teaspoon allspice**	
1 large egg white	
1 pound chicken tenders (or boneless, skinless chicken breast, sliced into strips)	**4** Bake 15 to 20 minutes, turning once halfway through baking.

Per serving: Calories 240 (From Fat 110); Fat 12g (Saturated 1g); Cholesterol 63mg; Sodium 669mg; Carbohydrate 6g; Dietary Fiber 3g; Protein 28g.

Note: You can also make these chicken fingers without the almond meal if you're trying to minimize your nut intake. Just roll the chicken tenders in the spice blend and follow baking instructions.

Vary it! To make spicy chicken fingers, add ¼ to ½ teaspoon ground cayenne pepper to the almond meal or give them a smoky spin with smoked paprika. You can also substitute pieces of firm, white fish for the chicken to make fish sticks or use beef strips for chicken-fried steak.

Tip: Serve with Ranch Dressing (Chapter 14) for dipping along with Mashed Cauliflower, Classic Cole Slaw, or Sweet Potato Shoestring Fries (Chapter 12).

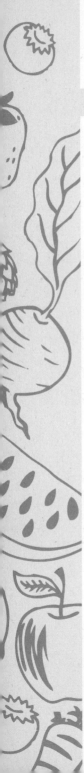

Orange Shrimp and Beef with Broccoli

Prep time: 15 min • **Cook time:** 10 min • **Yield:** 4 servings

Ingredients	*Directions*
1 tablespoon sesame seeds, optional	*1* Heat a large sauté pan or wok over medium-high heat. When the pan is hot, add the sesame seeds and stir constantly until they're lightly toasted, about 3 to 5 minutes. Remove from pan and reserve for later.
3 oranges	
3 tablespoons coconut aminos	
1 tablespoon rice vinegar	*2* With a vegetable peeler, peel wide strips of zest from half of one of the oranges. Cut the zest into 1-inch pieces and set aside.
2 tablespoons arrowroot powder (optional)	
1 teaspoon plus 2 teaspoons coconut oil	*3* Squeeze the juice from all the oranges into a small bowl; you should have about ¾ cup. Add coconut aminos and rice vinegar; stir to combine.
¾ pound beef sirloin, trimmed and sliced against the grain into ⅛-inch-thick slices	
½ pound shrimp, peeled, deveined, and halved	*4* In another small bowl, mix the arrowroot powder with 2 tablespoons of water to form a paste; whisk into the orange juice and set aside.
1 large onion, thinly sliced	*5* Heat 1 teaspoon coconut oil in the pan over high heat until very hot, about 2 minutes. Add beef, shrimp, and onion. Stir-fry until the beef is no longer pink on the outside, about 1 minute. Transfer to a plate and cover loosely with foil.
8 cloves garlic, minced	
¼ teaspoon dried ginger	
¼ teaspoon ground cayenne pepper	
2 pounds broccoli, cut into small florets	*6* Add remaining 2 teaspoons coconut oil to the pan and heat until very hot. Add garlic, ginger, cayenne, and reserved orange zest. Stir-fry until fragrant, about 30 seconds. Add the broccoli, red pepper, and water. Cover and steam, stirring occasionally, until the water has evaporated and the broccoli is tender, about 3 to 4 minutes.
2 red bell peppers, seeded and thinly sliced	
⅓ cup water	
½ cup scallions, green parts only, thinly sliced	*7* Whisk the stir-fry sauce and pour into the pan. Bring to a boil and cook until the sauce is slightly thickened, about 1 to 2 minutes. Add the beef and shrimp, stirring to coat with the sauce. Remove from heat and sprinkle with scallions and toasted sesame seeds.

Per serving: Calories 551 (From Fat 164); Fat 18g (Saturated 8g); Cholesterol 146mg; Sodium 462mg; Carbohydrate 62g; Dietary Fiber 14g; Protein 36g.

Caraway Pork with Cabbage and Apples

Prep time: 15 min • **Cook time:** 1 hr • **Yield:** 4 servings

Ingredients	*Directions*
1 pound ground pork	**1** Preheat the oven to 350 degrees.
1 teaspoon salt	
½ tablespoon caraway seeds	**2** In a large bowl, mix the pork, salt, caraway seeds, paprika, and mustard until combined. Set aside.
½ tablespoon ground paprika	
½ tablespoon grainy mustard	**3** In a large skillet, heat the coconut oil over medium-high heat, and then add the onion, stirring until soft, about 5 to 7 minutes. Add the garlic and cook until fragrant, about 30 seconds. Crumble the pork into the pan and cook, breaking up the meat with a wooden spoon until browned, about 5 minutes.
½ tablespoon coconut oil	
1 medium onion, diced	
1 clove garlic, minced	
1 large head green cabbage (about 2 pounds), cored and thinly sliced	**4** Spread half the cabbage in a large casserole dish that's at least 4 inches deep. Spread half the apples on top of the cabbage and cover with all the meat. Add the remaining cabbage and top with the rest of the apples. Sprinkle with Morning Spice.
2 Granny Smith apples, cored and thinly sliced	
1 teaspoon Morning Spice (see recipe in Chapter 14) or cinnamon	**5** Cover tightly with foil and bake until the cabbage is tender, about 1 hour. Allow to rest 5 minutes before serving.

Per serving: Calories 381 (From Fat 184); Fat 21g (Saturated 8g); Cholesterol 76mg; Sodium 714mg; Carbohydrate 28g; Dietary Fiber 10g; Protein 25g.

Vary It! Substitute beef or ground turkey for the pork.

Tip: Leftovers make for a warming breakfast; add a few fried or scrambled eggs to increase the protein and make it even more breakfast-y.

Zucchini Lasagna

Prep time: 30 min • **Cook time:** 1 hr • **Yield:** 8 servings

Ingredients	Directions
4 pounds zucchini	**1** Preheat the oven to 400 degrees.
Salt and ground black pepper to taste	**2** Cut zucchini lengthwise into slices about ½-inch thick. Place in a colander and toss generously with salt to coat each slice. Allow zucchini to sweat for 30 minutes. Pat the slices dry with paper towels. Set aside.
2 pounds ground beef	
1 ½ tablespoons Italian Seasoning (see recipe in Chapter 14)	**3** Heat a large sauté pan over medium-high heat. Crumble the beef into the pan and sprinkle with Italian Seasoning. Break up large chunks with a wooden spoon and cook until the beef is browned, about 7 to 10 minutes.
1 tablespoon coconut oil	
2 cloves garlic, minced (about 2 teaspoons)	**4** Remove the meat to a bowl — drain excess fat, if necessary — and return the pan to the stove. Reduce the heat to medium, and then add the coconut oil and garlic to the pan. Cook until the garlic is fragrant, about 30 seconds.
Three 14.5-ounce cans diced fire-roasted tomatoes	
8 large basil leaves, slivered (about 2 tablespoons)	**5** Add the tomatoes and 1 tablespoon of the basil. Stir to combine, increase heat, and bring to a boil. Reduce heat to low and simmer until slightly thickened, about 10 minutes. Season with salt and pepper to taste. Remove from heat and allow to cool to room temperature.
4 eggs	
Garnish: 2 teaspoons extra-virgin olive oil, fresh basil leaves	
	6 When the tomato sauce is cool, scramble the eggs in a small bowl and blend them into the tomato sauce with a wooden spoon.

7 To assemble the lasagna, place a single layer of zucchini in the bottom of a 13-x-9-inch pan. Sprinkle half of the cooked meat on top of the zucchini, and then top with ⅓ of the sauce. Repeat for second layer. Build your final layer with zucchini and spread the remaining sauce evenly over the top.

8 Place the pan in the center of the oven and bake for 30 minutes. Remove the pan from the oven and let it rest for at least 30 minutes before slicing or eating. Before serving, lightly brush the top of the lasagna with the olive oil and sprinkle with additional basil.

Per serving: Calories 366 (From Fat 174); Fat 19g (Saturated 8g); Cholesterol 197mg; Sodium 592mg; Carbohydrate 15g; Dietary Fiber 4g; Protein 33g.

Note: This dish tastes even better on the second day, and it freezes well. Just reheat, covered, in a 300-degree oven before serving.

Snacks in seconds

What follows is a list of quick and tasty snacks. You can mix and match the snacks to help you get through a hungry patch between meals.

- Kipper snacks with raw veggies or a piece of fruit
- Boneless, skinless sardines packed in olive oil with raw veggies or a piece of fruit
- Sugar-free beef jerky with raw veggies or a piece of fruit
- Hard-boiled eggs with raw veggies or a piece of fruit
- Paleo-approved lunch meats with raw veggies or a piece of fruit
- Unsweetened coconut flakes mixed with berries and nuts
- Mashed avocado or guacamole with raw veggies

- Olives and raw veggies
- Cooked chicken with salsa and avocado
- Cooked beef slices wrapped around cucumber spears
- Celery sticks and almond butter
- Diced tomato and avocado mixed with diced cooked shrimp
- Prosciutto wrapped around melon slices
- Diced hard-boiled eggs, tomato, and avocado tossed with lemon or lime juice
- Berries topped with a few tablespoons of coconut milk
- Smoked salmon wrapped around cucumber spears or alongside berries

Berry-Nice Chicken Salad

Prep time: 2 hr • **Cook time:** 20 min • **Yield:** 4 servings

Ingredients	Directions
4 cups plus 2 cups water	**1** Place a 1-gallon zipper storage bag inside a large bowl. Pour in 4 cups water, and add salt, peppercorns, garlic, and lemon juice. Stir to dissolve salt, and add the chicken. Seal the bag and refrigerate for 2 hours.
2 tablespoons salt	
1 teaspoon whole peppercorns	
3 cloves garlic, lightly smashed	**2** Rinse the chicken well under running water and place in a single layer in a large pot. Add 2 cups water, bring to a boil, and then reduce heat to a gentle simmer. Cover and cook 10 minutes
2 tablespoons lemon juice	
1 pound boneless, skinless chicken breasts	
⅓ cup Homemade Mayonnaise (see recipe in Chapter 14)	**3** Turn off heat, allowing the chicken to sit, covered, another 15 to 20 minutes. When the chicken is cooked, place chicken in a large bowl and use two forks to shred it. Allow the chicken to cool while you prepare the rest of the salad.
½ tablespoon red wine vinegar	
¼ teaspoon ground cayenne pepper	**4** In a small bowl, mix the Homemade Mayonnaise, vinegar, and cayenne pepper with a fork until just combined.
½ cup fresh raspberries	
¼ cup pecans, coarsely chopped	**5** To the chicken, add the raspberries, pecans, scallions, and parsley. Toss gently with a rubber scraper to combine and then add the Homemade Mayonnaise dressing. Toss until evenly coated. Allow flavors to meld for 10 to 20 minutes before serving.
2 scallions, green only, thinly sliced	
¼ cup fresh parsley leaves, minced	

Per serving: Calories 324 (From Fat 211); Fat 24g (Saturated 2g); Cholesterol 75mg; Sodium 475mg; Carbohydrate 4g; Dietary Fiber 2g; Protein 24g.

Note: Brining ensures that the chicken is flavorful and tender. If you don't have the time to brine, skip that step and add the peppercorns, garlic, and lemon juice to the water when you poach the chicken.

Vary It! In a pinch, you can use defrosted frozen berries in place of fresh. In winter, use dried cranberries or cherries.

Club Sandwich Salad

Prep time: 10 min • **Cook time:** 4 min • **Yield:** 4 servings

Ingredients	*Directions*
4 strips high-quality, nitrate-free bacon	*1* Cut the bacon crosswise into ¼-inch wide pieces and place in a large, cold skillet; turn the heat to medium-high, and fry the bacon until it's crisp, about 3 to 4 minutes. Remove bacon from pan with a wooden spoon and drain on a paper towel.
1 head green or red leaf lettuce, torn	
2 large cucumbers, peeled and thinly sliced	*2* Divide lettuce among four plates and line rim with cucumber slices.
12 ounces cooked boneless, skinless chicken breast, diced	
2 ripe tomatoes, diced	*3* In a large bowl, gently toss chicken, tomatoes, avocado, red onion, and parsley. Divide on top of lettuce-cucumber bed.
1 ripe avocado, diced	
½ medium red onion, thinly sliced	*4* Drizzle each serving with Ranch Dressing, sprinkle with bacon, and serve immediately.
½ cup fresh parsley leaves, coarsely chopped	
⅓ cup Ranch Dressing (see recipe in Chapter 14)	

Per serving: Calories 309 (From Fat 120); Fat 13g (Saturated 3g); Cholesterol 78mg; Sodium 972mg; Carbohydrate 17g; Dietary Fiber 8g; Protein 33g.

Tip: This dish travels well for packed lunches. Package the chicken and dressing separately from the vegetables and assemble just before eating.

Chinese Chicken Salad

Prep time: 2 hr • **Cook time:** 20 min • **Yield:** 4 servings

Ingredients	*Directions*
4 cups plus 2 cups water	*1* Place a 1-gallon zipper storage bag inside a large bowl. Pour in 4 cups water; add salt, peppercorns, 3 cloves smashed garlic, and jalapeño. Stir to dissolve salt and add the chicken. Seal the bag and refrigerate for 2 hours.
2 tablespoons salt	
1 teaspoon whole peppercorns	
3 cloves garlic, lightly smashed, plus 1 clove garlic, minced	*2* Rinse the chicken well under running water and place in a single layer in a large pot. Add 2 cups water, bring to a boil, and then reduce heat to a gentle simmer. Cover and cook for 10 minutes.
1 fresh jalapeño, cut into rings	
1 pound boneless, skinless chicken breast	
¼ cup coconut aminos	*3* Turn off heat, allowing the chicken to sit, covered, another 15 to 20 minutes. When the chicken is cooked, place chicken in a large bowl and use two forks to shred it.
¼ cup rice vinegar	
1 tablespoon sesame oil	
1 teaspoon mustard powder	
½ teaspoon ground black pepper	*4* In a small bowl, whisk coconut aminos, rice vinegar, sesame oil, 1 clove minced garlic, mustard powder, ground black pepper, red pepper flakes, and ginger until combined. Continue whisking and add oil in a slow, steady stream until combined.
½ teaspoon crushed red pepper flakes	
¼ teaspoon dried ginger	
¼ cup light-tasting olive oil (not extra-virgin)	
1 pound Napa cabbage, cored and very thinly sliced	*5* Place cabbage, snow peas, bell pepper, scallions, carrots, cilantro, and chicken in a large bowl. Toss to combine, and then add dressing and toss well for 2 to 3 minutes until evenly coated. Allow the flavors to meld for 10 minutes before eating. Sprinkle with almonds and sesame seeds; serve immediately.
½ pound snow peas, cut into slivers	
1 red bell pepper, thinly sliced	
3 to 4 scallions, green and white, thinly sliced	
2 carrots, grated	
½ cup loosely packed cilantro leaves, chopped	
¼ cup sliced almonds, toasted (optional)	
2 tablespoons sesame seeds, toasted (optional)	

Per serving: Calories 463 (From Fat 72); Fat 8g (Saturated 2g); Cholesterol 96mg; Sodium 811mg; Carbohydrate 49g; Dietary Fiber 5g; Protein 40g.

Chapter 11

One-Pot Meals

In This Chapter

▶ Warming up to the Paleo lifestyle with soups and stews

▶ Getting egg-cited about the enticing possibilities with eggs

▶ Taking your time with delicious slow cooker meals

Spices are 100 percent Paleo approved and can take your taste buds on an international tour, without leaving your kitchen. Enjoying a variety of flavors and textures is essential for fighting food boredom, and one-pot meals mean less time in the kitchen for you and more time to enjoy the other things in your life.

In this chapter, you find recipes that bring a world of flavors to your kitchen in easy one-pot meals, including soups and stews, egg dishes, and slow cooker recipes. Finding inspiration in traditional dishes, these recipes from Italy, Asia, India, Thailand, Mexico, and more are adapted for a modern Paleo lifestyle.

Sitting Back with Soups and Stews

Something is undeniably comforting about a steaming mug of soup or deep bowl of stew. And making soups and stews is so easy! Most of the work is done during simmering, so after a short investment of time to prep the ingredients, you can walk away and let the stove do the work.

Here are a few tips for making and serving soups and stews:

✔ **Try 'em for breakfast.** Leftover soups and stews make for a warm, hearty breakfast. Top with poached or fried eggs to add a little extra protein and increase the breakfast quotient.

✔ **Make a double batch.** You can easily double and freeze all the soups and stews recipes we include in this chapter.

Exploring Easy Egg Dishes

Whether it's a lazy brunch on Sunday morning or breakfast for dinner on a random Thursday night, eggs are a delicious comfort food, and they're packed with Paleo nutrition. Partner them with vitamin-rich vegetables and seasonings, and they taste great any time of day and any time of year.

Add even more vegetables to these dishes by serving them on top of a bed of raw baby spinach leaves — or make a quick salad of arugula or spinach tossed with extra-virgin olive oil, lemon juice, salt, and pepper and pile on top of the eggs.

Keeping It Simple with Slow Cooker Meals

The slow cooker is the ultimate hands-off, meal-making machine! These recipes take advantage of its slow-roasting capabilities to produce meat that's fall-off-the-bone tender and very flavorful. And thanks to the slow cooker, you can use inexpensive cuts of meat, which means these recipes are economical, too.

Here's a foolproof way to roast large, tough cuts of beef, lamb, and pork — no recipe required. Pat the meat dry with paper towels and generously sprinkle the meat with salt, pepper, and garlic powder. Place the meat in the slow cooker with ½ cup broth or water. Cover and cook on high for 4 to 5 hours, until fork tender.

Teriyaki-Turkey Meatball Soup

Prep time: 10 min • **Cook time:** 15 min • **Yield:** 4 servings

Ingredients	Directions
1 pound ground turkey	*1* In a large bowl, mix the turkey with the cayenne pepper, salt, pineapple, coconut aminos, dried ginger, garlic, and egg. Measure a level tablespoon of turkey and roll into a meatball shape. If the meat sticks to your hands, wet your hands with water between rolling. Set meatballs aside.
½ teaspoon ground cayenne pepper	
¼ teaspoon salt	
½ cup canned crushed pineapple (sugar-free, packed in its own juice), drained well	
1 tablespoon coconut aminos	*2* With the bottom of a glass or the handle of a heavy knife, smash the ginger slices to release their flavor. Place them in a large pot and add the broth; bring to a boil over medium-high heat.
½ teaspoon dried ginger	
1 clove garlic, minced	
1 large egg, lightly beaten	*3* Reduce the heat to simmer and add the meatballs. Simmer, covered, until the meatballs are cooked through, about 8 minutes. Season with salt and pepper to taste and add the spinach. Cook uncovered until the spinach is just wilted, about 2 minutes.
2-inch piece fresh ginger, cut into ½-inch slices	
8 to 10 cups chicken broth	
8 cups fresh spinach leaves, coarsely chopped	*4* Serve in deep bowls and sprinkle with scallions and sesame seeds.
Salt and ground black pepper	
3 to 4 scallions, white and green, very thinly sliced	
1 tablespoon sesame seeds, toasted (optional)	

Per serving: Calories 333 (From Fat 182); Fat 20g (Saturated 5g); Cholesterol 139mg; Sodium 2,469mg; Carbohydrate 10g; Dietary Fiber 2g; Protein 28.

Vary It! Substitute ground pork for the ground turkey. You may also substitute other greens for the spinach. Collard greens, Swiss chard, kale, and escarole are all good choices.

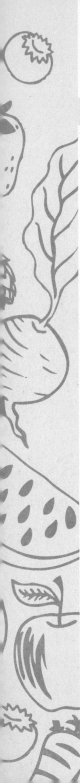

Thai Butternut Squash Soup

Prep time: 10 min • **Cook time:** 40 min • **Yield:** 4 servings

Ingredients	Directions
One 14.5-ounce can coconut milk	**1** Open the can of coconut milk and scoop out about 2 tablespoons of the coconut cream that has risen to the top. Place in a small bowl and mix with the red curry paste until combined. Cover and set aside. Reserve remaining coconut milk in can.
One 4-ounce jar Thai Kitchen red curry paste	
1 tablespoon coconut oil	
2 medium onions, finely chopped	**2** Heat a large, deep pot over medium-high heat, and add the coconut oil. When the oil is melted, stir in onions with a wooden spoon and cook until they're translucent, about 7 minutes.
4 cloves garlic, minced	
2 tablespoons minced fresh ginger	**3** Add garlic, fresh ginger, peppercorns, lemongrass, and cumin. Cook, stirring, for 30 seconds, and then add the squash, chicken broth, coconut milk, and chicken to the pot. Bring to a boil.
1 teaspoon peppercorns	
2 stalks lemongrass, trimmed, smashed, and cut in half crosswise	
1 tablespoon ground cumin	**4** Reduce heat to simmer and cook, covered, until the squash is tender and chicken is cooked through, about 30 minutes. Remove the lemongrass and chicken from the pot. Place the chicken in a bowl to cool; when cool enough to handle, shred with two forks and set aside.
1 large butternut squash, seeds removed and cut into 2-inch cubes	
6 cups chicken broth	
1 pound boneless, skinless chicken breasts	**5** Add the curry paste to the soup pot, along with the lime zest and lime juice. Stir to combine. Then, working in batches, carefully purée the soup in a food processor or blender and return to the pot until heated through.
Zest of 1 lime	
Juice of 1 lime	**6** Ladle the soup into bowls and sprinkle with shredded chicken, chopped cilantro, and additional fresh lime juice.
1 cup fresh cilantro leaves, coarsely chopped	

Per serving: Calories 515 (From Fat 311); Fat 35g (Saturated 25g); Cholesterol 70mg; Sodium 2,088mg; Carbohydrate 26g; Dietary Fiber 7g; Protein 29g.

Note: You can find Thai red curry paste in most grocery stores and online retailers. The Thai Kitchen brand is sugar free and Paleo friendly.

Hearty Chili

Prep time: 20 min • **Cook time:** 2 hr • **Yield:** 8 servings

Ingredients	*Directions*
2 tablespoons coconut oil 2 medium onions, diced 2 green bell peppers, diced 1 fresh jalapeño, diced	*1* Heat a large, deep pot over medium-high heat, and add the coconut oil. When the oil is melted, add onions, bell peppers, and jalapeño. Stir with a wooden spoon and cook until the vegetables are tender, about 7 minutes.
4 cloves garlic, minced (about 4 teaspoons) 1 pound ground beef 1 pound ground pork	*2* Add the garlic, and as soon as it's fragrant (about 30 seconds), crumble the ground meat into the pan with your hands, mixing with the wooden spoon to combine. Continue to cook the meat, stirring often, until it's no longer pink.
1 teaspoon dried oregano leaves 3 tablespoons chili powder 2 tablespoons ground cumin 1 teaspoon salt	*3* In a small bowl, crush the oregano between your palms to release its flavor, and add the chili powder, cumin, and salt. Combine with a fork, and then add to the pot, along with the tomato paste. Stir until combined, about 2 minutes.
One 6-ounce can tomato paste One 14.5-ounce can chopped tomatoes One 14.5-ounce can beef broth 1 cup water	*4* Add the chopped tomatoes with their juice, beef broth, and water to the pot. Stir well. Bring to a boil; reduce the heat and simmer, uncovered, for 2 hours.
Garnishes: diced red onion and avocado; minced fresh cilantro leaves	*5* Serve in deep bowls and top with garnishes.

Per serving: Calories 387 (From Fat 176); Fat 20g (Saturated 9g); Cholesterol 73mg; Sodium 670mg; Carbohydrate 12g; Dietary Fiber 4g; Protein 25g.

Note: This dish freezes well, so make a double batch for chili any time.

Classic Beef Stew

Prep time: 30 min • **Cook time:** 2½ hr • **Yield:** 8 servings

Ingredients	Directions

Ingredients

3 tablespoons arrowroot powder (optional)

Generous sprinkle of salt and ground black pepper

2 pounds beef stew meat

2 tablespoons coconut oil

2 medium onions, diced

3 ribs celery, thinly sliced

2 cloves garlic, minced

6 tablespoons tomato paste (half of a 6-ounce can)

1 cup beef broth

1 tablespoon coconut aminos

6 cups water

2 bay leaves

1 teaspoon salt

½ teaspoon ground black pepper

1 teaspoon dried thyme leaves

½ teaspoon ground paprika

Dash ground allspice

4 large carrots, peeled and cut into 1-inch dice

2 sweet potatoes, peeled and cut into 1-inch dice

Garnish: fresh parsley leaves; extra-virgin olive oil (optional)

Directions

1 In a small bowl, mix the arrowroot powder (if desired) with a generous sprinkle of salt and pepper. Place the meat in a large bowl and sprinkle with the arrowroot powder, tossing to coat.

2 In a large pot or Dutch oven, heat the coconut oil over medium-high heat; add the meat in batches and sear on all sides. With tongs or a slotted spoon, remove the browned pieces to a bowl to catch their juice. Repeat with the remaining cubes.

3 In the same pot, sauté the onions, celery, and garlic for about 2 minutes, stirring with a wooden spoon. Add the tomato paste and stir for about 1 minute.

4 Add the broth and coconut aminos, scraping up any brown bits at the bottom of the pan. Keep stirring until the mixture starts to thicken.

5 Put the meat and its drippings back into the pot. Add the water, bay leaves, salt, black pepper, thyme, paprika, and allspice. Bring to a boil, and then reduce the heat to simmer with the pot only partially covered for about 90 minutes. Check the pot occasionally and add more broth or water if it gets too dry.

6 Add the carrots and sweet potatoes to the pot and simmer an additional hour, until the vegetables are tender. Serve immediately.

Per serving: Calories 283 (From Fat 103); Fat 12g (Saturated 6g); Cholesterol 71mg; Sodium 614mg; Carbohydrate 20g; Dietary Fiber 3g; Protein 24g.

Pizza Frittata

Prep time: 15 min • **Cook time:** 20 min • **Yield:** 4 servings

Ingredients	Directions
12 large eggs	**1** Preheat the oven to 400 degrees.
1 teaspoon Italian Seasoning (see recipe in Chapter 14)	**2** In a large bowl, beat the eggs, Italian Seasoning, salt, and pepper until blended.
¾ teaspoon salt	
½ teaspoon ground black pepper	**3** Heat a large oven-safe skillet over medium-high heat and add coconut oil. When it's melted, add the onion and sauté until translucent, about 5 minutes. Add the bell pepper and tomatoes; cook until tender, about 5 minutes.
2 tablespoons coconut oil	
1 medium onion, diced	
1 cup diced green bell pepper	
1 cup grape tomatoes, halved	**4** Pour the beaten eggs into the pan and add the basil. Using a spatula to stir, gently scrape the bottom of the skillet to form large curds, about 2 minutes. Shake the pan to evenly distribute the ingredients and allow to cook undisturbed so the bottom sets, about 30 seconds.
8 large fresh basil leaves, coarsely chopped	
One 5-ounce package Applegate Farms Natural Pepperoni	
	5 Arrange the pepperoni slices on top of the frittata. Place the pan in the oven and bake until the top is puffed and beginning to brown, about 13 to 15 minutes. Remove the skillet from the oven and allow to set for 5 minutes, and then cut into wedges to serve.

Per serving: Calories 412 (From Fat 277), Fat 31g (Saturated 14g); Cholesterol 583mg; Sodium 956mg; Carbohydrate 9g; Dietary Fiber 2g; Protein 25g.

Tip: This dish is wonderful hot, straight out of the oven. It's also good at room temperature for a quick snack or lunch.

Vary It! Replace pepperoni with cooked ground beef or pork. Add variety with your other favorite pizza topping vegetables, like zucchini or eggplant slices, mushrooms, or artichoke hearts. Serve the frittata at lunch or dinner with a quick topping of arugula salad. Just toss fresh arugula with a little red wine vinegar, extra-virgin olive oil, salt, and pepper, and pile the greens on top of the hot or room temperature frittata.

Breakfast Sausage Scramble

Prep time: 10 min • **Cook time:** 20 min • **Yield:** 6 servings

Ingredients	Directions
1 pound ground pork	*1* Place pork in a large mixing bowl and add the applesauce, marjoram, thyme, nutmeg, ginger, cayenne pepper, salt, black pepper, and allspice. Knead with your hands until combined.
½ cup unsweetened applesauce	
¼ teaspoon ground marjoram	
½ teaspoon dried thyme leaves	*2* Heat a large skillet over medium-high heat and add the coconut oil. When it's melted, crumble the pork into the pan, using a wooden spoon to break up large clumps. Sauté the pork until it's browned and cooked through, about 10 minutes. Remove the pork to a bowl with a slotted spoon; set aside.
¼ teaspoon ground nutmeg	
¼ teaspoon ground ginger	
¼ teaspoon cayenne pepper	
¼ teaspoon salt	*3* Drain all but 1 tablespoon of fat from the pan. Add the onion and sauté until translucent, about 5 minutes. Add the bell pepper and cook until tender, about 5 minutes.
¼ teaspoon ground black pepper	
⅛ teaspoon allspice	
1 tablespoon coconut oil	*4* Add the pork back to the pan and stir to combine. Pour in the eggs and cook, stirring frequently, until set. Season with salt and pepper to taste. Serve immediately.
1 medium onion, diced	
1 large red bell pepper, diced	
10 large eggs, scrambled	
Salt and ground black pepper to taste	

Per serving: Calories 301 (From Fat 182); Fat 20g (Saturated 8g); Cholesterol 299mg; Sodium 319mg; Carbohydrate 6g; Dietary Fiber 1g; Protein 23g.

Vary It! Substitute ground turkey or chicken for the pork.

Tip: This sausage works great as patties, too. Just form 2-inch patties with the pork and cook in a hot skillet until evenly browned. They're an excellent accompaniment for Pumpkin Pancakes or Anytime Waffles (Chapter 13).

Huevos Rancheros

Prep time: 10 min • **Cook time:** 20 min • **Yield:** 4 servings

Ingredients	Directions
½ **tablespoon coconut oil**	*1* Heat a large skillet over medium-high heat and add coconut oil. When it's melted, add the onion and sauté until translucent, about 5 minutes. Add the garlic, cumin, cocoa, and cayenne pepper; cook until fragrant, about 30 seconds.
1 **medium onion, diced**	
2 **cloves garlic, minced**	
1 **teaspoon ground cumin**	
1 **teaspoon unsweetened cocoa**	*2* To the pan, add the tomatoes, green chiles, and chipotle chile. Stir to combine, taste, and season with salt and black pepper. Bring to a boil, and then reduce heat to simmer and cook until slightly thickened, about 15 minutes.
¼ **teaspoon cayenne pepper**	
Two 14.5-ounce cans diced fire-roasted tomatoes	
One 6-ounce can diced green Anaheim chiles	*3* Working in batches, if necessary, carefully purée the sauce in a food processor or blender. Return to the skillet.
1 **canned chipotle chile in adobo sauce, chopped**	
Salt and ground black pepper to taste	*4* With the back of a large spoon, make eight shallow wells in the sauce. Break an egg into a cup, and then carefully pour the egg into the well in the sauce; repeat with the rest of the eggs. Sprinkle each egg with salt and pepper, and then cover the pan and cook over medium-low heat until the eggs are cooked: 4 to 5 minutes for runny yolks, 6 to 7 minutes for set yolks.
8 **fresh eggs**	
Garnishes: minced fresh cilantro, diced avocado, fresh lime juice (optional)	
	5 Serve immediately, dividing the sauce and eggs among four plates. Sprinkle with cilantro, avocado, and a squeeze of lime juice.

Per serving: *Calories 235 (From Fat 108); Fat 12g (Saturated 5g); Cholesterol 372mg; Sodium 837mg; Carbohydrate 15g; Dietary Fiber 3g; Protein 15g.*

Vary It! If you prefer fried eggs to poached, fry the eggs separately in a little coconut oil and then top them with the ranchero sauce.

Note: The sauce can be made ahead of time and frozen or stored in the refrigerator for a quick weekday breakfast.

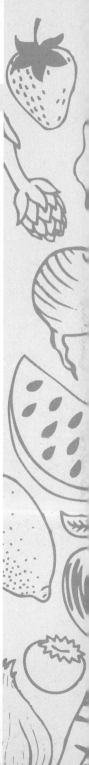

Slow Cooker Pork and Sauerkraut

Prep time: 15 min • **Cook time:** 8–10 hr • **Yield:** 8 servings

Ingredients	*Directions*
2 pounds boneless pork shoulder, trimmed of excess fat and blotted dry	*1* Cut the pork shoulder into 3- to 4-inch chunks and season generously with salt and pepper. Heat a large skillet over medium-high heat and add coconut oil.
Salt and ground black pepper to taste	
½ tablespoon coconut oil	*2* When oil is melted, add the pork, browning on all sides. You'll probably need to cook the pork in two batches so you don't overcrowd the pan. Transfer pork to the slow cooker.
2 medium onions, thinly sliced	
3 cloves garlic, minced	*3* In the same pan, cook the onions until translucent, about 5 minutes. Add the garlic and cook until fragrant, about 30 seconds. Transfer the onions and garlic to the slow cooker. Add the bay leaf.
1 bay leaf	
Three 14.5-ounce cans sauerkraut	*4* Place the sauerkraut in a colander and rinse with cold water. Squeeze out excess moisture and pile the sauerkraut on top of the pork. Cover the slow cooker and cook on low until the pork is fork tender, about 8 to 10 hours.

Per serving: Calories 203 (From Fat 98); Fat 11g (Saturated 4g); Cholesterol 66mg; Sodium 831mg; Carbohydrate 6g; Dietary Fiber 3g; Protein 20g.

Note: You can use sauerkraut from a can or bag; just check the ingredient label for non-Paleo ingredients.

Tip: Serve with unsweetened applesauce and Mashed Cauliflower (Chapter 12).

Slow Cooker BBQ Pulled Pork

Prep time: 15 min • **Cook time:** 8–10 hr • **Yield:** 4 servings

Ingredients	Directions
2 tablespoons smoked paprika	**1** In a small bowl, mix the paprika, black pepper, cumin, cocoa, and salt with a fork.
2 tablespoons ground black pepper	
2 tablespoons ground cumin	**2** Cut the pork into 2-inch chunks and place in a large bowl.
1 tablespoon unsweetened cocoa powder	**3** Add the spices to the pork and toss until evenly coated.
1 tablespoon salt	
2 pounds boneless pork shoulder, trimmed of excess fat and blotted dry	**4** Transfer the pork to the slow cooker, cover, and cook for 8 to 10 hours, until the pork is browned and fork tender.

Per serving: Calories 370 (From Fat 191); Fat 21g (Saturated 7g); Cholesterol 132mg; Sodium 1,862mg; Carbohydrate 6g; Dietary Fiber 3g; Protein 39g.

Tip: Use two forks to shred the pork and toss with Tangy BBQ Sauce (Chapter 14). Serve with Classic Cole Slaw and Sweet Potato Shoestring Fries (Chapter 12).

Vary It! Use this spice blend on baby back ribs, beef roast, beef short ribs, or chicken. You can mix and match various meats in the same slow cooker for a BBQ feast.

Slow Cooker Moroccan Apricot Chicken

Prep time: 1 hr • **Cook time:** 5½ hr • **Yield:** 8 servings

Ingredients	Directions
4 cloves garlic, minced	**1** In a large bowl, combine garlic, ginger, coriander, cumin, pepper, and salt. Add chicken and toss to coat.
½ tablespoon dried ginger	
2 teaspoons ground coriander	**2** Heat a large skillet over medium-high heat and add coconut oil. When it's melted, add the chicken in batches and brown on all sides. Transfer chicken to slow cooker.
1 teaspoon ground cumin	
1 teaspoon ground black pepper	
¾ teaspoon salt	**3** To the slow cooker, add the chicken broth, lemon juice, and cinnamon stick. Cover and cook on low for 4 to 5 hours, until the chicken is tender.
2 pounds boneless, skinless chicken thighs	
1 tablespoon coconut oil	
¾ cup chicken broth	**4** Add apricots and lemon zest to the slow cooker. Cover and cook on high for 30 minutes to allow flavors to meld.
¼ cup lemon juice	
1 cinnamon stick	
16 pitted, dried apricots (about ½ cup)	**5** To serve, sprinkle with almonds and chopped cilantro (if desired).
1 tablespoon grated lemon zest (about 2 lemons)	
¼ cup sliced almonds, toasted	
Garnish: chopped fresh cilantro leaves (optional)	

Per serving: Calories 224 (From Fat 108); Fat 12g (Saturated 4g); Cholesterol 76mg; Sodium 377mg; Carbohydrate 6g; Dietary Fiber 1g; Protein 22g.

Tip: Serve over Cauliflower Rice or Mashed Cauliflower (Chapter 12).

Vary it! Replace the chicken thighs with cubed, boneless lamb. You can also substitute dried prunes or dates for the apricots.

Chapter 12

Vegetable Side Dishes

In This Chapter

▶ Making the most of fresh vegetables in delicious salads

▶ Discovering exciting, flavorful side dishes to replace your favorite grains

Although vegetables are often called a side dish, they move to center stage when you're eating Paleo — and with the recipes in this chapter, you'll be glad they do. Eating too many vegetables is nearly impossible, so dig into these recipes and fill your plate.

In this chapter, you find recipes that are healthy, tasty stand-ins for some of your non-Paleo favorites, like rice, mashed potatoes, and noodles. These options have more flavor and tongue-pleasing texture than their traditional counterparts, and they're chock-full of vitamins and minerals.

Satisfying Your Paleo Palate with Cool Side Salads

Nothing says picnic or potluck like a big bowl of bright, fresh salad tossed with a flavorful dressing. And a colorful chopped salad brings that same sense of fun to your dining table any time of year.

 TIP

If you're cooking for one or two, you may want to cut the salad recipes in half to ensure that they taste fresh and crisp each time you eat them. Also, all the salad recipes work well when doubled. These salads hold up for about three days in the refrigerator.

Evolving Past Starches: Paleo-Friendly Hot Side Dishes

The right side dish can elevate a boring pork chop or bunless hamburger to favorite-dinner status. The hot vegetable side dishes in this chapter are ambitious and step away from the norm of steamed-and-buttered to deliver lots of flavor and interesting texture. We cover all the favorite variations of the starch family — mashed, fries, fritters, noodles, and rice — without a problematic grain in sight.

If your family is skeptical about replacing grains with vegetables, try a new spin. Instead of telling them that you're substituting their old favorites with vegetables, promote the new side dish as the latest gourmet invention. If your family ate Cauliflower Rice or Zucchini Noodles in a restaurant, they'd probably be impressed. So put on your chef's hat and talk up your new menu like a pro.

Shopping locally

When shopping for high-quality ingredients to use in the recipes in this book, you may be surprised to find them right under your nose at the following local food shops:

- **Traditional grocery stores:** Many grocery stores stock at least a small assortment of grass-fed, pastured meat, cage-free eggs, and wild-caught seafood, organic produce, and many alternative pantry items, such as coconut oil. If you don't see what you need, ask an employee; the store may stock items on request.

- **Big-box retailers:** A lot of large-scale retailers and membership stores carry grass-fed meat and organic produce in bulk. That means lower prices and larger quantities (so you can shop less often). Just stock up and sock away extras in the freezer.

- **Natural food markets:** No longer the domain of hippies, natural food markets are a great option for quality meats, organic produce, and bulk pantry items like coconut flakes and nuts. Explore your options locally to find the mix of stores that works for you.

- **Farmers' markets:** Produce at the farmers' market is fresher than anything you'll find in the grocery store. Most of the produce in a traditional store is at least several days old, but when you shop at the farmers' market, the produce is fresh, and you know you're eating what's in season. The produce at the market is often riper than its store counterparts because it's picked at its peak. And because you're cutting out the middleman, produce — especially organic produce — is usually priced lower. You can also feel great about supporting your local family farm while you're enjoying how much better the fruits and vegetables taste.

Chopped Salad with Tahini Dressing

Prep time: 15 min • **Yield:** 6–8 servings

Ingredients	Directions
⅓ cup tahini sauce	*1* Place tahini sauce, lemon juice, water, and garlic in a food processor. Blend until smooth, taste, and season with salt and pepper. Set aside.
⅓ cup lemon juice	
⅓ cup water	
1 garlic clove, crushed	
Salt and ground black pepper to taste	*2* Place the minced parsley in a large bowl. Dice all the vegetables into ¼-inch cubes and add to the parsley. Slice the olives and add to the bowl. Drizzle olive oil over the vegetables, season with salt and pepper, and toss until coated.
1 cup fresh parsley leaves, minced (about ¼ cup)	
2 medium cucumbers, peeled	
1 medium red bell pepper, seeded	*3* Pile vegetables on individual salad plates and drizzle with 2 tablespoons of the tahini dressing. Store leftover salad and tahini dressing in the refrigerator, covered, for up to three days.
1 medium green bell pepper, seeded	
3 medium tomatoes	
½ medium red onion	
1 bunch radishes	
One 6-ounce can large black pitted olives	
½ tablespoon extra-virgin olive oil	

Per serving: Calories 166 (From Fat 103); Fat 11g (Saturated 1g); Cholesterol 0mg; Sodium 267mg; Carbohydrate 15g; Dietary Fiber 3g; Protein 4g.

Note: You can find tahini sauce (ground sesame seeds) in the international section of most grocery and health food stores.

Vary It! Just about any raw vegetable works great in this salad. Try adding slivered red cabbage, fresh fennel, or a few hot peppers.

Tip: This salad is a big hit at potluck dinners — just double the recipe and serve the dressing on the side. No one will even notice that it's Paleo.

Vietnamese Cucumber Salad

Prep time: 2 min • **Yield:** 4–6 servings

Ingredients	*Directions*
2 English (seedless) cucumbers	*1* Cut cucumbers in half lengthwise, and slice into very thin half-moons. Place in a large bowl.
2 medium carrots	
4 medium radishes	*2* Finely dice the carrots, radishes, and jalapeño; add to cucumbers and toss until combined.
1 small jalapeño	
1 clove garlic, minced	*3* In a medium bowl, place the garlic, cashews, basil, mint, lime juice, rice vinegar, olive oil, and coconut aminos. Whisk until combined.
2 tablespoons dry roasted cashews, finely chopped	
6 to 8 large basil leaves, finely chopped (about 2 tablespoons)	*4* Pour dressing over vegetables and toss until evenly coated, about 2 minutes. Taste and season with salt and pepper. Allow flavors to meld for 10 minutes and serve.
10 fresh mint leaves, finely chopped (about 1½ tablespoons)	
1 tablespoon lime juice	
1 tablespoon rice vinegar	
½ teaspoon olive oil	
1 tablespoon coconut aminos	
Salt and ground black pepper to taste	

Per serving: Calories 109 (From Fat 23); Fat 3g (Saturated 1g); Cholesterol 0mg; Sodium 255mg; Carbohydrate 18g; Dietary Fiber 3g; Protein 3g.

Tip: Add cooked chicken, pork, or shrimp to make this salad a complete meal.

Vary It! Make spring rolls by spreading a butter lettuce leaf with ½ teaspoon Homemade Mayonnaise (Chapter 14). Place a large spoonful of cucumber salad in the leaf and roll to form a spring roll shape.

Classic Cole Slaw

Prep time: 15 min • **Yield:** 4 servings

Ingredients	Directions
⅔ **cup Homemade Mayonnaise (see recipe in Chapter 14)**	**1** In a small bowl, whisk together the Homemade Mayonnaise, red onion, lemon juice, vinegar, honey (if desired), salt, and pepper. Set aside.
2 tablespoons grated red onion	
1 tablespoon lemon juice	**2** In a large bowl, toss the cabbage, carrots, and parsley with two wooden spoons. Add the dressing and toss vigorously for 2 minutes to ensure that the vegetables are evenly coated. Cover and refrigerate for at least 1 hour before serving.
1 tablespoon white wine vinegar	
½ **tablespoon honey (optional)**	
½ **teaspoon salt**	
¼ **teaspoon ground black pepper**	
1 head green cabbage, very thinly sliced	
3 large carrots, shredded	
½ **cup loosely packed parsley leaves, roughly chopped**	

Per serving: Calories 392 (From Fat 287); Fat 32g (Saturated 2g); Cholesterol 21mg; Sodium 513mg; Carbohydrate 23g; Dietary Fiber 8g; Protein 5g.

Note: To cut the cabbage, slice in half through the stem end. Remove and discard the tough inner core, and then thinly slice the cabbage into long, thin shreds.

Vary It! Add 1 to 2 teaspoons of caraway seeds for a traditional German touch, or make it a little sweeter by adding 1 cup shredded canned pineapple (unsweetened, packed in its own juice) or ⅓ cup raisins. You can also replace the whole head of green cabbage with half a head of green and half a head of red for colorful variety.

Tip: This recipe is easy to double for a potluck or cut in half for a dinner-for-two serving. This slaw tastes better the second day, so make it in advance if time permits.

Ambrosia Salad with Whipped Coconut Cream

Prep time: 25 min • **Yield:** 8 servings

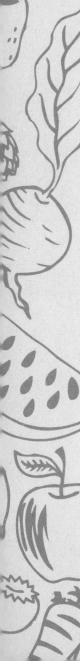

Ingredients	*Directions*
¾ **cup unsweetened shredded coconut, toasted**	**1** Heat a large sauté pan over medium-high heat. When the pan is hot, add the shredded coconut and pecans and stir constantly until lightly toasted, about 3 to 5 minutes. Sprinkle with salt and toss to coat. Remove from the pan and reserve for later.
¾ **cup pecans, toasted and coarsely chopped**	
⅛ **teaspoon salt**	
2 large seedless oranges	**2** Peel the oranges with a sharp knife and remove all the bitter white pulp. Separate the sections and cut into 1-inch pieces. Place in a large bowl.
One 14.5-ounce can crushed pineapple, unsweetened and packed in its own juice	
1 cup fresh cherries, pitted and halved	**3** Drain the juice from the pineapple and add the pineapple to the oranges. Add the coconut, pecans, and cherries to the bowl, and toss gently with a rubber scraper to combine.
Whipped Coconut Cream (see the following recipe)	
	4 Gently fold the Whipped Coconut Cream into the fruit with the rubber scraper and mix until just combined. Chill for at least 15 minutes before serving.

Whipped Coconut Cream

One 14.5-ounce can coconut milk, chilled in the refrigerator overnight

1 teaspoon almond or vanilla extract

1 Remove the can of coconut milk from the refrigerator and place in the freezer for 10 minutes, along with a mixing bowl and beaters from a stand or hand mixer.

2 When the coconut milk is cold, flip the can upside down and open the bottom with a can opener. Pour off the liquid that's accumulated at the bottom. Scoop out the thickened coconut milk into the chilled mixing bowl.

3 Add the almond extract and whip on your mixer's highest setting until the milk is fluffy and has the texture of whipped cream, about 5 to 7 minutes.

Per serving: Calories 296 (From Fat 215); Fat 24g (Saturated 15g); Cholesterol 0mg; Sodium 46mg; Carbohydrate 21g; Dietary Fiber 4g; Protein 3g.

Making foods look fun

Getting some kids to eat healthy can be a chore, and you may have trouble convincing your kids to try some of the veggie side dishes in this chapter. Have you ever had a meal with a kid who examines his plate as if he was the lead investigator of a crime scene? Texture is important to kids but so is presentation. Kids are visual when it comes to food.

When your brain see's something colorful and yummy, you get a desire for that food and immediately begin to release enzymes, which help in breaking your food down. You may be able to get your kids to eat something just by cutting the food in to the shape of a heart or adding a smiley face. Here are some other tools to make food look fun and appealing.

- **Cookie cutters:** Pick some shapes your kids like and use them on any foods you can. Keep a bunch on hand.

- **Ladle:** Use a ladle to put foods in mounds, to look like mountains. You can use different sizes for different effects.

- **Food for faces:** Use whatever foods you can, like raisins, olives, baby carrots, or apple slices, to add eyes, noses, and mouths or other designs on foods. Make it funny — kids love humor!

- **Lunchbox beauty:** Make packed lunches look as attractive as possible. Use lunchboxes with compartments to make lunch look colorful and attractive.

- **Fun plates and cups:** Invest in plates or cups in shapes or colors that your kids find fun and adventurous to eat from.

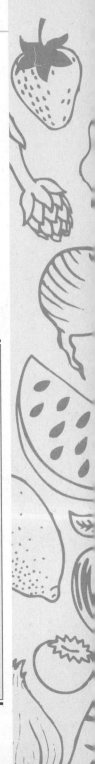

Sesame Kale

Prep time: 15 min • **Cook time:** 12 min • **Yield:** 4 servings

Ingredients	Directions
1 tablespoon sesame seeds	**1** Heat a large sauté pan or wok over medium-high heat. When the pan is hot, add the sesame seeds and stir constantly until they're lightly toasted, about 3 to 5 minutes. Remove from pan and reserve for later.
1 bunch fresh kale, washed, ribs removed, coarsely chopped	
⅓ cup water	**2** Wash the kale and remove any tough and/or thick ribs, and then roughly chop or tear the leaves. Place the water in the skillet and bring to a boil over high heat.
1 tablespoon sesame oil	
½ teaspoon ginger	
Dash cayenne pepper	**3** Add half the kale to the boiling water and stir with a wooden spoon until it begins to wilt, and then add the rest of the leaves. Cover and allow the kale to steam until tender, about 5 to 6 minutes.
Salt and ground black pepper to taste	
	4 Remove the lid and allow any remaining water to evaporate. Turn off the heat and drizzle the kale with the sesame oil, tossing to coat. Sprinkle with ginger, cayenne pepper, salt, and black pepper; toss again. Sprinkle with sesame seeds just before serving.

Per serving: Calories 76 (From Fat 44); Fat 5g (Saturated 1g); Cholesterol 0mg; Sodium 174mg; Carbohydrate 8g; Dietary Fiber 3g; Protein 3g.

Vary It! This basic recipe works well with other greens, like collards, beet tops, and spinach. You can also vary the flavors with different oils. For Italian flair, use olive oil in place of sesame oil, and replace the ginger with crushed garlic.

Sweet Potato Shoestring Fries

Prep time: 10 min • **Cook time:** 40 min • **Yield:** 4 servings

Ingredients	*Directions*
2 large sweet potatoes	***1*** Preheat the oven to 450 degrees. Cover two baking sheets with parchment paper.
1 tablespoon arrowroot powder	
2 tablespoons coconut oil	***2*** Cut sweet potatoes into ⅛- to ¼-inch strips. Place in a large bowl, add the arrowroot powder, and toss until the fries are lightly coated.
½ tablespoon ground cumin	
1 teaspoon chili powder	***3*** In a small bowl, combine the coconut oil, cumin, chili powder, cinnamon, thyme, salt, and pepper. Heat in the microwave for 15 to 20 seconds, until the coconut oil is melted. Stir with a fork to combine.
¼ teaspoon ground cinnamon	
¼ teaspoon dried thyme	
¼ teaspoon salt, plus more to taste	***4*** Add the seasoned coconut oil to the sweet potatoes and toss with two wooden spoons to evenly coat the fries with the oil.
¼ teaspoon ground black pepper	
	5 Arrange coated fries on the baking sheets, making sure the fries aren't touching. Bake for 15 minutes, and then flip and bake an additional 15 to 20 minutes, until desired crispness.
	6 Remove from the oven, sprinkle with additional salt, and serve immediately.

Per serving: Calories 164 (From Fat 65); Fat 7g (Saturated 6g); Cholesterol 0mg; Sodium 164mg; Carbohydrate 24g; Dietary Fiber 3g; Protein 2g.

Note: If using organic sweet potatoes, keep the skin on. If using conventionally grown potatoes, peel them.

Tip: These fries are great with bunless burgers, Slow Cooker BBQ Pulled Pork (Chapter 11), or eggs for a fun and fancy brunch. Dip them in Cave Man Ketchup, or eat them the Belgian way with seasoned Homemade Mayonnaise (both recipes in Chapter 14).

Vary It! Change the seasonings! Try Garam Masala or Morning Spice (both recipes in Chapter 14), smoked paprika, or a little garlic powder for extra zing.

Spaghetti Squash Fritters

Prep time: 10 min • **Cook time:** 5 min • **Yield:** 4 servings

Ingredients	*Directions*
½ onion, finely minced	**1** In a large bowl, mix onion, almond flour, eggs, salt, and pepper with a whisk until combined. Squeeze any excess moisture from the squash with a clean dish towel or paper towels, add to the bowl, and mix well. Allow the batter to rest 10 minutes.
½ cup almond flour	
3 large eggs	
½ teaspoon salt	
½ teaspoon ground black pepper	**2** Place ½ tablespoon coconut oil in a nonstick skillet and heat over medium-high heat until the oil is melted and shimmers. Swivel the pan to coat the bottom.
1 spaghetti squash, roasted and shredded (about 4 cups)	
1 to 2 tablespoons coconut oil	**3** Drop ¼-cup servings of batter into the pan, making sure they don't touch. Cook until browned on the bottom and starting to set, about 4 to 5 minutes. Flip gently and cook the other side until browned, an additional 3 to 4 minutes.
	4 Cook in batches, adding more coconut oil to the pan as necessary. Serve hot.

Per serving: Calories 197 (From Fat 130); Fat 14g (Saturated 5g); Cholesterol 140mg; Sodium 359mg; Carbohydrate 8g; Dietary Fiber 3g; Protein 9g.

Note: See the Spaghetti Squash and Meatballs recipe in Chapter 10 for instructions on how to roast the spaghetti squash.

Tip: These fritters are great topped with browned ground beef or lamb, served with Hearty Chili or enjoyed alongside grilled meats and Slow Cooker Moroccan Apricot Chicken (see recipes in Chapter 11).

Vary It! Substitute shredded zucchini for the spaghetti squash; just follow the instructions for Zucchini Noodles (later in this chapter) to prep the zucchini.

Mashed Cauliflower

Prep time: 5 min • **Cook time:** 5 min • **Yield:** 2–4 servings

Ingredients	Directions
2 garlic cloves	*1* Peel the garlic and cook along with the cauliflower, following the package directions, until the cauliflower is very soft but not waterlogged.
One 16-ounce bag frozen cauliflower florets	
1½ tablespoons coconut oil	*2* In a microwave-safe bowl or small saucepan, heat the coconut oil, coconut milk, thyme, salt, and pepper about 1 minute.
½ cup coconut milk	
2 teaspoons dried thyme leaves	*3* Meanwhile, purée the cauliflower in a food processor, scraping down the sides. Add the coconut milk and process about 10 seconds. Taste and adjust seasonings.
Salt and ground black pepper to taste	

Per serving: Calories 289 (From Fat 227); Fat 25g (Saturated 22g); Cholesterol 0mg; Sodium 356mg; Carbohydrate 16g; Dietary Fiber 7g; Protein 6g.

Note: You can use fresh cauliflower for this recipe, but frozen cauliflower packs the same nutritional punch and reaches a creamy texture faster and easier than fresh.

Vary It! Try substituting parsley or chives for the dried thyme. You may also use chicken broth in place of the coconut milk.

Zucchini Noodles

Prep time: 35 min • **Cook time:** 3 min • **Yield:** 4 servings

Ingredients	Directions
6 medium zucchini, sliced with a julienne peeler (about 6 cups)	**1** Place the julienned zucchini in a colander or wire strainer and toss generously with salt until the strands are lightly coated. Allow the zucchini to sit for 20 to 30 minutes. Rinse with running water, drain well, and squeeze dry in a clean dish towel.
2 tablespoons extra-virgin olive oil	
1 clove garlic, minced (about 2 teaspoons)	**2** Heat a large skillet over medium-high heat. Sauté the zucchini noodles in the dry pan until they're just tender, stirring them constantly with a wooden spoon, about 2 minutes. Push the noodles to the side of the pan, and reduce the heat to low.
Salt and ground black pepper to taste	
	3 Add the olive oil and garlic to the pan, stirring with a wooden spoon until the garlic is fragrant, about 20 seconds. Push the zucchini noodles into the oil and stir gently until they're coated. Turn off the heat and season the noodles with salt and pepper.

Per serving: Calories 102 (From Fat 65); Fat 7g (Saturated 1g); Cholesterol 0mg; Sodium 154mg; Carbohydrate 9g; Dietary Fiber 4g; Protein 4g.

Note: Sweating the zucchini noodles with salt is essential so they don't become watery and limp during cooking. If you use this technique, the result is zucchini noodles with the texture of al dente pasta.

Tip: Substitute Zucchini Noodles in the Spaghetti Squash and Meatballs recipe (Chapter 10), or add fresh herbs to the noodles and enjoy as a side dish with grilled or roasted meats and seafood. You can also put Zucchini Noodles in a deep bowl with cooked protein and cover with hot broth for a quick soup.

Cauliflower Rice

Prep time: 10 min • **Cook time:** 10 min • **Yield:** 4–6 servings

Ingredients	Directions
1 large head fresh cauliflower	**1** Break the cauliflower into florets, removing the stems. Place the florets in a food processor and pulse until the cauliflower looks like rice, about ten to fifteen 1-second pulses. You may need to do this step in two batches.
1½ tablespoons coconut oil	
½ medium onion, diced (about ½ cup)	
1 clove garlic, minced (about 1 teaspoon)	**2** Heat a large skillet over medium heat, about 3 minutes. Add the coconut oil and allow it to melt. Add the onion and garlic, and cook gently until the onions are translucent, about 7 minutes.
Salt and ground black pepper to taste	
	3 Add the riced cauliflower to the pan and sauté until the cauliflower is tender, about 5 to 7 minutes. Taste and season with salt and pepper.

Per serving: Calories 106 (From Fat 50); Fat 6g (Saturated 5g); Cholesterol 0mg; Sodium 209mg; Carbohydrate 13g; Dietary Fiber 6g; Protein 5g.

Vary It! Make curry fried rice by adding 1 teaspoon of curry powder to the cooked Cauliflower Rice, along with 2 tablespoons each of sliced almonds and raisins.

The power of cauliflower

Generally speaking, the brighter or darker the color of the vegetable, the better it is for you. But don't be fooled by cauliflower's pale color; it packs a nutritional wallop.

Loaded with vitamin C, cauliflower is a rich source of antioxidants, including beta carotene and other phytonutrients. It also helps fight inflammation, thanks to high amounts of vitamin K and omega-3 fatty acids, and it's a good source of thiamine (B1), riboflavin (B2), folic acid (B9), phosphorus, and potassium.

Creamy Spiced Broccoli

Prep time: 5 min • **Cook time:** 10 min • **Yield:** 4 servings

Ingredients	*Directions*
1 large bunch broccoli, broken into small florets	*1* Heat a large skillet over medium-high heat, and add the broccoli and water. Bring to a boil and cover, steaming the broccoli until bright green and beginning to soften, about 5 to 7 minutes.
¼ cup water	
2 teaspoons Garam Masala (see recipe in Chapter 14)	*2* In a small bowl, mix the Garam Masala, garlic, and salt with a fork. Set aside.
2 cloves fresh garlic, minced	
Pinch of salt	*3* Remove the lid from the broccoli and allow any remaining water to evaporate. When the pan is mostly dry, push the broccoli to the side and add the coconut oil. Let the oil warm up, and then pour the spices directly into the pool of oil to release their fragrance and flavor, about 20 seconds.
1 teaspoon coconut oil	
½ cup coconut milk	
	4 Pour the coconut milk into the pan, stirring to combine the broccoli, seasonings, and liquid. Sauté until the sauce begins to thicken and serve immediately.

Per serving: Calories 105 (From Fat 78); Fat 9g (Saturated 7g); Cholesterol 0mg; Sodium 60mg; Carbohydrate 7g; Dietary Fiber 3g; Protein 3g.

Tip: Make this dish a complete meal by adding cooked chicken, beef, lamb, pork, or seafood during the last step.

Vary It! Substitute green beans or braising greens, such as chard, kale, or collards, for the broccoli.

Chapter 13

Snacks and Treats

In This Chapter

▶ Staying on track with healthy snacks and treats

▶ Discovering delicious recipes that make living Paleo easy

The foods on the Paleo "yes" list (see Chapter 2) are among the tastiest we can eat, but every once in a while, even the most devoted cave man (or woman) wants a treat with that little something extra. The key to living Paleo is choosing treats that are based on healthful, natural ingredients that don't make you feel like you swallowed a bowling ball.

In this chapter, you discover recipes for healthy snacks that satisfy your craving for a salty crunch or a sweet treat. From toasty coconut chips and a fresh take on deviled eggs to a classic apple crisp and chocolaty fudge balls, you see how deliciously easy it is to adapt tasty snacks and treats to fit into your new lifestyle.

Making Sure Your Snacks Are Healthy

When you eat foods from the Paleo "yes" list, you most likely find avoiding snacks between meals effortless, because Paleo foods are more filling and satisfying. But if a workout leaves you particularly hungry or your stomach is growling between lunch and dinner, the snack and treat recipes in this chapter will help ensure that you treat your body — and your taste buds — right.

 Remember the Paleo Big Three: proteins, fats, and carbs. Snacks should be half the size of your standard meals and, ideally, should include protein, healthy fats, and veggie or fruit to maintain steady blood sugar levels. In a pinch, combine at least two of the three, but avoid eating fruit on its own. For more on the Paleo Big Three, see Chapter 4.

Indulging with fruit and desserts

Nothing's wrong with enjoying something a little sweet from time to time. But when you do decide to indulge, make sure to savor every bite and to choose treats that include nutritious ingredients.

The fruit and nut flour–based recipes in this chapter are best enjoyed with protein and fat, so eat them as part of your meal rather than as a snack between meals or before bed.

To make the most of your dessert, keep your serving sizes small and relish every single bite.

Enjoying Paleo-friendly, grain-free goodies

The grain-free treats in this chapter (pancakes, waffles, and coffee cake) are technically Paleo but are higher in natural sugars and fats than standard meals of protein, vegetables, and fat. These recipes are much healthier options than traditional pancakes, waffles, and coffee cake, but they're still treats, which means they're meant for occasional indulgences, special occasions, and celebrations. Why not designate one Sunday a month as "Waffle Brunch Day" or plan a "Breakfast for Dinner" night once a week to turn an ordinary day into something special!

To make the most of your grain-free goodies, always eat them with high-quality protein, savor every bite, and throughout the rest of the day, try to minimize your intake of nuts and fruit.

Cocoa-Cinnamon Coconut Chips

Prep time: 1 min • **Cook time:** 3 min • **Yield:** 1 cup

Ingredients	Directions
¼ teaspoon salt	*1* In a small bowl, mix the salt, cocoa, and cinnamon with a fork; set aside.
¼ teaspoon unsweetened cocoa powder	
¼ teaspoon ground cinnamon	*2* Heat a nonstick skillet over medium-high heat, about 2 minutes. Add the coconut flakes and distribute evenly so that they form a single layer in the bottom of the pan. Stir frequently. When the flakes start to golden, remove the pan from the heat.
1 cup unsweetened coconut flakes	
	3 Sprinkle the spices on the hot coconut flakes and toss until evenly seasoned. Transfer to a plate, arrange in a single layer, and allow them to cool and crisp. Store in an air-tight container.

Per serving (1 teaspoon): Calories 40 (From Fat 33); Fat 4g (Saturated 3g); Cholesterol 0mg; Sodium 38mg; Carbohydrate 1g; Dietary Fiber 1g; Protein 0g.

Tip: These chips are great on their own for a snack, or you can sprinkle them over fresh fruit for a dessert treat.

Vary It! Tickle your taste buds by seasoning these chips with other flavors. Just replace the cocoa and cinnamon with ¼ teaspoon of another spice. Other tempting options include garlic powder, chili powder, or Morning Spice or Garam Masala (recipes in Chapter 14). Toss these savory chips in a salad for a healthy alternative to croutons.

Coconut's super powers

Coconut is one of our favorite Paleo foods because it provides so many luscious options for eating: coconut flakes, coconut milk, coconut oil, coconut butter, and coconut aminos.

But coconut is also a superfood with plenty of health benefits. It helps with digestion, which aids in the absorption of vitamins and minerals to build healthy bones and tissues. Coconut also improves your body's insulin management and use of blood sugar, while also supporting the immune system and thyroid function. Delicious and nutritious, coconut is an excellent choice for snacks and meals.

Crispy Kale Chips

Prep time: 2 min • **Cook time:** 10–12 min • **Yield:** 3 servings

Ingredients	Directions
4 cups raw kale, washed, dried, and torn into 2-inch pieces	*1* Preheat the oven to 350 degrees.
1 tablespoon coconut oil, melted	*2* Place kale in a large bowl and pour the coconut oil over the top. Toss the leaves with two wooden spoons until completely coated with oil, about 2 minutes.
Salt to taste	*3* Spread the kale on a baking sheet in a single layer and sprinkle generously with salt.
	4 Bake for 10 to 12 minutes until crispy and lightly browned on the edges. Keep an eye on the kale chips! They can change from brown to burnt quite quickly.
	5 Remove baking sheet and allow to cool on cooling rack for 3 minutes. The chips are crispier after they cool.

Per serving: Calories 84 (From Fat 46); Fat 5g (Saturated 4g); Cholesterol 0mg; Sodium 232mg; Carbohydrate 9g; Dietary Fiber 2g; Protein 3g

Tip: Eat these chips fairly soon after baking — they can begin to wilt after about 30 minutes out of the oven.

Vary It! Adapting your favorite potato chip flavors to kale chips is easy! Just add additional spices along with the salt before baking. For barbecue flavor, add ½ teaspoon chili powder mixed with ½ teaspoon paprika. For onion flavor, replace the plain salt with onion salt.

Kale packs a punch — of nutrients, that is

Kale is one of the healthiest vegetables you can eat! As a member of the cabbage family, kale is loaded with antioxidants, anti-inflammatory properties, and nutrients, including folic acid, manganese, potassium, and vitamins B6, C, and K. Kale also includes a chemical called *glucosinolates* that's metabolized by your body into powerful cancer-fighting molecules called *isothiocyanates.*

Because it's high in fiber, kale helps you feel satisfied after a meal or snack, so kale chips not only taste good, but they're also good for you. Unlike traditional snacks, kale helps manage your appetite in a positive way.

Nutty Fruit Stackers

Prep time: 2 min • **Yield:** 2 servings

Ingredients	Directions
1 raw apple	*1* With a sharp knife, cut the apple into six equal slices.
2 tablespoons almond butter	
¼ teaspoon pure vanilla extract	*2* In a small bowl, mix almond butter, vanilla, cinnamon, and salt with a fork until combined.
¼ teaspoon ground cinnamon	*3* Spread each slice of apple with 1 teaspoon of almond butter. Pile slices to form stacks of three slices each. Sprinkle the top of each stack with ½ tablespoon raisins.
Dash of salt	
1 tablespoon raisins	
	4 Chill in the refrigerator for 5 minutes before eating.

Per serving: Calories 159 (From Fat 88); Fat 10g (Saturated 1g); Cholesterol 0mg; Sodium 73mg; Carbohydrate 18g; Dietary Fiber 3g; Protein 3g.

Tip: This snack is also a sweet treat, so be sure to serve it with some protein to balance the sugars. A piece of grilled chicken breast or a hard-boiled egg is a good accompaniment.

Vary It! This recipe also works great with pears! Or change the flavor by swapping out the almond butter with another Paleo-friendly option, such as sunflower seed butter with a few sunflower seeds sprinkled on with the raisins. You may also like cashew or pecan butter. Or try coconut butter and add a sprinkle of shredded, unsweetened coconut to the top.

Southwest Deviled Eggs

Prep time: 25 min • **Yield:** 12 egg halves

Ingredients	*Directions*
6 large eggs	**1** Place the eggs in a saucepan and cover with water. Bring to a boil over high heat. Remove the pan from the heat, cover, and let sit for 10 minutes.
2 tablespoons Homemade Mayonnaise (see recipe in Chapter 14)	
½ teaspoon white wine vinegar	**2** Drain the water from the eggs and shake the pan to lightly crack the shells. Fill the pan with cold water and allow the eggs to cool for 5 minutes.
¼ teaspoon dry mustard	
¼ teaspoon chipotle pepper powder	**3** Peel the eggs and slice in half lengthwise. Using a spoon, gently remove the yolks and place in a mixing bowl. Add the Homemade Mayonnaise, vinegar, mustard, chipotle pepper powder, salt, and black pepper. Mix well with a fork, mashing until the yolks form a smooth paste.
⅛ teaspoon salt	
⅛ teaspoon ground black pepper	
¼ ripe avocado, finely diced	
½ ripe tomato, finely diced	**4** Arrange the egg whites on a serving platter and fill the wells with the seasoned yolk, making a small mound about half an inch above the whites. Top with a little avocado, tomato, and scallion. Serve immediately.
1 scallion, green only, thinly sliced	

Per serving: Calories 63 (From Fat 46); Fat 5g (Saturated 1g); Cholesterol 94mg; Sodium 65mg; Carbohydrate 1g; Dietary Fiber 0g; Protein 3g.

Note: You can find chipotle pepper powder in many grocery stores and through online spice vendors. If you have trouble finding it, chili powder is a good replacement. You can also substitute 1 teaspoon finely minced canned chipotle pepper; be sure to check the label for non-Paleo ingredients.

Tip: Very fresh eggs are difficult to peel. For success with hard-boiled eggs, buy a dozen and let them rest in the refrigerator for about a week before hard boiling; just keep an eye on their expiration date.

Tropical Mango Parfait

Prep time: 15 min • **Yield:** 4 servings

Ingredients	Directions
2 to 3 ripe mangoes	*1* Peel and core the mangoes and cut into ½-inch dice and place in a small bowl. You should have about 2 cups of diced mango. Add the lime zest and juice, and toss lightly to combine.
1 teaspoon lime zest	
1 teaspoon fresh lime juice	
Whipped Coconut Cream (see recipe in Chapter 12)	*2* To serve, spoon ¼ cup mango into a parfait glass or bowl. Top with 1 to 2 tablespoons Whipped Coconut Cream (see Chapter 12); repeat layers. Sprinkle with ½ tablespoon macadamia nuts.
2 tablespoons dry roasted macadamia nuts, finely chopped	

Per serving: Calories 302 (From Fat 229); Fat 25g (Saturated 20g); Cholesterol 0mg; Sodium 16mg; Carbohydrate 21g; Dietary Fiber 3g; Protein 3g.

Vary It! This dessert is also delicious with other fruits and nuts. Replace the mango with berries, omit the lime, and substitute almonds for the macadamia nuts to make another summery sweet treat.

Classic Apple Crisp

Prep time: 15 min • **Cook time:** 40 min • **Yield:** 4–6 servings

Ingredients	Directions
1 pound apples, cut into half-moon slices (about 4 cups)	**1** Preheat the oven to 350 degrees.
½ teaspoon lemon zest	**2** In a medium bowl, mix the apples, lemon zest, and lemon juice with a wooden spoon. Allow to rest at room temperature while you prepare the topping.
½ tablespoon lemon juice	
⅓ cup almond flour	
4 dried dates, pitted	**3** Place almond flour, dates, cinnamon, nutmeg, and salt in food processor. Pulse until combined.
¼ teaspoon ground cinnamon	
⅛ teaspoon nutmeg	**4** Sprinkle the chilled coconut oil chunks over the flour mixture. Pulse about 10 times, and then process on high for 5 to 10 seconds until there are no more lumps. Pour the topping into a bowl and use a fork to mix in the chopped nuts.
⅛ teaspoon salt	
1 tablespoon coconut oil, chilled until solid, then diced	
¼ cup chopped walnuts or pecans	**5** Pour the fruit into an 8-inch square pan, pressing it gently into place with the back of a wooden spoon. Sprinkle the nut topping over the fruit and lightly press it into the fruit with the back of the spoon.
	6 Cover the crisp lightly with foil and bake for 30 minutes. Remove foil and bake 5 to 10 more minutes, until browned.

Per serving: Calories 220 (From Fat 120); Fat 13g (Saturated 4g); Cholesterol 0mg; Sodium 77mg; Carbohydrate 24g; Dietary Fiber 5g; Protein 4g.

Note: You can also bake this dish in individual ramekins. Place four ramekins on a baking sheet covered with parchment paper. Spoon generous ½-cup servings into each ramekin, press about 2 tablespoons of topping onto each, and then follow baking instructions above.

Tip: This crisp is yummy topped with Whipped Coconut Cream (see recipe in Chapter 12) or with a drizzle of coconut milk.

Vary It! Substitute pears for the apples and sliced almonds for the walnuts or pecans. For extra zing, add ½ teaspoon dried ginger along with the lemon juice to the pears.

Ginger-Fried Pears

Prep time: 10 min • **Cook time:** 5 min • **Yield:** 4 servings

Ingredients	Directions
2 tablespoons blanched, sliced almonds	*1* Heat a nonstick skillet over medium-high heat. Add the sliced almonds and stir with a wooden spoon until toasted, about 3 to 4 minutes. Remove from pan.
1 tablespoon coconut oil	
2 large, ripe pears, cored and sliced (about 2 cups)	*2* In the same skillet, heat the coconut oil over medium-high heat. Add the pear slices and sauté until the pears begin to soften, about 3 to 4 minutes.
¼ teaspoon powdered ginger	
½ teaspoon lemon zest	*3* In a small bowl, mix the ginger, lemon zest, and salt with a fork, and then add to the pears. Continue cooking until the pears are golden and fragrant, about 5 minutes.
Generous pinch of salt	
	4 To serve, spoon the pears into dessert dishes and sprinkle with the sliced almonds.

Per serving: Calories 109 (From Fat 48); Fat 5g (Saturated 3g); Cholesterol 0mg; Sodium 72mg; Carbohydrate 17g; Dietary Fiber 3g; Protein 1g.

Tip: To make this dish even more decadent and to increase the healthy fats, drizzle each serving with 1 or 2 tablespoons of warm coconut milk.

Vary It! Substitute apples for the pears and replace ginger with cinnamon.

Soothing ginger

In addition to being tasty, ginger has been used in healing for centuries. A natural anti-inflammatory, ginger is also soothing for motion sickness, upset stomachs, and menstrual cramps.

Fudge Bombs

Prep time: 15 min • **Chill time:** 30–60 min • **Yield:** 32 servings

Ingredients	Directions
1 cup whole pecans	**1** Place pecans, dates, vanilla, and cocoa in a food processor. Process on high until the mixture forms a paste, about 5 to 7 minutes.
18 pitted dates	
1 teaspoon pure vanilla extract	**2** Wet your hands with water and shake off the excess, and then roll the dough into 1-inch balls. Set on a baking sheet.
4 tablespoons unsweetened cocoa powder	
Garnishes: coarse sea salt, unsweetened shredded coconut, very finely chopped pecans (optional)	**3** Top the balls with a few grains of sea salt or roll them in either coconut flakes or additional nuts (if desired).
	4 Place the fudge bombs in the refrigerator until firm, about 30 to 60 minutes. Allow the fudge bombs to come to room temperature before eating, but store them covered in the refrigerator.

Per serving: Calories 39 (From Fat 23); Fat 3g (Saturated 0g); Cholesterol 0mg; Sodium 0mg; Carbohydrate 4g; Dietary Fiber 1g; Protein 1g.

Note: These fudge bombs are essentially Paleo candy and should be reserved for special occasions — and they're definitely meant to be shared with friends. This recipe also works well when cut in half (if you have a problem resisting the temptation of a whole batch).

Vary It! Give these bombs a spicy bite by adding ¼ teaspoon cayenne pepper to the dough.

Pumpkin Pancakes

Prep time: 5 min • **Cook time:** 10 min • **Yield:** 4 servings

Ingredients	*Directions*
4 large eggs	*1* Place eggs, pumpkin, and almond butter in a large bowl and beat with a wire whisk until smooth. Add the cinnamon, vanilla, and nutmeg, and then whisk again to incorporate the seasonings.
1 cup canned pumpkin	
⅔ cup almond butter	
1 teaspoon ground cinnamon	*2* Place ½ tablespoon coconut oil in a nonstick skillet and heat over medium-high heat until the oil is melted and shimmers. Swivel the pan to coat the bottom.
½ teaspoon pure vanilla extract	
¼ teaspoon nutmeg	
2 to 3 tablespoons coconut oil, divided	*3* Drop ¼-cup servings of batter into the pan, making sure they don't touch. Cook until bubbles begin to appear and the edges are set, about 2 minutes. Flip gently and cook the other side until golden, about 2 minutes.
	4 Cook in batches, adding more coconut oil to the pan as necessary. Serve hot with Paleo-friendly sausage or eggs and a small amount of honey or pure maple syrup.

Per serving: Calories 462 (From Fat 358); Fat 40g (Saturated 12g); Cholesterol 185mg; Sodium 71mg; Carbohydrate 18g; Dietary Fiber 6g; Protein 14g.

Tip: Make these pancakes in advance and freeze for quick breakfasts and snacks. Just cook and cool the pancakes, and then stack them with pieces of cooking parchment in between them to prevent sticking. Wrap tightly in plastic wrap and pop into the freezer.

Vary It! Replace the canned pumpkin with 1 cup unsweetened applesauce for another tasty treat.

Anytime Waffles

Prep time: 15 min • **Cook time:** 5 min • **Yield:** 4 servings

Ingredients	Directions
⅓ cup unsweetened shredded coconut	*1* Preheat the oven to 350 degrees. Spread the coconut on a baking sheet in a single layer and toast until golden, about 4 minutes. Remove from oven and set aside to cool.
1½ cups almond flour or almond meal	
½ teaspoon baking soda	*2* In a medium bowl, mix the almond flour, baking soda, salt, and cinnamon with a fork. Set aside.
½ teaspoon salt	
½ teaspoon ground cinnamon	*3* In a large bowl, whisk together the eggs, coconut milk, sweet potato, and vanilla until smooth. Add the toasted coconut and dry ingredients to the wet ingredients and whisk until combined.
5 large eggs	
¼ cup coconut milk	
¾ cup cooked sweet potato, mashed	*4* Allow the batter to rest for 10 minutes. Meanwhile, preheat the waffle iron.
1 teaspoon pure vanilla extract	*5* Pour ½ to 1 cup of batter onto the waffle iron, depending on the size of your model. If you're not sure, use the smaller amount. Close the lid and allow the batter to cook, about 2 to 3 minutes.
	6 Remove waffle to a baking sheet and place in the warm oven while you prepare the rest of the waffles. Serve waffles hot with eggs or other protein and a small amount of honey or pure maple syrup.

Per serving: Calories 450 (From Fat 321); Fat 36g (Saturated 11g); Cholesterol 233mg; Sodium 258mg; Carbohydrate 10g; Dietary Fiber 7g; Protein 18g.

Note: You may substitute unsweetened, canned sweet potatoes for fresh sweet potatoes.

Tip: Almond meal and almond flour are simply very finely ground almonds. You can find almond flour in the baking aisle of most grocery or health food stores; you can also purchase it online.

Vary It! Substitute a ripe, mashed banana for the sweet potato and add ¼ cup chopped pecans for banana-nut waffles.

Lime-Blueberry Poppy Seed Coffee Cake

Prep time: 10 min • **Cook time:** 40 min • **Yield:** 12 servings

Ingredients	Directions
½ cup coconut flour	**1** Preheat the oven to 350 degrees.
½ teaspoon salt	**2** In a small bowl, mix coconut flour, salt, and baking soda with a fork. Set aside.
¼ teaspoon baking soda	
6 eggs	**3** In a large bowl, whisk eggs, coconut oil, honey, vanilla, lime zest, and lime juice until smooth. Stir in the flour mixture, poppy seeds, and blueberries until just combined.
½ cup coconut oil, melted	
¼ cup honey	
½ tablespoon pure vanilla extract	
Zest of 1 lime	**4** Grease an 8-x-8-inch square pan with coconut oil, and then dust with coconut flour. Pour batter into pan and spread into corners with a rubber scraper. Bake until lightly golden and a toothpick inserted in the center comes out clean, about 35 to 40 minutes.
2 tablespoons lime juice	
1½ tablespoons poppy seeds	
1¼ cup fresh blueberries (or frozen, defrosted)	**5** Cool the cake in the pan, and then cut into 12 squares. Store covered in the refrigerator or at room temperature.

Per serving: *Calories 170 (From Fat 115); Fat 13g (Saturated 9g); Cholesterol 106mg; Sodium 165mg; Carbohydrate 11g; Dietary Fiber 3g; Protein 4g.*

Tip: Serve this coffee cake alongside Berry-Nice Chicken Salad (Chapter 10) for brunch.

Vary It! Substitute raspberries or strawberries for the blueberries — or replace the lime juice and zest with lemon.

Snack attack

Some people do great on three meals per day, and others need a small snack to get them through the morning or afternoon. Living Paleo is flexible enough to support whatever your body needs. Your snacks should be about half the size of your meals and should always include protein and fat.

If you work out, you need to add two special snacks into your day. You should eat these snacks in addition to your regular meals:

✔ **Pre-workout fuel:** For your strongest workout, eat a small snack of protein and fat about 30 to 90 minutes before your workout. By avoiding carbs just before exercise, you help your body tap into stored fat as fuel during your workout.

✔ **Post-workout fuel:** Within 30 minutes of finishing your workout, refuel with Paleo-approved, nutrient-dense carbohydrates, like a sweet potato or butternut squash, along with lean protein, like eggs, chicken breast, or salmon. Fat slows the absorption of food in your digestive system, and that usually works in your favor. Post-workout is the one time when you want to minimize fat so your muscles can quickly absorb the carbohydrates they need to recover from your workout.

If you're doing long-duration activities or are preparing for a race or fitness contest, you may need more. Use these guidelines and adjust them to meet your personal activity levels and lifestyle. Some days, you'll need more; other days, you'll need less.

Chapter 14

Sauces and Seasonings

In This Chapter

▶ Using condiments and spices to dress up meals

▶ Discovering easy recipes for sugar-free condiments and spice blends

The right sauces and seasonings can mean the difference between a delectable and dull meal. Simple ingredients like chicken, beef, and vitamin-rich vegetables become exciting when they're dipped into something creamy or dusted with something spicy — and the right seasonings can take your taste buds on a world tour.

In this chapter, you find recipes for salad dressings, condiments, and spice blends that add personality and flavor to every dish on your table. Think living Paleo means giving up creamy ranch dressing or luscious Asian dipping sauce? Think again.

Making Your Own Dressings and Condiments

Most commercial condiments include added ingredients that make them poor choices for living Paleo. Sweet-tasting favorites like ketchup and BBQ sauce often contain high-fructose corn syrup and other sweeteners, while classics like mayonnaise and bottled salad dressing are usually based on poor quality industrial oils.

But homemade condiments can be a good source of healthy, Paleo-approved fats and naturally occurring sugars that don't wreak havoc on your blood sugar levels — and the homemade versions taste even better than the factory-produced varieties found in the grocery store.

Adding Flavor with Sugar-Free Spice Blends

The fastest way to liven up a meal is to add the right amount of spice. A sprinkle of Garam Masala or Italian Seasoning can make a standard weeknight meal feel like a weekend feast. But many spice blends include sneaky forms of sugar or wheat, along with preservatives that make them decidedly unfriendly to Paleo cooks.

Homemade spice blends take less than five minutes to throw together, and they last almost indefinitely in your pantry. Doubling or tripling batches of your favorites is easy and in your favor because then you always have some on hand. And a jar of a homemade spice blend, along with a recipe for how to use it, makes a great gift for a friend or family member who's considering the Paleo lifestyle.

Buy spices in bulk to save money and to ensure that you never run out of your favorites!

Read those food labels carefully

Beware of sneaky names and hidden ingredients on food labels. MSG, soy, corn, and sugar can camouflage themselves with aliases. MSG hides under names like *glutamate, yeast extract, soy protein,* anything *hydrolyzed,* and *autolyzed yeast.*

Soy shows up with names like *soya, soy protein, soy isolate, vegetable protein, textured soy flour (TSF)* and *textured vegetable protein (TVP). Monodiglyceride* is soy, too.

Corn or *maize* is found in just about all packaged foods with a wide variety of names: *maltodextrins, sorbitol, high-fructose corn syrup, corn syrup solids, corn flour, corn starch (mazena), dextrose, food starch, vegetable starch, dextrin, vegetable gum, modified gum starch,* and *vegetable protein.*

Cashew Butter Satay Sauce

Prep time: 5 min • **Yield:** 1 cup

Ingredients	Directions
½ cup cashew butter (no sugar added)	**1** Place all the ingredients except the coconut milk in a food processor or blender and process until smooth.
3 tablespoons coconut aminos	
2 tablespoons lime juice	**2** Scrape down the sides of the bowl with a rubber scraper, and then add the coconut milk. Process until blended.
1 clove garlic, minced (about 1 teaspoon)	
1 teaspoon crushed red pepper flakes	**3** Allow flavors to meld for 10 minutes before serving. Store covered in the refrigerator for up to five days.
½ teaspoon powdered ginger	
Dash of ground cayenne pepper (optional)	
½ cup coconut milk	

Per serving (1 tablespoon): Calories 97 (From Fat 52); Fat 6g (Saturated 2g); Cholesterol 0mg; Sodium 66mg; Carbohydrate 9g; Dietary Fiber 0g; Protein 2.

Tip: Serve Cashew Butter Satay Sauce along with grilled meats, like chicken, pork, and beef, or with seafood, like shrimp, scallops, and white fish. This sauce is especially nice with kabobs! Cashew Butter Satay Sauce is also a tasty addition to a raw vegetable and fruit platter.

Vary It! Try substituting sunflower butter or almond butter in place of cashew butter for a slightly different but still deliciously creamy flavor.

Classic Stir-Fry Sauce

Prep time: 5 min • **Cook time:** 10 min • **Yield:** ⅔ cup

Ingredients	Directions
1 clove garlic, minced (about 1 teaspoon)	**1** In a small saucepan, mix the garlic, red pepper flakes, five-spice powder, ginger, and rice vinegar with a fork to form a smooth paste. Stirring continuously with the fork, add the applesauce and coconut aminos.
1 teaspoon crushed red pepper flakes	
1 tablespoon Chinese five-spice powder	**2** In a small bowl, whisk the arrowroot powder and water together until smooth; set aside.
¼ teaspoon ground ginger	
1 teaspoon rice vinegar	**3** Place the saucepan over medium-high heat and bring to a boil. Add the arrowroot paste to the saucepan, stirring to combine. Return to a boil, and then reduce heat and simmer gently, uncovered, until slightly thickened, about 5 minutes.
¼ cup unsweetened applesauce	
¼ cup coconut aminos	
½ tablespoon arrowroot powder	**4** Use immediately in a stir-fry or store covered in the refrigerator for up to five days.
½ tablespoon water	

Per serving (1 tablespoon): Calories 69 (From Fat 2); Fat 0g (Saturated 0g); Cholesterol 0mg; Sodium 127mg; Carbohydrate 14g; Dietary Fiber 0g; Protein 0g.

Note: This stir-fry sauce works well with just about any combination of meat and vegetables. One batch is enough for about 4 servings.

Tip: Keep your freezer stocked with grab-and-go Classic Stir-Fry Sauce. Just double or triple the recipe, and then freeze the sauce in flexible plastic ice cube trays. Pop the sauce cubes into a freezer-safe bag so you'll always have fast access to individual portions of Classic Stir-Fry Sauce whenever you need them.

Vary it! If you can't find Chinese five-spice powder, you can substitute a combination of cinnamon, cloves, ginger, and nutmeg.

Homemade Mayonnaise

Prep time: 5 min • **Yield:** 1½ cups

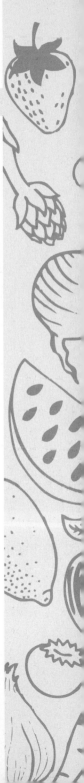

Ingredients	Directions
1 large egg **1 tablespoon lemon juice** **1 tablespoon white wine vinegar** **¼ cup plus 1 cup light-tasting olive oil (not extra-virgin)** **½ teaspoon dry mustard** **½ teaspoon salt**	*1* In a blender or food processor, place the egg, lemon juice, and vinegar. Put the lid on and allow the liquids to come to room temperature together, about 20 to 30 minutes.
	2 Add ¼ cup of oil to the canister and blend on medium until the ingredients are combined.
	3 With the motor running, drizzle the remaining 1 cup of oil into the canister by pouring in a steady stream, about 2 to 3 minutes. If you're using a blender, you'll hear the pitch change as the liquid begins to form the emulsion.
	4 Transfer the mayonnaise to a container with a lid and store in the refrigerator. It will slightly thicken as it chills. Mark a calendar with your egg expiration date; that's the expiration date for the mayo, too.

Per serving (1 tablespoon): Calories 29(From Fat 28); Fat 3g (Saturated 0g); Cholesterol 8mg; Sodium 51mg; Carbohydrate 0g; Dietary Fiber 0g; Protein 0g.

Tip: Don't use extra-virgin olive oil to make mayonnaise; the olive flavor is overpowering. Use an inexpensive, light-tasting olive oil instead for the most neutral flavor.

Note: Mayonnaise is an emulsion — when the oil and egg combine with the acid in the lemon juice and vinegar, they create what's known as a colloid, a substance in which one substance is dispersed throughout another substance. To help this process along, all the ingredients should be at room temperature.

Vary It! For a light, lemony flavor that's similar to aioli, use 2 tablespoons lemon juice and omit the vinegar.

The obligatory warning about raw eggs

To reduce the risk of salmonella and other food-borne illnesses, use only fresh, properly refrigerated, clean, cage-free, organic eggs with intact shells. You may also use an egg substitute in this recipe, but most brands contain trace amounts of non-Paleo ingredients.

Cave Man Ketchup

Prep time: 5 min • **Cook time:** 10 min • **Yield:** 1 cup

Ingredients	*Directions*
One 6-ounce can tomato paste	**1** Place all ingredients in a saucepan and whisk to combine. Place on high heat and bring to a boil. Reduce heat to low and simmer gently, uncovered, for 5 minutes.
⅓ cup water	
2 tablespoons cider vinegar	
2 teaspoons honey	**2** Cool the ketchup to room temperature before using. Transfer to a container with a lid and store in the refrigerator.
¼ teaspoon dry mustard	
¼ teaspoon ground cinnamon	
Pinch of cloves	
Pinch of allspice	

Per serving (1 tablespoon): Calories 13 (From Fat 0); Fat 0g (Saturated 0g); Cholesterol 0mg; Sodium 7mg; Carbohydrate 3g; Dietary Fiber 0g; Protein 1g.

Note: To avoid the unhealthy compound Bisphenol A (BPA) found in most canned goods, look for tomato paste in a tube or use Muir Glen brand, which uses BPA-free cans.

Tangy BBQ Sauce

Prep time: 5 min • **Cook time:** 25 min • **Yield:** 1½ cups

Ingredients	*Directions*
1 cup Cave Man Ketchup (see previous recipe)	**1** In a large bowl, whisk the Cave Man Ketchup, water, applesauce, vinegar, coconut aminos, honey (if desired), mustard, hot pepper sauce, and black pepper until smooth.
½ cup water	
⅓ cup unsweetened applesauce	
2 tablespoons cider vinegar	**2** Heat the coconut oil in a saucepan over medium heat until shimmering. Add the garlic, chili powder, and cayenne pepper, and cook until fragrant, about 30 seconds.
2 tablespoons coconut aminos	
1 tablespoon honey (optional)	
1 teaspoon dry mustard	**3** Add the ketchup mixture to the saucepan, and whisk to combine. Bring to a boil, and then reduce the heat to medium-low and simmer gently, uncovered, until the sauce thickens, about 20 minutes.
1 teaspoon hot pepper sauce	
¼ teaspoon ground black pepper	
1 tablespoon coconut oil	**4** Enjoy warm or at room temperature. Store in the refrigerator for up to a week.
1 medium clove garlic, crushed	
1 teaspoon chili powder	
¼ teaspoon cayenne pepper	

Per serving (1 tablespoon): *Calories 30 (From Fat 6); Fat 1g (Saturated 1g); Cholesterol 0mg; Sodium 39mg; Carbohydrate 5g; Dietary Fiber 0g; Protein 1g.*

Tip: Use this BBQ sauce to spice up grilled chicken, to toss with Slow Cooker BBQ Pulled Pork (Chapter 11), or to dollop on top of a freshly cooked beef burger.

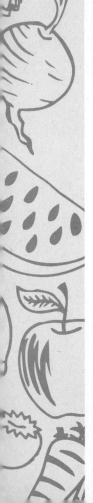

Ranch Dressing

Prep time: 5 min • **Yield:** ½ cup

Ingredients	Directions
½ cup **Homemade Mayonnaise (see recipe earlier in this chapter)**	*1* In a small bowl, use a fork to blend the Homemade Mayonnaise and the garlic.
1 clove **garlic, minced**	
¼ teaspoon **paprika**	*2* Add the rest of the ingredients to the bowl, and mix gently with a fork until just combined. Add water or additional lemon juice a little bit at a time to reach desired thickness.
¼ cup **fresh parsley leaves, minced**	
1 tablespoon **dried chives**	*3* Allow flavors to meld about 10 minutes before using. Store covered in the refrigerator for up to a week.
¼ teaspoon **dried dill**	
¼ teaspoon **onion powder**	
Salt and ground black pepper to taste	
1 teaspoon **lemon juice**	
Water (optional)	

Per serving (1 tablespoon): Calories 32 (From Fat 29); Fat 3g (Saturated 0g); Cholesterol 8mg; Sodium 125mg; Carbohydrate 1g; Dietary Fiber 0g; Protein 0g.

Aromatic Vinaigrette

Prep time: 10 min • **Yield:** 1½ cups

Ingredients	Directions
2 tablespoons finely minced onion	*1* Combine all ingredients except the olive oil in a medium bowl. Whisk to combine.
1 clove garlic, crushed	
½ cup lemon juice	*2* While whisking continuously, drizzle the olive oil into the bowl in a slow, steady stream until combined.
2 tablespoons water	
2 tablespoons Cave Man Ketchup (see recipe earlier in this chapter)	*3* Allow the flavors to meld about 10 minutes before using. Store covered in the refrigerator for up to a week.
1 teaspoon salt	
½ teaspoon dry mustard	
½ teaspoon dried oregano leaves	
½ teaspoon paprika	
¼ teaspoon hot sauce	
⅔ cup extra-virgin olive oil	

Per serving (1 tablespoon): Calories 57 (From Fat 55); Fat 6g (Saturated 1g); Cholesterol 0mg; Sodium 99mg; Carbohydrate 1g; Dietary Fiber 0g; Protein 0g.

Tip: Toss this dressing with a green salad, or use in place of the tahini dressing in the Chopped Salad with Tahini Dressing recipe in Chapter 12. You can also use Aromatic Vinaigrette to marinate chicken and pork before grilling or roasting.

Grilling Spice Rub

Prep time: 5 min • **Yield:** ⅓ cup

Ingredients	*Directions*
2 tablespoons cumin	**1** Place all the spices in a medium bowl and mix with a fork until combined.
2 tablespoons chili powder	
1 tablespoon salt	**2** Transfer the spice blend to an airtight container.
½ tablespoon dry mustard	
½ tablespoon ground black pepper	
1 teaspoon cayenne pepper	

Per serving (1 teaspoon): Calories 9 (From Fat 4); Fat 1g (Saturated 0g); Cholesterol 0mg; Sodium 448mg; Carbohydrate 1g; Dietary Fiber 1g; Protein 0g.

Tip: Use this spice blend liberally as a rub on steaks, chops, or chicken parts. You can also mix 1 tablespoon per pound into ground beef, pork, lamb, or turkey for burgers or meatballs.

Basic grilled chicken

The secret to fast weeknight meals is having cooked protein on hand, and nothing is quite as versatile — or satisfying — as grilled chicken. Eat it on its own, or use it in stir-fries, sautés, and salads.

1. Coat boneless, skinless chicken thighs and/or breasts with Grilling Spice Rub.

2. Wrap the chicken tightly in plastic wrap and allow it to marinate in the refrigerator for 2 hours, or overnight.

3. To cook, preheat a gas grill on high with the lid closed, about 10 minutes.

4. Place the chicken smooth side down on the preheated grill, close the lid, and cook for 4 to 5 minutes.

5. Flip the chicken, cook for an additional 3 to 4 minutes with the lid closed, until the chicken is browned and cooked through. Allow to rest 5 minutes before serving.

Italian Seasoning

Prep time: 5 min • **Yield:** ⅓ cup

Ingredients	Directions
1 tablespoon dried oregano leaves	**1** Mix all the spices with a fork until combined.
1 tablespoon dried basil leaves	**2** Transfer the spice blend to an airtight container.
1 tablespoon dried parsley leaves	
1 tablespoon dried rosemary	
2 teaspoons coarse (granulated) garlic powder	
1 teaspoon salt	

Per serving (1 teaspoon): Calories 4 (From Fat 1); Fat 0g (Saturated 0g); Cholesterol 0mg; Sodium 146mg; Carbohydrate 1g; Dietary Fiber 0g; Protein 0.

Note: When making the spice blend, toss the dried herbs gently to avoid crushing them. When using the spice blend to cook, crush the spice blend between your fingers to release the leaves' flavor.

Tip: Use the Italian Seasoning to make a quick salad dressing with extra-virgin olive oil and red wine vinegar, or sprinkle onto steamed vegetables tossed with coconut or olive oil and a freshly crushed garlic clove.

Quick marinara sauce

Why buy sauce from a jar, which usually has added sugar or high-fructose corn syrup, when you can make this tasty sauce in almost no time?

1. Heat a saucepan over medium-high heat and add 1 tablespoon coconut oil and 2 cloves crushed garlic.

2. Cook until the garlic is fragrant, about 30 seconds, and then add a 28-ounce can diced tomatoes and 1 tablespoon Italian Seasoning.

3. Stir to combine, increase heat, and bring to a boil.

4. Reduce heat to low and simmer until slightly thickened, about 10 minutes. Season with salt and pepper to taste.

5. Serve on a bed of Zucchini Noodles (Chapter 12) with your favorite protein on the side or simmered in the sauce.

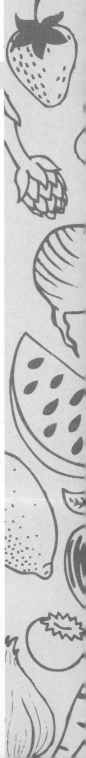

Garam Masala

Prep time: 5 min • **Yield:** ⅓ cup

Ingredients	*Directions*
1 tablespoon ground cumin	*1* Place all the spices in a medium bowl and mix with a fork until combined.
1 tablespoon ground coriander	
1 tablespoon ground cardamom	*2* Transfer the spice blend to an airtight container.
1 tablespoon ground black pepper	
1 tablespoon ground cinnamon	
1 teaspoon ground cloves	
1 teaspoon ground nutmeg	
½ teaspoon chili powder	

Per serving (1 teaspoon): Calories 8 (From Fat 3); Fat 0g (Saturated 0g); Cholesterol 0mg; Sodium 2mg; Carbohydrate 1g; Dietary Fiber 1g; Protein 0g.

Tip: Mix 1 tablespoon per pound into ground beef, pork, lamb, or turkey for burgers or meatballs. It's also delicious mashed with baked sweet potatoes or roasted butternut squash.

Quick curry for two

This recipe is a great way to use leftovers!

1. Heat a saucepan over medium-high heat, and then add 1 tablespoon coconut oil, 2 cloves crushed garlic, and 1 tablespoon Garam Masala.

2. Cook until fragrant, about 30 seconds, and then add ⅔ cup coconut milk.

3. Stir to combine; add 4 cups of cooked vegetables (broccoli, red peppers, green beans, eggplant, and sweet potatoes are good choices) and 8 ounces of cooked protein (grilled or roasted chicken, pork, beef, or shrimp).

4. Increase heat and bring to a boil. Reduce heat to low and simmer until slightly thickened, about 10 minutes.

5. Serve on a bed of Cauliflower Rice (Chapter 12) or braised greens, such as kale, collards, or spinach.

Morning Spice

Prep time: 5 min • **Yield:** ¼ cup

Ingredients	*Directions*
1 tablespoon ground cinnamon	*1* Measure all the spices into a medium bowl and mix with a fork until combined.
2 teaspoons ground marjoram	
1 teaspoon ground nutmeg	*2* Transfer the spice blend to an airtight container.
1 teaspoon coarse (granulated) garlic powder	
1 teaspoon salt	
½ teaspoon ground black pepper	

Per serving (1 teaspoon): Calories 4 (From Fat 1); Fat 0g (Saturated 0g); Cholesterol 0mg; Sodium 194mg; Carbohydrate 1g; Dietary Fiber 0g; Protein 0.

Note: This spice blend is cozy and spicy-sweet. Based on traditional Russian sausage seasonings, it adds warmth to burgers, meatballs, soups, stews, and hearty vegetables.

Tip: Mix 1 tablespoon per pound into ground beef, pork, lamb, or turkey for instant "sausage." Just shape into patties or brown loose in a skillet. It also livens up baked sweet potatoes, cooked carrots, fried plantains, and roasted butternut or acorn squash.

Quick breakfast scramble for two

A hot, nutritious breakfast doesn't have to be time consuming or complicated. You can make the following egg dish with a minimum of thought or effort. Feel free to change up some of the ingredients if you need to get rid of leftovers or vegetables that are about to go bad.

1. Heat a skillet over medium-high heat, and then add 1 tablespoon coconut oil and 1 tablespoon Morning Spice.

2. Cook until fragrant, about 30 seconds, and then add 1 cup diced baked sweet potato and 1 diced fresh apple.

3. Sauté until the apples soften and the sweet potatoes begin to caramelize.

4. Scramble 4 eggs in a small bowl and add to the pan, stirring until eggs are cooked through.

5. Divide onto two plates and sprinkle with chopped fresh parsley.

Part IV
Making Paleo Practical in a Modern World

The 5th Wave
By Rich Tennant

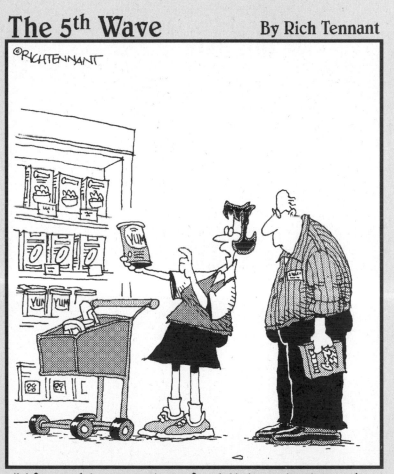

"After this long list of additives, it lists the expiration date. Does that pertain to the product or the person who eats it?"

In this part . . .

Modern life is filled with challenges that can make staying on the Paleo path difficult. But with planning and perseverance, living Paleo can become second nature. We take a look at some common obstacles and health issues and how you can overcome them. Then we tackle practical tips for eating in restaurants, traveling, and navigating special occasions. We also explore how to help your family make the transition to the Paleo lifestyle without inciting a revolution.

Chapter 15

Dealing with Potential Pitfalls

· ·

· ·

Your mindset is everything! The perception you have of any situation makes it real to you. That's why training your subconscious with thoughts and patterns that serve you and help you create the body, health, and *life* you're looking for is so important.

When you experience roadblocks, hurdles, or challenges of any kind, sometimes you just need to take a step back and look at the situation from a different angle or perspective. That's what this chapter is about: Helping you identify a possible roadblock you've had, or are currently experiencing, and take a look from a different perspective so you can lean into the changes of eating Paleo.

If you feel as though you've tried to eat better or live healthier before and it didn't work long-term, don't let that get you down. Every time you've tried something and didn't succeed, understand that you didn't really fail; you just came one step closer to success. Forget about any hurdles you've had in the past and get ready to figure out how to address those concerns and make living Paleo a way of life.

Long-term success is where Paleo really shines. When you address your roadblocks and jump over hurdles, you begin to embrace the power of what eating Paleo can add to your life. This chapter walks you through any potential setbacks and helps you remove doubts or excuses to succeed with your Paleo transition.

Clearing Diet-Related Hurdles

How and what you eat has a direct relationship to how you feel. Sometimes, you may eat something and feel lousy. Certain foods may even make you feel tired all the time. You may find that your eating patterns make you shaky. The foods you eat elicit a chemical response in your body, and you feel those effects, whether good or bad.

Sometimes, those effects are short-term means to a greater purpose. For example, if you start eating a clean and healthy diet, such as the Paleo diet, your body may go through some metabolic changes or shift in a way that may make you uncomfortable for a short time. Or you may find that you need to tweak the amount you're eating of a particular food to customize your personal eating plan.

In the following sections, we talk about what your body may be experiencing during a change in diet, what diet-related hurdles may get in your way, and how you can get back on track.

The carb flu

Ah, the carb flu. This term describes the unpleasant symptoms your body may experience when you begin your journey of cutting out the sugars and sugary carbohydrates. It's called the *carb flu* because the symptoms are often similar to how you feel when you have the flu. Riding the wave and being patient as these symptoms pass is probably the most common hurdle in transitioning to a Paleo diet. For many, simply understanding what the carb flu is helps lead them to a successful outcome. When you're going through dietary changes that cause you to feel differently and you don't understand what's happening or what to expect, you may start to believe that you need to change course. However, in the case of the carb flu, staying on track is definitely the right move.

The degree to which your body experiences the carb flu symptoms is purely individual. Some people snap out of this phase in a couple of days; for others, it takes closer to three weeks. Here are the symptoms commonly associated with the carb flu:

- Mental fuzziness, like you're in a mental fog
- Headaches, not like a sharp pain headache but more like a hangover headache that's a dull, annoying kind of discomfort
- Moodiness
- Shakiness
- Fatigue × 10
- Achy joints

Experiencing these systems as you begin the Paleo diet means nothing more than your body is transitioning. Think of your body pushing the compost button and trying to start over with cleaner, more efficient fuel. Your body is going through a good detox and flipping the switch to the more efficient fat-burning system of using fats (dietary and body fat) and proteins to create the energy it needs, rather than the sugarary carbs it was accustomed to using.

If you feel a little shaky during a workout, give your body time to adjust and try eating some protein and fat before you train. A piece of protein and a handful of nuts works well for most, but you have to adjust to what works best for you.

The goal is for you to understand what's happening to your body so you can deal with these symptoms with as much smarts as possible and not trick yourself into feeling like this way of eating just makes you feel bad and cranky. This transition is part of the process and a small ticket for admission to what you'll get in the end, so hang in there! Try to ease off any intense training when you're dealing with the carb flu and let your body recalibrate.

Bottom line: Stay the course. You've come too far too give up now! Tell yourself it's worth it and white knuckle through this one.

Cravings

Your cravings in the beginning can be intense. You may even *dream* about foods when you're making the transition to Paleo. These cravings are easy to confuse with hunger. Your brain causes these cravings as it adjusts to going without the sugary stuff and the sugary spikes that it's used to.

You've removed all the carbohydrate-dense, nutrition-poor foods, such as packaged, processed, sugary carbs, grains, and legumes. Often, being hungry is your body recalibrating to a new system, and these carbs may have been the source of most of your calories. Replacing these calories with healthy fats from grass-fed animal fats, coconut, or avocado fuels your body efficiently and sustains you so your hunger diminishes with healthy raw material.

Be sure to drink enough water. Your body can often confuse the low signal for water as a low signal for food. Drink a minimum of half your body weight in ounces of water.

Also be in check with your protein and fat and make sure you're getting enough (as we talk about in Chapter 2), which can help sustain you. Building your plate with proteins, fats, and non-starchy carbs is critical. You want to give your body the rest and the right raw material to start this process of change and to curb cravings.

Your brain and cravings

Don't forget about serotonin, the feel-good guy we discuss in Chapter 3. When you have cravings, your body is looking for some kind of chemical change to make it feel better — that "something" your brain is scanning for is often the chemical that affects mood: serotonin. Self-medicating with sugary foods to answer these cravings isn't the answer. Try exercising, thinking good thoughts, or building yourself a healthy, well-balanced Paleo plate, and you can kick those cravings to the curb!

If you're eating enough proteins, fats, non-starchy carbs (see Chapter 2) and drinking enough water, you're doing everything right. Relax, think good thoughts, and move your body to balance your serotonin, which will diminish these cravings and replace them with feelings of balance and satiety. Hang tight; the magic will happen.

Accelerating Through Eight Common Roadblocks to Living Paleo

Most people encounter roadblocks at some point in their life. These roadblocks are the frustrations you may go through when you know what you have to do but feel apprehension to accelerate. They're the out-of-the-gate fears you have when you know change is closing in. They're the stories you tell yourself that make eating Paleo difficult to endure.

The Paleo lifestyle is about you. It's about changing your life for the better and saying goodbye to illness, weight gain, and fatigue. If there was ever a time where you needed to be in charge of what you allow yourself to buy into, it's now.

We know that figuring out all this stuff when you're busy (and for many, even overwhelmed) isn't easy. That's why we wrote this book. We want to make this transition simple for you and help you accelerate through roadblocks by providing the tools (and answers) you need to push forward.

If you can relate to some of the roadblocks in the following sections, you're not alone. Many people have the same fears and frustrations as you and have jumped over their hurdles, and *so can you!* Your job is to keep an open mind, clear out all your past experiences with food, and look at this change as a fresh start.

In the following sections, we cover eight common roadblocks and share with you how to push past each roadblock to get results.

"It's just too hard"

Telling yourself this one is easy. But think about something for a moment: Have you ever tried to recover from surgery? Heal from a disease? Been through the treatment or recovery process with someone with cancer? Or just tried to deal with a progressive disease that no one can diagnose and feel hopeless that you'll ever return to "the real you" again? Now that's hard. Real hard.

 Don't think of living Paleo as being hard but rather liberating! Finally, you're getting a road map to a healthy you that actually works. For many, it means thinking differently, behaving differently, and changing a lot of patterns. It's new; it's scary; and it takes guts. But don't let yourself think it's too hard. Without question, you're capable of living Paleo.

When you begin to discover the ropes of living Paleo, your body starts getting what it needs to be fuelled with energy. You literally begin the process of de-aging, you have more charge in your body, and you're able to get more done. As your brain chemistry becomes more balanced, you feel better and everything you do gets easier. So stick with the plan; it gets easier the longer you do it.

"I'm too busy; I don't have time for this"

Boy do we know busy, so we really feel you on this one. Preparing whole foods from scratch definitely takes some time investment.

When you face this roadblock, you really have to be honest about your time and time management. Do you have time sucks throughout the day? You know, things that you do that maybe you can give up or do less of. For example, do you watch movies or TV shows? Or do you watch the news, play a video game here and there, or surf the web or social media sites?

We're not trying to pin you against the wall about what you do with your time; instead, we're trying to help you evaluate your *time allocation*. Consider reallocating your time, just a couple hours a week, to get big gains. Figure out where you can trade a little time doing something else to organize yourself for success.

Really, when you get down to the nitty-gritty of the matter, the issue is more about your *organization* than your *time*. Organize your time and your meals so that eating Paleo isn't a big deal. When you organize, you get in and out of the grocery store faster, make your meals faster, and don't spend time fumbling around aimlessly. When you're not clear or organized (this goes for anything), it costs you time.

Here are some quick tips to organize your way into more time and, ultimately, better health:

1. **Talk it out.**

   Make a list of your family's 20 or 30 favorite meals; if you don't know where to even start, peruse the recipes in Part III of this book or check out coauthor Melissa Joulwan's cookbook *Well Fed: Paleo Recipes for People Who Love to Eat* (Smudge Publishing, LLC) for some great family recipes. Bookmark your favorites.

2. **Turn into a planner.**

   Plan out your meals for the week based on the meals you picked.

3. **Make your grocery list.**

   When you pick your meals for the week, put the ingredients for those recipes right onto your list.

4. **Go shopping!**

   Stick to your list and don't be tempted by non-Paleo food traps.

5. **Batch it out.**

   Pick two days a week to precook as many staple or convenience foods as you can. Prepare foods like hard-boiled eggs, cut and chop veggies, precook some meat (super valuable), make some salads, and prepare dips or sauces, like guacamole. Prepare anything your family uses for staples. After you do this step a couple of times, you get super quick and it's no big deal.

The more access you have to real foods, the better you'll feel and the more you'll get done regardless of time crunches.

"I'm not losing any weight"

If you're eating a true Paleo diet and following the guidelines in Chapter 2, it's nearly impossible for your weight not to shift. You're introducing so many benefits to your health that your weight should naturally normalize. If you're not getting results, it may be attributed to one of these causes:

✔ **Eating too much fruit:** Eating too much fruit is easy to do. You push all the junk off your plate in your new eating regime and replace it with an overload of fruit. Just because fruit is natural doesn't mean you can go to town. Fruit has fructose, and although some fruit can be very nutritious, consuming too much fruit creates an insulin response that causes your body to lay down fat.

✔ **Not getting enough sleep:** You can lose 14.3 pounds a year by getting one more hour a night of sleep. Sleep deprivation causes you to gain weight while decent sleep helps you lose weight. Not sleeping enough causes you and your body systems (including important hormones) to run sluggish and inefficient. When your body slows down, you gain weight.

✔ **Not getting organized:** If you don't get organized with meals and perhaps some batch cooking of convenience foods, you're asking for trouble. A starving body can convince you of almost anything and can even rationalize the benefits of a Twinkie. Be careful here to avoid setting yourself up for grabbing foods that are surely going to put on those pounds.

✔ **Expecting results too quickly:** If you expect results fast or even at a moderate pace, you may be disappointed. For some, it may take a while for weight to normalize. Living Paleo is by no means a red-carpet, quick-fix diet. It's a lifestyle diet, leading to forever results. Trust us on this one. It *will* happen.

✔ **Eating too many nuts:** Yes, nuts are on the "yes" list, but the serving size is a closed handful. Period. Not half a bag. Nuts will pile on the pounds if you crunch away on them mindlessly, not to mention a lot of nuts have an off balance omega-6 to omega-3 ratio, which won't help you move toward health.

✔ **Keeping foods on the "no" list hanging around:** I think you know where we're going with this. Don't hang on to stuff in your pantry or fridge for a rainy day. Donate, or, better yet, toss it. No need to explain this one.

✔ **Indulging in Paleo treats:** We're super glad you're eating foods with much better ingredients. Bravo! If you want to use the Paleo packaged cookies, breads, treats, and sweets once in a while, go for it. Just don't make it routine or the pounds will start creeping on.

✔ **Skipping the fat:** Many people have ingrained in their minds that fat is evil. Some fats may be, but healthy fats on the Paleo "yes" list are anything but evil. Having the right quantities of fat actually helps you *lose* fat. Try it; you'll see.

✔ **Not measuring your food properly:** You probably don't need to think about portion control all the time, but you should get used to how to glance at your food and make sure you're not getting three times what your body needs. Figuring out how much food you actually need is a real eye opener for most people. (See some at-a-glance portion examples in Chapter 2.)

✔ **Falling into automatic eating:** After you start feeling better and begin looking better, you may start to relax a little too much and fall into some of your old patterns. Remember why you started this new lifestyle in the first place and make sure that you're eating Paleo as a rule, not an exception. When you realize you're having a gelato or a martini one too many times, be intuitive about it. Ask yourself why you're doing what you're doing, and shift back on plan.

✔ **Not completely letting go:** For some people, letting go of a lot of foods may be pretty easy, but clutching onto that *one* food or drink you struggle to let go of may be making it hard for your body to dump the weight. People commonly hold onto drinks and snacks with artificial sugars.

These foods and drinks are destructive to your weight loss (and health) efforts. It's time to let go!

✔ **Not managing stress:** Chronic stress activates your stress hormones. If you or anyone you know is thin yet still has that "tire" around the waist, chances are it's a *cortisol tire*. Too much stress means too much cortisol is released, giving you a middle-aged gut no matter how old you are! If your goal is weight loss, make stress management part of your plan.

"I feel like I can't eat anything on this diet"

You may feel like you're trapped in a small fishbowl of Paleo foods, probably because many of the ingredients and produce are new to you. Most of the people who decide to follow the Paleo diet have become so accustomed to eating grains that eliminating that alone can be enough to make them feel at a complete loss as to what to eat. You just have to get on the other side of the learning curve and give yourself time to adapt to all the foods and variety you have living Paleo.

For almost every SAD (Standard American Diet) food, some kind of Paleo conversion exists, maybe not spot on but close. Mourning about giving up pasta is normal, but the Paleo "yes" list is more giving and more delicious than you think. The Paleo diet easily includes enough meats, vegetables, fruits, fats, nuts, and spices to make thousands of meals. Investigate your produce aisles and talk to your butcher or fishmonger. Get creative with pantry items. Consult cookbooks, websites, and chefs. Loads of resources and options are available within the Paleo framework.

The biggest difference with eating Paleo is that instead of dissecting food labels, you're using real foods as your raw material, and this change may take time to organize. You'll find Paleo meals ridiculously easy to prepare (one of the reasons so many people love eating Paleo), and eating out on Paleo is nearly foolproof.

Be patient, use this book as a reference, step outside your comfort zone, get creative, and acquaint yourself with as many spices as you can to really put a zing in your meals.

"My friends and family think I've gone mad"

Everyone wants support from family and friends. Some people will support you unconditionally. Others will give their support after they see you transform.

But some people may despise your enthusiasm, efforts, or transformation and won't give you an inch of support. Just be prepared for the different ways people may react by arming yourself with the following tips and let yourself be okay with it. It's about you and your health, anyway.

- ✔ **Some folks may surprise you.** Some people who you never expected to be intrigued and supportive, will be. Others who you thought would be supportive, won't. Be calm and at peace with either scenario. Remember that your health and what you choose to eat is *your* deal and your responsibility and leave it at that.

- ✔ **They'll come when they're ready.** People who are resistant will come to you with questions and support when they're ready. You can't strong-arm your way into changing their beliefs. When people are ready for change, they'll see your success and will come to you for answers.

- ✔ **Understand the phycology.** Getting your stuff together and eating clean even though you could easily succumb to the excuses of the busy perils of life reminds people of what they *can* and *should* be doing. Tread lightly and don't embarrass people at dinner parties or in front of spouses or colleagues. Speak in private and let them come to you when they're ready.

- ✔ **Don't preach.** Always remember dignity and grace are much more effective ways of influencing others. Getting in someone's face and launching into everything you're doing and your profound results (no matter how much you want everyone around you to share in your experience) may be counterproductive. We love enthusiasm, but measure what you say to make a bigger impact.

- ✔ **Be prepared.** Educate yourself and be prepared for questions like "no grains? Huh. Now I *know* beans are healthy, what's the problem there?" Plan on people asking questions, so get your shtick down because as sure as you're standing, they'll challenge you. Refer to Part I of this book to help explain why you're doing what you're doing. Gather information from websites or other resources to help you explain that you really are making an intelligent decision for your health.

You may not want to base your argument too heavily on science, unless you're ready for some tough, "heady" questions. As sure as you can throw out a landmark study, someone will overturn a stone on another study that refutes your evidence. Real people with real results are more impressive to others, anyway. Let that be your launch pad.

- ✔ **Keep a smile on when under attack.** Smile, smile, smile. Smiling defuses a lot. So smile, take a deep breath, and remember this sentence: "Glad what you're doing is working for you. This diet is working for me right now, so I'm going to stay the course." End with another smile. Then wait. Eventually they'll come to you. One thing for sure: The one with the most certainty is always the one who walks away having the most influence. So get your ego out of it, stay strong and certain, and, most importantly, just let it go.

"I can't afford to eat Paleo"

We respect being on a budget or having tight funds. We want you to know that, without question, you can do Paleo on a budget.

Having said that, if you're used to buying nutritionally void, supersized junk foods and eating fast food a couple times a week, eating Paleo will cost a little more. In the long run, though, you end up spending money on the healthcare you will most certainly need in the future. So if you compare Paleo foods to *frankenfoods* (fake foods with artificial ingredients made to look like real foods) and fast foods, you've got us. Paleo eating is going to cost you more. The goal, however, should be *how can I eat the healthiest way possible within my budget?* Eating Paleo can be done on budget and keep your engine going far longer and stronger than supersized French fries.

Here are some tips to save you some of that hard-earned cash and crush any financial excuses that you can't afford to do Paleo:

- ✔ **Shop at farmers' markets and Community Supported Agricultures (CSAs).** If you buy meat at a farmers' market, you can often save a bundle, even on grass-fed meats. You can also save on produce. Not only that, but the meat and produce you buy from farmers' markets is often fresher than what you can buy in a traditional grocery store.

- ✔ **Buy your produce local (when you can) and in season:** Local, in-season produce is always the freshest and often sold at a reasonable price point because not a lot of travel is involved. You also get a lot of variety by choosing seasonal produce.

- ✔ **Download the Environmental Control Group's Dirty Dozen and Clean 15 lists.** These lists help you decide what produce is safe to purchase non-organic versions of and have the least amount of toxins.

- ✔ **Go in on a cow (or half of a cow).** You can pitch in with a friend or family member to buy a cow or part of a cow directly from a farmer through a meat share and stock up. (You may need some extra freezer space if you get a lot of meat, so plan accordingly and go in with a few friends or family members if needed.)

- ✔ **Buy in bulk.** Big-box retailers, like Sam's Club, Wal-Mart, and Costco, continue to get better in quality and definitely have the best prices. They're pretty much unbeatable and, when you're on a tight budget, worth their weight in gold.

- ✔ **Go to a local butcher shop or fishmonger.** Want to buy fresh meats and fish from knowledgeable people at fair price points? Check out your local butcher shop or fishmonger.

✔ **Look for lean cuts of meat that are on sale and stock up.** This tip is key for purchasing meats. When you buy conventional meats, remember to buy leaner cuts, such as skinless turkey or chicken breast, eye of round roast, top sirloin, or low-fat ground beef. These leaner meats reduce the omega-6 you get and still allow you to benefit from the great protein source.

✔ **Do an honest evaluation.** Take an honest look at where you can cut back on less important items (such as wine, expensive lotions and other beauty products, video games, cellphone services, and "fancy" clothes or shoes), freeing up more money for your more important cause — good quality food.

We mention throughout this book that grass-fed meat is a superior quality protein. But if you just can't swing the usually higher price, it's okay. Grass-fed protein is certainly not a requirement for eating Paleo. Health is your goal, not following hyper-specific rules. Just do the best you can and remember that you've already shed a lot of unhealthy foods, so give yourself a break and know that you're making major headway regardless. You're still eating far better than the SAD. Just eat the cleanest food you can afford and feel good about the strides you're making.

"I can't find healthy meats or vegetables where I live"

You don't have to have a gourmet grocer or Whole Foods nearby to eat Paleo. Eating Paleo doesn't require following hyper-specific rules. You just need to find meat, vegetables, fruits, nuts, seeds, and some good oil. If you don't have a Whole Foods, Trader Joe's, or a gourmet grocer nearby, no big deal whatsoever.

In fact, the buying clubs, like Sam's Club, Costco, and Wal-Mart, and any of your local grocery chains, farmers' markets, CSAs, and local butcher shops have most of what you need. For some of the pantry items, like coconut oil or almond flour, you may have to seek out a natural foods store or an online source, but every year, more conventional and club stores are expanding their stock to healthier, more natural foods.

If you want to buy pasture-raised, grass-fed, or organic and you can't find it in your area, refer to Chapter 7 for recommended online resources to help you find everything you need.

"I don't know how to cook"

Cooking Paleo is about the easiest way to prepare meals that you can possibly imagine. You're working with basic foods, and you can access an overwhelming number of amazing resources to get started. The best part is you can create super nutritious, wonderfully easy dishes in a snap.

Finding out that many of the foods you've become accustomed to eating no longer have a place in your diet can be intimidating. Especially when these foods make up a large portion of your meals. Cooking new Paleo foods is just another layer that may seem daunting in your transition. Turning cereal for breakfast, a sandwich for lunch, and pizza for dinner into Paleo-friendly meals that you look forward to becomes easy in no time.

Start out basic and work your way into more sophisticated meals. You'll find that Paleo dishes can be tasty *and* healthy, and they provide you with a road map to create tasty and nutritous Paleo meals. Before long, you'll begin to experiment and alter recipes that are traditionally non-Paleo and make them Paleo. Sometimes, you'll hit a home run; other times, not so much. But either way, you'll find cooking Paleo to be easy and fun.

A basic Paleo dish is as easy as putting some healthy oil in a pan, browning up some meat, adding in herbs or spices, adding a vegetable, and cooking for about 10 minutes. Voilà! You've got a wholesome, Paleo-friendly meal. Leftover protein from the night before and a handful of nuts are a rock-solid Paleo breakfast. Toss a giant salad, top it with some meat, add a drizzle of extra-virgin olive oil, and you're good to go. If you start with the basics and progress from there, you'll find tons of variety and super easy cooking.

Eating Paleo means you have to cook, at least some of the time. If you try to go about it doing just salads, you'll fall into a dark hole of boredom. It won't be pretty. So grab a pan and start with super easy meals and see where they take you.

Incorporating Paleo into Vegetarian and Vegan Lifestyles

Eating Paleo does recommend the inclusion of animal protein. However, you can enjoy eating Paleo and gain considerable health benefits without making animal protein a part of your Paleo plan. Whether you choose not to eat meat because of ethical, religious, or spiritual beliefs, we respect your choice and help you make the best vegetarian or vegan choices within the framework of your obligations.

If you don't eat meat because you feel that it's the healthier way to go, we ask that you give the foods on the Paleo "yes" list a try. Here's why: We truly believe that your body is the most nutritionally sufficient and balanced with the inclusion of meat products. Countless stories of folks who took on the vegetarian way of life because they were trying to take the very best care of their body have found that their health declined over time on that plan, only to discover that their health skyrocketed after they started eating animal products again.

If you choose not to eat animal products because you're concerned about the treatment of animals or global issues, thankfully, there are now ways to source meat, fish, and eggs responsibly. Here's one such source: `www.sustainable table.org/home.php`.

Perhaps you just don't like the taste of meat or have been a vegetarian for so long that eating meat just turns you off. Or perhaps you do eat some eggs and fish. Whatever scenario fits you, we help you embrace the Paleo lifestyle in the following sections, from making sure you're getting adequate protein to showing you why eating real, quality food is the best lifestyle choice you can make.

Getting enough protein

If you eat some eggs and fish, try to build your plate with these foods as your protein and use the plant-based proteins only as the exception, not the rule. Eating plenty of eggs and fish along with veggies, fruits, and nuts ensures that you get the protein you need.

On the other hand, if you choose not to eat any meat, fish, or eggs, you have to look to other vegetarian protein to get your nutrition. The most optimal choices are organic, dense protein sources, like non-GMO plant-based foods, including the following:

- Beans: Lentils, black beans, pinto beans, and red beans
- Edamame
- Full-fat pasture-raised yogurt and kefir
- High-quality protein powders, hemp, or pea protein
- Natto
- Tempeh
- Tofu

TIP

The beans we recommend have the lowest impact on blood sugar. Having your blood sugar spike up and down causes you to become unhealthy and overweight. If you buy canned beans, be sure to rinse them a couple of times before eating, which rinses off the starch and salt and reduces the gassiness that beans cause for many. If you're preparing dried beans, soak them for at least 12 hours.

Don't look to string cheese, cottage cheese, or conventional yogurt or dairy products as your protein sources. These foods may cause congestion or inflammation in the body. In fact, a lot of people are finding that they're intolerant to dairy. If your body shows signs of a dairy sensitivity, such as feeling tired after eating any dairy products, constant sniffles, coughing, or acne or skin rashes, then making dairy your protein source is definitely not going to move you toward health.

Avoiding frankenfoods

Whether you decide to eat a little meat, eggs, or fish or stick with plant-based proteins, avoiding what we call *frankenfoods* is of upmost importance. Frankenfoods are made to look like real foods but are nothing more than fake foods from head to toe. They're the worst of the worst of processed foods. These foods are genetically engineered and full of allergens, preservatives, additives, and flavor enhancers. In a word, yuck!

Frankenfoods are processed soy and meat alternatives. Unlike soy foods, such as edamame, tempeh, and traditional miso, which are closer to their natural state, these foods are a far cry from anything real. We understand that some vegetarians don't eat any eggs or fish and are looking for ways to expand their protein sources. You do have to get your protein somewhere. But look past these food products for your options. This stuff just isn't healthy for anyone. Period. In fact, these options aren't even foods. They're *food products,* usually a mixture of a wheat protein with a subpar oil. The frankenfoods we strongly urge you to avoid include the following:

- ✔ Soy milk
- ✔ Tofu hot dogs
- ✔ Veggie bacon
- ✔ Veggie chicken
- ✔ Veggie chicken wings
- ✔ Veggie loafs
- ✔ Veggie "sausage" links

All these "food" items should be in a landfill and not in your kitchen!

We hope that you're inspired to reconsider adding some animal protein to your diet. However, if you're holding steadfast on vegetarianism or veganism, make sure your protein sources are as healthy and as natural as can be. Also, make sure you're getting plenty of healthy fats and loads of fruits and veggies. People who take the vegetarian approach tend to have intestinal, inflammatory, and autoimmune types of problems and healthy fats help reduce that inflammation.

Chapter 16

Dining Out and Traveling

· ·

In This Chapter

▶ Selecting the right restaurants for your Paleo lifestyle

▶ Figuring out what to order from restaurant menus

▶ Traveling without sacrificing your good habits

· ·

When you've made the commitment to follow a Paleo lifestyle, eating the Paleo Big Three becomes second nature, especially when you're cooking and eating at home. But if you're like most humans, you're a social creature who likes to get out and see the rest of the world once a while. In this chapter, you discover how to eat in restaurants — in your neighborhood or on vacation — without sacrificing your good habits or good taste.

Identifying the best restaurants for Paleo-friendly food and finding the best items on the menu is essential for happy dining outside the safety zone of your Paleo kitchen. With the tips in this chapter, you'll be able to find something to eat in just about any type of restaurant — without resorting to plain lettuce and ice water.

Travel feeds the soul and the imagination, but vacations can often be detrimental to good nutrition. This chapter shows you how to decide when to stray from your Paleo path to enjoy local culture, as well as how to stick to your guns when you're on the road.

Whether you're dining out to celebrate with friends, traveling to another city for a business trip, or taking an extended trip in exotic territory, this chapter provides all the info, tricks, and tips you need to feel great on your journey and when you return home.

Choosing the Right Restaurant

Research and preparation are the first steps to enjoying a successful restaurant experience. With a little bit of recon, you can review restaurant menus in advance to ensure that you can find food that fits into your eating plan. And by deciding in advance what to order, you can prevent temptation or confusion from derailing your good intentions.

National chain restaurants and most locally owned restaurants have websites that include their menus, and review sites, like Yelp.com, are another good way to gain insight into the menu and quality of the food.

Whenever possible, choose restaurants that serve locally sourced ingredients, like meat and organic produce from nearby farms. The phrase *farm to table* is usually a reliable indicator that the quality of the ingredients are top-notch, and restaurants concerned with serving only the best ingredients are also interested in responding to diners' requests, so you have free rein to be a "picky eater."

Living Paleo doesn't require you to be perfect but, instead, is meant to encourage you to make intentional food choices that make you feel good physically and emotionally. As we discuss in Chapter 9, you may choose to indulge in a non-Paleo treat occasionally. The guidelines for restaurant dining outlined in the following sections are meant to help you eat well when you're trying to remain true to your Paleo habits. When you decide to indulge in special occasion foods at restaurants, refer to the guidelines in Chapter 9 and choose only the most delicious options, and then savor every bite.

Keeping your expectations in check: Restaurants aren't perfect

When you cook in your kitchen, you know exactly what's going into your meals, and you're probably paying equal attention to the healthiness and tastiness of your food. In most restaurants, the number-one priority is to serve food that tastes good, and that philosophy means that professional chefs add sugars, fat, soy, and wheat to their food in ways that you probably don't at home.

Now that you've adopted the Paleo lifestyle, you need to decide how much wiggle room you can accept in restaurant food. For example, during your 30-Day Reset, you should avoid brown-sugar crusted ribs at your favorite barbecue joint, but when you've accomplished your 30 days and you're "just living Paleo," it's up to you to decide whether a little added sugar, a splash of soy sauce, or canola oil is acceptable.

Avoiding foods that cause a severe negative reaction in your body should be a no-brainer. If you have a painful bowling ball in your stomach for three days after eating cheese or gluten, you probably don't want to indulge in those foods, no matter how delicious they are. But if a little extra sugar interrupts the quality of your sleep for one night, is it worth it to you? Only you can answer that question, and your answer may change under different timing and circumstances. The goal is not to be perfect but to find the guidelines that work for you.

This chapter is packed with tips and tricks to help you successfully navigate eating in restaurants. But even when you order carefully and verify ingredients, non-Paleo ingredients can sneak into your food, despite the best intentions of the cook or your server. If you have serious ailments or allergies, choose your dining opportunities carefully.

Making friends with the server and chef

Now that you're a Paleo aficionado, you're going to develop some serious detective skills and become an expert at asking questions about food. Your first task when you arrive at the restaurant is to enlist the server as your ally in understanding everything that may end up on your plate. This task is easier when you've done your homework by reviewing the menu in advance (see previous section).

Asking for what you need can sometimes be uncomfortable, but remember: At a restaurant, you're a paying customer and have the right to get exactly what you want on your plate (within reason).

Here are some tips to help you win over your server and get the information you need to make Paleo-friendly choices:

- ✔ **Call ahead.** Particularly in fine-dining or family-owned restaurants, the proprietors are dedicated to making your dining experience a pleasant one. In many cases, you can call ahead to ask questions and make special requests. Don't be afraid to ask for what you need; people are often happy to accommodate you, especially if it means repeat business.

- ✔ **Ask about gluten.** Many restaurants have become more sensitive to the need for gluten-free options for diners' allergies and conditions like celiac disease. Although gluten-free options may still involve grains, a gluten-free menu is a good starting point for asking questions and finding meals that don't include glutinous grains.

- ✔ **Say "no" to the pre-meal freebies.** Nothing is "free" about a bread basket, bowl of peanuts, or basket of tortilla chips that tempt you to eat their unhealthy contents. When the server delivers these snacks with your menu, smile and say, "no, thank you."

- ✔ **Ask about oils.** Most restaurants use canola oil for their griddles, pan frying, deep frying, and salads. If you know you're sensitive to oils high in omega-6 fatty acids, skip any foods cooked in canola oil.

  Canola oil is a highly-processed oil used in just about every restaurant, from fast food joints, to family-owned diners, to upscale restaurants. It's inexpensive, flavorless, and can withstand high temperatures, so it's the ideal choice for a restaurant kitchen concerned with profit and taste, but it's a terrible choice for people concerned about their health. If you eat in a restaurant, canola oil is almost unavoidable. Don't panic! Make healthy choices at home, select the best options you can in a restaurant, and then stop worrying about it and enjoy your food.

✔ **Make substitutions.** You can always swap side dishes — request a side of fruit instead of potatoes at breakfast, for example — or ask for a double order of good things like vegetables. In some cases, you may be charged a little extra, but it's worth the investment to get the food your body needs.

✔ **Get creative.** Mix and match from the choices on the menu to create new combos. Request that sauces be served on top of vegetables instead of pasta or ask for sandwich fillings on a bed of lettuce instead of between slices of bread.

The best choice for butter is clarified butter from grass-fed, organically raised cows. Most restaurants don't use this highest quality butter in cooking. Broiled fish and steak is often finished with butter, so be sure to ask your server to have the chef broil your food dry.

✔ **Check the dressing.** The majority of restaurants in the United States are serviced by one food supply company, from frozen foods to produce and everything in between. Factory-made salad dressings are notorious for including hidden sugars, soy, and corn, so ask your server about the ingredients in the salad dressing. If it's commercially made, opt instead for vinegar or lemon juice and extra-virgin olive oil for your salad.

Managing the Restaurant Menu

If you're diligent and ask lots of questions, eating in a restaurant can be a fun, pleasurable experience. *Remember:* You're not aiming for perfection. Just do your best, and then relax and savor your food.

In the following sections, we walk you through selecting the best options from restaurant menus, including what to look for when partaking of American and international cuisines, so you can dine out with confidence no matter where your taste buds take you.

The "yes" list: Paleo-friendly cooking methods

As customers like you become more savvy about the healthfulness of the food they eat in restaurants, chefs are broadening the options on their menus to include better options.

Look for these cooking methods and descriptions to find the most Paleo-friendly choices on the menu — and remember to ask clarifying questions of your server to verify ingredients and cooking.

- ✔ **Broiled:** Broiled fish, seafood, steak, chicken, and all kinds of chops are a great choice. Be sure to ask whether the meat is basted with anything before, during, or after broiling.

- ✔ **Steamed:** Steaming is just about the most ideal way to cook vegetables. Ask whether the vegetables are dressed with seasoning or fat after cooking and ask for them plain with extra-virgin olive oil on the side.

- ✔ **Poached:** Fish and chicken poached in water or broth is flavorful, tender, and Paleo-approved. Ask the server whether wine is included in the poaching broth so you can make an informed decision about whether you want to make an exception to your rules for the added flavor.

- ✔ **Braised:** This is another great Paleo-friendly cooking method that should make you feel confident about the food. Wine or soy may be involved in the braising liquid, so clarify with the server.

- ✔ **Roasted:** Roasted meats and vegetables are almost always a good choice; get details about dry rubs or marinades to verify the ingredients.

- ✔ **Grilled:** Grilling may be the favored Paleo cooking method! Remember to double-check the marinade and dry rub ingredients, and ask whether the grilled meat is finished with a sauce or oil when it comes off the grill.

- ✔ **Sous vide:** Sous vide is becoming more popular, and it's a great choice for Paleo people. The meat or seafood is cooked in a hot water bath then finished over or under a high heat source to brown the outside. Ask your server whether anything is added to the meat before it's served.

- ✔ **Sautéed:** Sautéed food can go two ways; if it's sautéed in a quality form of fat without added sugar, soy, or grains, it gets a green light. If it's drenched in non-Paleo ingredients, it's a definite stop sign.

- ✔ **Smoked:** Like grilling, smoking is a Paleo-friendly cooking method. Sugar is often included in the rubs used on meat, but the amounts are usually minimal and not worth too much worry. Verify with the server how much, if any, is used.

Beware of soups and stews. They can be a satisfying one-stop source of quality protein and vegetables, unless the chef thickens them with a flour-based roux or adds cream for a smooth texture. Ask lots of questions about soups and stews, including whether they contain soy, flour, other grains, or dairy.

Be inquisitive! Terms like *salsa* and *relish* usually indicate fresh vegetables diced and tossed together with seasonings to add zing to meats and vegetables, which means they can be Paleo friendly. But these condiments can also include added sugar, soy, and wheat, so ask plenty of questions before you dig in.

The "no" list: Cooking methods and terms to avoid

Words like *crispy* and *battered* can make food sound appetizing, but now that you're living Paleo, those words should also sound an alarm of caution. Anything battered and crispy is most likely rolled in flour and deep-fried in canola oil, which means it's out of consideration for a Paleo eater.

When you see the following terms on menu descriptions, ask lots of questions and be prepared to take a pass on foods that don't meet your standards:

- ✔ Battered
- ✔ Breaded
- ✔ Coated
- ✔ Crispy
- ✔ Deep fried
- ✔ Dumpling
- ✔ Fritter
- ✔ Meatballs/Meatloaf/Croquettes
- ✔ Sauced
- ✔ Sausage

Most restaurants use commercial mayonnaise, which is almost always made from inflammatory, industrial seed oils like canola, safflower, sunflower, or a blend. Avoid restaurant mayo unless you're choosing it as a treat. And this applies to creamy dressings, too. Even if the restaurant's salad dressing is homemade, it may be based on commercial mayo.

American restaurants, diners, and cafés

Diners and cafés are among the easiest restaurants to find Paleo-friendly meals because their menus often offer fresh salads, burgers, and stick-to-your-ribs fare, like roast poultry or meat, steaks, chops, and vegetables. Here are some tips for finding the gems on the menu.

- ✔ **Look for the eggs.** From scrambled and omelets to poached and fried, eggs are a protein-packed choice that can be found just about everywhere. Be sure to ask whether the chef includes dairy, wheat, or soy in the scrambled eggs and omelets. Most kitchens will honor your request to make eggs without added ingredients. When in doubt, order poached eggs because the only ingredients are eggs and water.

✔ **Go bunless.** With a salad and a side of vegetables, a burger (without the bun) makes a great meal. Some restaurants have gotten hip to the trend and offer burgers wrapped in fresh lettuce leaves instead of buns.

✔ **Stick with protein and vegetables.** When in doubt, a steak and a salad is always a safe bet. Other good options are salmon, grilled or roasted chicken, roasted turkey, grilled or broiled pork chops, pot roast, or any variety of fish or seafood. Ask questions about the preparation and then dig in!

✔ **Watch the barbecue grub.** Smoked beef, pork, chicken, and turkey are all good choices at your favorite barbecue joint. Although most barbecue rubs contain sugar, it's usually a trace amount, so probably not worth too much concern. Beware of barbecue sauce, however, which usually includes a lot of sugar as an ingredient; enjoy your meat plain instead. For side dishes, look for braised greens and tossed salad, but avoid the Paleo no-nos of potato salad and cole slaw.

✔ **Mix it up with salads.** A big salad is another reliable choice — lots of fresh veggies topped with protein and drizzled with quality fat. Be on the lookout for sneaky ingredients like croutons or cheese, and verify the ingredients in the dressing to be sure they comply with your Paleo standards. You can get creative with salads by combining toppings from different salad options into your own combos.

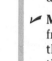

Salads can quickly turn from a great choice to a problematic one with the addition of a few unhealthy ingredients. Always request dressings on the side so you can control the amount that's added to your vegetables, or discretely bring a small container of homemade dressing with you. Don't forget to ask your server whether the salad includes grated cheese and/or croutons and request that yours be served without them.

Breakfast food isn't just for breakfast! Many diners and cafés offer breakfast any time. A serving of eggs with a side of fruit and vegetables or a side salad is an easy, reliable way to eat deliciously and healthily away from home.

International cuisine

One of the most enjoyable aspects of eating out is a restaurant's ability to introduce you to the tastes of other cultures. And even as a Paleo eater, you can enjoy some of your favorite international dishes. With these guidelines for the following cuisines, you can eat your way around the world without damaging your good habits.

✔ **Mexican:** Olé! Mexican food can be Paleo-friendly when you focus on meat, salsa, and guacamole. Take a pass on the chip basket and avoid tortillas, gorditas, enchiladas, and other dishes that may be wrapped in tortillas or buried under cheese. In place of rice and beans, request a side of vegetables or grilled jalapeños, if you like it hot. Look for dishes like steak, shrimp, or chicken fajitas; carnitas; carne asada; barbacoa; and rotisserie-roasted chicken. You can even enjoy tacos — just eat the middles and leave the tortilla.

✔ **Italian:** You're not eating pasta or garlic bread, but that doesn't mean you can't enjoy Italian food. Look for roasted chicken, veal piccata, grilled fish, and beef dishes like pot roast. Remember to ask questions about preparation because pan-sautéed meats are often dusted in flour before cooking; the chef can probably make your order without flour, so ask nicely. A big antipasto platter with olives, peppers, and Italian meats is a good choice, along with a side salad dressed with olive oil and vinegar. As a side, order grilled vegetables or a green vegetable, like broccoli or spinach, topped with marinara sauce.

Bad news: Restaurants don't have a Paleo-friendly choice for pizza. Although a gluten-free crust topped with sauce and vegetables (and no cheese) is a better choice than traditional pizza, you're better off making a Paleo-friendly pizza at home. If you find that your system can handle the grains included in gluten-free flours — or even cheese, on occasion — you may opt to enjoy pizza as a treat. But do so consciously and savor every bite.

✔ **Thai:** Avoid stir-fries, which often contain soy, noodle dishes that usually include noodles and added sugar, and the rice that comes standard as a side. Opt, instead, for curries made with coconut milk, protein, and vegetables — and request that the chef double the vegetables in your serving.

✔ **Indian:** Grilled and roasted meats and vegetables — especially those made in the Tandoori oven — are usually a safe bet. Avoid curries in rich sauces because they're based on yogurt and may also include flour. Take a pass on the naan and rice.

✔ **Japanese and sushi:** Sushi restaurants can be a great place to eat Paleo with a little preparation and by making special requests. Bring a bottle of coconut aminos with you and use them in place of soy sauce. When ordering maki or hand rolls, ask that they be made without rice — and sashimi is always an excellent option. Avoid tempura rolls and ask about sauces that may be included in rolls or drizzled over the top, because they most likely include soy and/or sugar. Appetizers, like dumplings and edamame, aren't Paleo options, but seaweed salad can be a delicious choice.

When dining on Asian cuisine, ask that your food be prepared without MSG.

✔ **Chinese:** Unless you have a relationship with the chef or management of your local Chinese restaurant, eating Chinese food in a restaurant can be difficult. Most Chinese foods include soy, cornstarch, rice and rice flour, and added sugars. If you find yourself in a Chinese restaurant and have no other options, the *cleanest* choices are steamed vegetables and roasted meats, like barbecued spareribs or chicken wings, but even those meats will probably include a small amount of soy sauce. If you're particularly sensitive to gluten and/or soy, you should probably avoid Chinese restaurants and reserve stir-fries for home cooking.

✔ **Middle Eastern:** Although living Paleo means you have to say "no" to pita bread, rice, and hummus, other delicious Middle Eastern choices fit into the Paleo lifestyle. Look for beef, lamb, pork, and chicken shawarma, baba ghanoush (eggplant purée), and shish kebabs made from lamb, beef, chicken, and vegetables. Tahini dressing — made from lemon juice, sesame seed paste, and olive oil — is a great choice for dipping or drizzling over salads.

✔ **Greek/Mediterranean:** Grilled fish, Greek salad (minus the feta cheese), gyro meat (as long as it doesn't contain grains as fillers), roasted chicken, shish kebabs, and olives are all delicious, Paleo-approved choices. Take a pass on pita bread, as well as casseroles like moussaka, which include dairy and flour.

Part of the fun of dining out is eating foods you don't usually enjoy at home and luxuriating in the experience of someone else doing the cooking and serving. If you adhere to our Paleo guidelines when you cook at home 80 to 90 percent of the time, loosening up your standards to enjoy restaurant experiences is perfectly okay.

Taking Paleo on the Road

Finding high-quality, Paleo-friendly food while traveling away from home — whether for business or pleasure — can be difficult. The situation is further complicated when you're tired or stressed by the challenges of traveling. Plus that old saying, "When in Rome . . . ," may tempt you to stray from Paleo practices. How do you balance the desire to experience local culture with your need to feed yourself well for mental and physical health?

Here are some guidelines to ensure that a few special treats don't ruin your entire vacation with gastrointestinal distress, lethargy, or moodiness:

✔ **Eat very clean before you go.** In preparation for your trip, follow the Paleo eating guidelines as closely as you can. You may even want to be super strict and repeat your 30-Day Reset (Chapter 8) to prep your body before you go.

✔ **Choose only the best.** If you're traveling to France, for example, you'll probably want to try the wine, the cheese, and the bread. Do research to find the very best and then hold out until you can enjoy it. Don't settle for the mediocre baguette on the plane or the cheese from the super-marché. Set your standards high and treat yourself with only the best version of the special foods you choose.

✔ **Set parameters.** Will you allow yourself one treat per day? One treat per meal? Maybe you'll eat clean at breakfast and lunch, but make dinner a special meal. Decide in advance how you want to manage your meals so you're not caught off guard or overtaken by cravings during your trip.

✔ **Savor every bite.** When you've selected a treat, eat it slowly and experience every bite with all your senses — the taste, the smell, the texture, the environment. All of them add up to an experience that makes an indulgence a special memory that can sustain you when you're back to eating clean protein and vegetables.

✔ **Refocus when you get home.** When you return from your trip, your cravings may be a bit fired up from the indulgences you enjoyed on your vacation. Now isn't the time for self-recrimination! Instead, enjoy your memories of your special dining experiences and get right back into your Paleo groove. Again, you may want to follow the rules of the 30-day reset; even just a week of eating strict Paleo can help ease you back onto your healthy path.

Finding or bringing airport-friendly snacks

Let's face it: The food options at most airports are pretty terrible, and airplane food is not only junky, but it's also not very tasty. You'll be happier and healthier if you eat well before your flight, make a plan for where you'll eat at your destination, and pack Paleo-friendly snacks for the travel time in between. Arm yourself with a small, insulated cooler food bag to carry foods that need to be kept cool, and stuff non-perishables into your carry-on for snacks any time.

What follows are some foods that won't send the TSA into a panic and will travel well without refrigeration.

Pack the following in your cooler bag:

✔ Sugar-free, high-quality deli meats

✔ Smoked salmon

✔ Hard-boiled eggs

✔ Cooked chicken, cut into easily managed pieces

✔ Cooked meatballs or burger patties

✔ Cooked sweet potatoes

✔ Raw veggies, cut into easily managed pieces

✔ Fresh fruit, cut into easily managed pieces

✔ Avocado or guacamole

✔ Olives

Take these items in your carry-on bag:

- ✔ Sugar-free beef jerky
- ✔ Coconut flakes
- ✔ Nuts
- ✔ Dried fruit
- ✔ Canned sardines, tuna, or salmon
- ✔ Snack bars that contain only dried fruit and nuts
- ✔ Squeeze packs of nut butter and/or coconut butter

Snacking while driving: The "emergency" car cooler

A road trip (or train travel) lets you take your good Paleo habits to go. With some advance cooking and a well-stocked cooler, you're all set for Paleo eating wherever your wanderlust takes you.

Put together the following items in your toolkit to keep with you while on the road:

- ✔ Small cutting board
- ✔ Paring knife
- ✔ Can opener
- ✔ Empty BPA-free storage containers
- ✔ Ziploc bags in a variety of sizes
- ✔ Salt, pepper, and other spices in travel-sized jars
- ✔ A small sponge and dish soap
- ✔ Toothpicks

For perishable items, pack the following in your cooler:

- ✔ Sugar-free, high-quality deli meats
- ✔ Smoked salmon
- ✔ Hard-boiled eggs
- ✔ Cooked chicken, cut into easily managed pieces
- ✔ Cooked meatballs or burger patties
- ✔ Cooked sweet potatoes

- ✔ Whole raw veggies
- ✔ Whole fresh fruit
- ✔ Salsa
- ✔ Baba ghanoush
- ✔ Homemade salad dressing (see recipes in Chapter 14)

These items are great for the road; keep them in your dry goods bag:

- ✔ Sugar-free beef jerky
- ✔ Coconut flakes
- ✔ Nuts
- ✔ Dried fruit
- ✔ Canned sardines, tuna, or salmon
- ✔ Snack bars that contain only dried fruit and nuts
- ✔ Jars of nut butter and/or coconut butter

Chapter 17

Enjoying Special Occasions

In This Chapter

▶ Celebrating holidays and special occasions the Paleo way

▶ Enjoying treats on occasion

Sticking to your Paleo habits in a primarily non-Paleo world can be challenging. Well-meaning family members and friends may try to tempt you with foods that don't fit into your Paleo guidelines. In this chapter, you discover how to enjoy an active social life and take part in holiday celebrations without feeling deprived — and without compromising your healthy new habits. With a few easy-to-implement tricks, you'll be able to attend dinner parties, holiday celebrations, work commitments, weddings, and potlucks without stress, and when your family and friends see how much you're enjoying yourself, you just may convince them to try the Paleo lifestyle.

Especially on holidays or significant occasions, like a wedding, food is more than just nourishment for the body; it's a way to bring people together in celebration. This chapter shows you how to balance treats with your Paleo commitment so you have the best of both worlds.

Whether you're closing a big deal over a five-course dinner — with wine! — or strapping on heels as a bridesmaid for the third time this year, this chapter gives you all the skills and details you need to truly celebrate.

Planning Ahead for Social Events

Planning and preparation make living Paleo much easier. This principle definitely applies to making the most of social situations. With just a little prep — and a willingness to actively change your public behavior — you can enjoy parties as much as ever without sacrificing your Paleo principles.

Following your Paleo guidelines will eventually feel like second nature in the comfort of your house and familiar surroundings, but socializing can present a new world of challenges. Here are some suggestions to help you carry your Paleo habits with you wherever your social life takes you:

✔ **Do your research.** As we discuss in Chapter 16, a quick review of a restaurant's menu in advance can mean the difference between a relaxing, enjoyable meal and a gluten-infused nightmare. Read all the options on the menu and decide what you're going to order before you go. Then, when you arrive at the restaurant, don't even open the menu — just revel in the knowledge that you know exactly what you're ordering and sip on a glass of water while your dining companions make their decisions.

✔ **Bring your own food.** This trick isn't always applicable or appropriate, but in many cases, it works like a charm. Are you going to a casual event, like a picnic? There's no harm in packing your own food in a cooler bag. And believe it or not, you can even pack your own food for a wedding, if you do it with class and care. Between the ceremony in the church and the reception, there's usually a lull of at least an hour. That's the perfect opportunity to eat a Paleo-friendly snack or mini meal to nourish your body. At the reception, when your stomach is full of good food and your blood sugar is stable, avoiding non-Paleo foods that may show up on your plate or the buffet table is easier. Take advantage of vegetables and salads — and even protein if it's served without sauces or breading. Or simply avoid the food altogether.

✔ **Eat before you go.** If your big night out is dinner in a restaurant with friends, you probably don't want to eat before you go. But a party at a friend's house, an afternoon of window shopping, or a movie night doesn't need to derail your good habits. Eat a solid Paleo meal before you go and bring Paleo-friendly snacks with you to sustain you if you get hungry or to give you something to eat when your companions indulge in a snack along the way.

If socializing is your priority, your snack or pre-meal doesn't have to be the best you've ever eaten. It just needs to be nutritious and satisfying enough to carry you through. Every meal doesn't need to be a sit-down feast that feeds your soul and all your senses. Sometimes you just need to eat.

✔ **Enlist help.** Tell your family and friends that you're sticking to your new Paleo habits to explain why you're not gulping beer, noshing on Grandma's sugar cookies, or diving face first into the plate of nachos you usually order while watching the playoffs. They may tease you a bit, but when they realize that you're serious and that eating Paleo is important to you, they'll probably also encourage you. And maybe they'll be curious enough about what you're doing to try it themselves. Don't be shy about creating an army of support to help you get over challenging humps.

✔ **Be firm.** You may be surprised to discover that, for the most part, no one else will really notice when you change your habits. And if they do, they most likely won't care too much. If someone gives you a hard time — a waiter, a co-worker, a friend — simply look him in the eye and say with as much steel (and patience) in your voice as possible, "Eating this way is important to me. I'm sure you understand my desire to be as healthy as possible." It's virtually impossible for anyone to argue with that.

> ✔ **Eat when you get home.** Congratulations! You did it! You went to happy hour after work and avoided chicken wings and 2-for-1 cocktails. When happy hour turned into dinner, you ordered a salad with grilled chicken while everyone else ate burgers and fries. Now, back at home, you're feeling proud, but also a little hungry. Now is the time to celebrate with a Paleo snack. Perhaps some Cocoa-Cinnamon Coconut Chips (see recipe in Chapter 13), an egg scrambled with some chives, or a hard-boiled egg topped with a dollop of Homemade Mayonnaise (Chapter 14). Then you can put on your pajamas and snuggle in to enjoy a restful sleep, knowing that the next morning you won't be plagued by a hangover.

When spending time with friends and family, you want your focus to be on the conversation, laughter, and camaraderie of your favorite people. Don't fall into the trap of thinking that a party is *primarily* about the food and the cocktails; it's really about enjoying social interaction with people you like. If you take the focus off the food and drink and redirect your attention to the people you're with, you'll enjoy the occasion, and following your Paleo guidelines will feel effortless.

Eating Paleo During Celebrations and Holidays

Living Paleo doesn't mean that you'll never eat your mom's legendary coffee cake or a piece of comforting lasagna ever again. But as we discuss throughout this book, choosing food indulgences carefully and intentionally is essential for optimal mental and physical health. In this section, we tell you how to enjoy holiday celebrations, from family dinners to big bashes, with Paleo-friendly food ideas; we provide some handy tips for managing cocktail hour and an open bar; and we share the magic words that can help you gently put off the food pushers who want you to break your rules.

Food traditions are some of the most cherished, and Thanksgiving may not seem like Thanksgiving without the green bean casserole you eat every year. But new traditions can be just as rewarding as old ones — and sometimes the old ones can be updated without anyone being the wiser. As you find out in this section, starting new traditions that make your family and friends healthier is easy and fun, and bringing old traditions into your Paleo lifestyle keeps that traditional feeling but in a new and improved way.

Creating Paleo-friendly celebratory meals

Take a moment and count up the number of holidays throughout the year: You have New Year's Day in January, Super Bowl Sunday (which is a major celebration for some people) and Valentine's Day in February, followed by

Easter, Memorial Day, Fourth of July, birthdays, weddings, anniversary parties, and graduation celebrations. Almost every month of the year has a reason to celebrate, and if you indulge on every holiday, you can seriously disrupt your healthy habits in a way that's counterproductive. In the following sections, we provide some tips for getting through all the celebrations and get-togethers without breaking your Paleo lifestyle.

Planning a Paleo party menu

To truly celebrate holidays, create menus that feature Paleo foods that nourish your body and taste great, and then on very special occasions, select a treat that's worth the compromise. Here are some suggestions to help with holiday menu planning when you're the host:

- ✔ **Make it fun.** If you make the food fun and engaging, chances are no one will notice how healthy it is. For a party, try setting up a burger bar with all the fixings and invite guests to build their own burgers. Put out colorful bowls of raw vegetables, guacamole, Tangy BBQ Sauce and Homemade Mayonnaise (see recipes in Chapter 14), pickles, and jalapeños, and shakers of spices and seasoned salts. Or set out a build-your-own taco bar with chicken and ground beef taco meat, salsas, avocado, and a variety of lettuce leaves for wrapping (see recipe for Leafy Tacos in Chapter 10). By encouraging everyone to play with their food, you amp up the fun as well as the nutrition.

- ✔ **Satisfy with side dishes.** For more formal dinners and holidays like Thanksgiving, Christmas, and Easter, serving some kind of roast meat or poultry is often tradition. That's perfect for a Paleo lifestyle! And the sides are where you can enjoy some special ingredients to make the meal memorable. Go-alongs, like roasted sweet potatoes with clarified butter and Mashed Cauliflower or Cauliflower Rice (recipes in Chapter 12), studded with dried fruit, are Paleo-friendly options that will delight your guests' taste buds.

- ✔ **Go with grain-free goodies.** There's no denying that the attachments to cookies on Christmas and a cake to celebrate a birthday are pretty strong. You can satisfy those yearnings with grain-free, gluten-free baked goods. These special occasion foods aren't recommended during your 30-Day Reset (Chapter 8), but they can be part of a healthy, balanced Paleo lifestyle. You can find excellent grain-free recipes in cookbooks and online; just be sure to verify that the ingredients conform to your Paleo guidelines. Then engage in the whole experience, from selecting the recipe, to baking the goodies, to savoring every bite.

- ✔ **Mix it up with finger foods.** Nothing says *party food* like fancy appetizers, and turning Paleo ingredients into finger foods that your friends and family won't be able to resist is easy. Raw vegetables become something special when they're cut into unusual shapes and dipped in homemade sauces, like Ranch Dressing or Cashew Butter Satay Sauce (see recipes in Chapter 14). Tuna salad turns into party food when you add apples and pecans then serve it on thin apple slices or cucumber rounds. Tuck a smoked almond inside a dried date for a salty-sweet treat. Toss green and black olives with Aromatic Vinaigrette (Chapter 14) and serve with frilly toothpicks. Simple, fresh ingredients can become memorable when you dress up their presentation and focus on bold flavors.

✔ **Don't forget the eye candy.** It's been said that we eat first with our eyes, and Paleo ingredients are beautiful: brightly colored fresh fruits and vegetables, toasty brown nuts, jewel-toned dried fruits. Take a little extra time to create enticing presentations of Paleo foods, and even the most devoted junk food junkie at your gathering won't be able to resist.

✔ **Indulge in really good dark chocolate.** High-quality, organic, dark chocolate is a not-too-sweet treat that satisfies the desire for something sweet without derailing all your hard work. Look for bars that are at least 70 percent cacao, and then break them into bite-size pieces, place on a beautiful serving dish with a few dry roasted nuts and a few unsweetened coconut flakes, and relish how no one complains that they're denied a gloppy, over-the-top dessert.

Picking up Paleo potluck ideas

Parties where you're asked to contribute to the spread are the best socializing option because you can bring food that supports your good habits and share that delicious food with others, potentially making new converts along the way. Plus, the looser social rules make it far easier to ask questions about ingredients and bring your own special food that maybe only you eat.

When preparing for a potluck, ask the host about protein options. If the party throwers aren't providing meat, be sure to bring your own so your meal has a solid nutritional foundation. You don't need to make a big fuss; just quietly bring some portable protein. Cold cooked chicken or meatballs travel well, as do hard-boiled eggs and smoked salmon. Use the guidelines in Chapter 16 to help you pack food that sets you up for success. You can also settle the protein question by cooking a potluck dish that includes adequate protein so you can simply eat your contribution to the buffet table.

Plenty of Paleo-friendly options are great to share on a potluck buffet, from hot and comforting to cool and crisp. Here are some ideas for you to contribute the next time you get an invitation:

✔ **Hearty salads:** Fresh produce tossed with quality protein and tangy dressing is always a crowd pleaser. Recipes like Berry-Nice Chicken Salad, Chinese Chicken Salad, and Club Sandwich Salad (see recipes in Chapter 10) have international flair and will surprise your non-Paleo friends with their bold flavors. You can also make a Chopped Salad (Chapter 12) and provide diced chicken or shrimp on the side, along with a sauce or dressing from Chapter 14.

✔ **Chili:** A slow cooker filled with chili is a potluck standby, but you can make it special by remembering to bring the condiments to top it off:

thinly sliced jalapeños, diced avocado, chopped scallions, raisins, shredded cabbage, and wedges of lime.

✔ **Veggies and dip:** A giant platter of fresh vegetables — carrot sticks, red pepper rings, cucumber rounds, jicama matchsticks, broccoli and cauliflower florets, mushrooms, and grape tomatoes — goes from humdrum to yum when you add a few special touches. After arranging the vegetables, add handfuls of black and green olives, then sprinkle the entire platter with minced fresh parsley and basil, and add pretty bowls of dipping sauces on the side.

✔ **Deviled eggs:** The classic picnic food, deviled eggs are a nice choice for potlucks because they pack high-quality protein into every fun bite. The Southwest Deviled Eggs recipe in Chapter 13 is a flavorful twist on the basic recipe. You can also use the ingredients to make a spicy egg salad and serve it on wedges of red bell pepper or cucumber slices. It's a fun, eye-pleasing way to add more veggies!

✔ **Nuts and berries:** When they're in season, nothing is more appealing than fresh berries. Gently toss raspberries, blueberries, and blackberries in a large bowl with pecan halves and unsweetened coconut flakes. You'll earn bonus points if you provide a squeeze bottle of coconut milk flavored with a little vanilla so people can drizzle their fruit with creamy coconut.

✔ **Fudge bombs:** These Paleo candies (see recipe in Chapter 13) are definitely in the *treat* category, but they're also an excellent way to demonstrate to skeptics that living Paleo doesn't mean giving up all food fun. And as sweet treats go, they're a far better choice than commercial candy made with corn syrup or baked treats that contain gluten. Fudge bombs are also a nice choice for potlucks because you can make them smaller than usual to increase the quantity — and they look pretty lined up on a serving dish with fresh strawberries and whole nuts.

Having the occasional drink

Drinking alcohol on a regular basis isn't part of the Paleo lifestyle, but enjoying a cocktail on occasion is okay, whether it's raising champagne in celebration, sipping a glass of red wine to relax, or cooling off at a hot fiesta with an icy margarita. The key to successfully imbibing alcohol while living Paleo is choosing the right adult beverages and consuming them in a responsible, intentional way. In the following sections, we share the secrets of enjoying the occasional alcoholic beverage (or looking like you are) while sticking to your Paleo plan.

The non-drink drink

Whether you're meeting friends at a local bar for happy hour, dancing the night away at a wedding reception, or meeting clients for a business dinner, you can enjoy the social scene without having to explain why you're not drinking like everyone else.

The NorCal Margarita

Made (in)famous by Paleo guru Robb Wolf, the NorCal Margarita is one of the tastiest and Paleo-friendly options you can find behind a bar. Based on tequila and lime juice, it has some interesting properties that make it a solid choice for cocktail time. The tequila, made from fermented agave, is naturally gluten and starch free, and the juice helps temper the release of insulin — plus it's refreshing on a hot day and goes great with Mexican food.

Just blend a shot of 100 percent agave tequila with the juice and pulp of one fresh lime. Shake with crushed ice, pour into a tall glass, and top off with club soda. Garnish with a fresh lime wedge and enjoy!

One way to manage social situations when you're not going to drink alcohol is to get a glass into your hand immediately upon entering the room. Simply walk up to the bartender and request a large club soda with two slices of lime and a few olives. With that glass in your hand, you look like everyone else in the room! You have a refreshing drink that appears to be a cocktail (so inquisitive friends are appeased), but it's not just a boring glass of water. Also, you can enjoy the added bonus of remaining clear-headed throughout the experience and wake feeling refreshed, instead of hung over, the following morning.

Smart indulgence

But what do you do if you want to enjoy a cocktail once in a while? Some choices for alcohol fit better into the Paleo lifestyle than others, and the cocktail you choose should be based on your taste preferences and what leaves you feeling your best. Here are the smartest options for when you want to indulge:

✔ **Wine and champagne:** Wine, especially red wine, may have some heart health benefits, and some evidence suggests that it even helps ward off infectious cold viruses. Wine includes antioxidants that help fight cancer and reduce the signs of aging, and organic wine is higher in antioxidants than conventionally produced varieties. Deep reds, like cabernet sauvignon, pack more power than red table wines — but white wine and champagne are also okay choices, because they're both also low in carbohydrates.

✔ **Vodka, gin, rum, and tequila:** Distilled spirits don't offer the health benefits of wine, but they don't include carbohydrates or gluten, either, so they're acceptable choices. They're best enjoyed chilled on their own or mixed with club soda and garnished with lemon and lime wedges or olives.

Paleo no-nos

Some alcoholic beverages aren't Paleo-friendly choices because of their problematic ingredients. Here are the ones you should avoid to feel your best:

- ✔ **Beer:** All regular beer includes gluten, which means you should steer clear of light beers, regular brews, stouts, and microbrews. Gluten-free beers may be an option if you want to occasionally enjoy the taste of beer, but some research shows that even gluten-free beers contain gluten. If you have a gluten-related illness, the safest bet is to avoid even gluten-free beers.

- ✔ **Whiskey, rye, and bourbon:** Conflicting opinions exist on whether grain-based spirits, like whisky, rye, and bourbon, include gluten, so if you're sensitive to gluten or have diagnosed gluten intolerance, avoid these types of liquor.

- ✔ **Sugary cocktails:** You can assume that if a cocktail has a cutesy name or is decorated with a paper umbrella, you should avoid drinking it. Cocktails based on multiple types of liquor and fruit juices are very sugary and produce a strong insulin response. Stick to the clean spirits listed in the previous section, but feel free to add an umbrella to your club soda cocktail if it makes you feel better.

Fighting temptation

The words you say to yourself and to others are important and can help you manage your eating habits when you face challenging social situations. You know that you're making choices to support good health and longevity. And you also know that your Paleo food choices don't mean you'll *never* eat some non-Paleo foods again; it means you choose Paleo foods most of the time. It means that when confronted with non-Paleo foods, you say in the sweetest, firmest voice you can, "Not right now."

These words come in handy when faced with overeager friends who want you to eat seconds or try a bite of their dessert. When you say "not right now," it defuses the situation. With those words, you avoid passing judgment on their food choices and make it clear that you're not on an austerity program for the rest of your life. Saying "not right now" is a demonstration of the choices you're making *now* for your health.

If these magic words don't work, here are a few other tips to help you deal with unsupportive people who may, even unwittingly, be trying to undermine your habits:

- ✔ **Address it head on.** Calmly confront your friends or family members when their behavior doesn't support your efforts. You're not expecting them to adopt your habits, but it's within your rights to expect that they'll get behind your efforts to improve your health or lose weight.

Point out to them that they're applying peer pressure in a way that's uncomfortable to you and ask them to stop. Remind them that you're not judging their food choices, and you'd like the same respect in return.

✔ **Change the subject.** You can stop the conversation in its tracks by simply refusing to engage in the conversation. Make it obvious that you're changing the subject and that your food choices aren't an acceptable topic of conversation. You may offer to explain the benefits of Paleo to them at another time, but you shouldn't feel like you need to defend your choices on the spot.

✔ **Ask for help.** Instead of responding to unsupportive comments or behavior with frustration or anger, you may try sincerely asking for help. Explain that your new habits are challenging, and that you'd welcome support. Your friends and family may surprise you.

As your lifestyle changes, you may need to find new ways to socialize — and maybe even some new friends who share your Paleo habits. You can invite old friends to try a new activity with you, like a leisurely walk to visit and catch up with each other, instead of the traditional drink after work. Or host the next holiday dinner at your house so you can control the menu and share your delicious Paleo foods with friends and family. Thanks to online meet-up groups, you may be able to add some new friends to your circle to find support and join you in your enthusiasm for Paleo.

Updating old traditions and creating new ones

One of the challenges of adopting the Paleo lifestyle is saying goodbye to favorite foods. You'll have an easier time of it if you embrace new possibilities, rather than trying to shoehorn your old eating habits into the Paleo framework. But especially on holidays or other special occasions, you may have family traditions or favorite recipes that you want to adapt or update so they can still be part of your life.

To do that successfully, you need to get to the root of why a tradition is important to you. Is it really that your grandmother's cake recipe is the best, or is it that you associate the cake with warm, loving times with your family? If it's the former, perhaps you can adapt the recipe to be more compliant with your new eating habits. If it's the latter, you can try to find other ways to re-create that family feeling.

The following sections provide some ways to help you update old family traditions and create new ones so that the food is *part* of the celebration without becoming the only reason to celebrate.

Adapting your favorite recipes

Many standard recipes can be updated with Paleo ingredients to make them comply with your new habits. It may take some experimentation, but you'll gain more confidence as you practice in your Paleo kitchen. Table 17-1 lists some common substitutions to help you rework your favorite recipes.

Table 17-1	Paleo-Friendly Ingredient Substitutions
Original Ingredient	*Paleo Substitution*
White flour	Almond flour, coconut flour
White or brown sugar	Honey
Milk, cream, or yogurt	Coconut milk
Red wine	Balsamic vinegar
White wine	Chicken broth
Soy sauce	Coconut aminos
White potatoes	Sweet potatoes, turnips
Pasta	Zucchini Noodles (Chapter 12), Spaghetti Squash (Chapter 10)
Rice	Cauliflower Rice (Chapter 12)
Shortening, vegetable oil, seed oils (canola, sunflower, rapeseed)	Coconut oil, clarified grass-fed butter
Butter	Clarified grass-fed butter

If your family is averse to the Paleo versions of their favorite recipes, you may consider making both versions of the recipe, just to keep the peace. You can enjoy the updated version, and maybe you'll entice some new Paleo converts in the process.

Sometimes the sentiment, not the food, makes a dish special. You can honor the spirit and memory of a recipe without eating it by encouraging gathered family and friends to tell stories and share their recollections of eating a family favorite. Or have a treasured recipe duplicated and framed as a keepsake.

Starting your own traditions

Sometimes recognizing a tradition is simply about having something you can look forward to, but every tradition had to start somewhere! Here are a few tips to help you create new traditions that make get-togethers special and Paleo-friendly:

  ✔ **Tag themes to your meals.** You can easily make a weeknight meal or weekend breakfast a memorable event by giving it a name and writing it on the calendar — for example, Tuesday Taco Night, Saturday Paleo

Pancake Breakfast, or Souper Sunday. By creating an event around Paleo-friendly meals, you can generate excitement, make new family memories, and ensure that your family enjoys healthy food. This kind of planning makes grocery shopping easier, too!

✔ **Get rid of grains.** There's no denying that sweet treats, like birthday cakes, muffins, cookies, and waffles, are baked into our culture. Grain-free, gluten-free recipes shouldn't be everyday foods, but they're a wonderful way to mark special occasions without damaging your health and the well-being of your loved ones. For decades, generations of family members have bonded over baking together, and thanks to grain-free recipes that use coconut or almond flour, honey, and other natural ingredients, you can share that tradition in your family with good health.

✔ **Go beyond the food.** It's unlikely that major holidays will ever exclude special foods — people have been celebrating over shared food for centuries. But you can enhance the fun of get-togethers with activities that shift some of the focus from the food to spending quality time together. You may institute a family walk around the neighborhood after Thanksgiving dinner or a rousing session of carols after a Christmas feast. Birthdays can be recognized with cake and a dance contest in the living room or a challenge to do ten jumping jacks for every year the honoree has been alive. Use your imagination to add non-food traditions that make the day special.

Indulging with Pleasure

One of the most important aspects of living Paleo is developing the ability to balance the times when you comply completely with the Paleo rules and when you loosen your standards to enjoy a special treat. After your 30-day Reset (covered in Chapter 8), your challenge will be deciding for yourself whether you'll be 80 percent compliant, 90 percent compliant, or even more stringent than that. Your ability to stray from the strict Paleo path is dependent on your goals and health concerns, like whether you have a disease that requires you to avoid certain foods.

Here are some questions you can ask yourself to help you decide when is a good time for a treat and whether that treat is worth the indulgence:

✔ Do you have a medical concern, such as a gluten sensitivity, allergy, celiac disease, or diabetes, that requires you to avoid this food?

✔ Will eating this food trigger a domino effect of overeating?

✔ Will this food satisfy your craving, or will it merely be a momentary distraction?

✔ Are you eating this food for the pleasurable taste, to satisfy true hunger, to comfort an unpleasant emotion, or as entertainment?

> ✔ Will eating this food cause you any discomfort, such as gastrointestinal distress, bloating, interrupted sleep, or moodiness, after you eat it? If so, is it worth it?
>
> ✔ Is this version of the food the best you can find?
>
> ✔ How will you feel after eating this food? For example, will you be satisfied, happy, remorseful, ashamed, or hungrier?

The goal of this exercise is to help you determine when and how you may enjoy special treats without causing yourself unnecessary discomfort. It comes in handy when you're considering how to handle a big night out, a holiday or special occasion, or even when you just want to curl up on the couch with some ice cream after a bad day. Revisit this page whenever you need some help determining whether it's a good time to stray from the Paleo path.

Managing office temptations

Is there a dietary pitfall as dangerous as the break room at work? Between the box of doughnuts that's supposed to make Monday less heinous and the assorted leftover candy from Halloween and Easter, it can sorely test your willpower. Not to mention the vending machines that taunt you with packaged cookies and potato chips when your will weakens mid-afternoon. But the new-and-improved Paleo you is stronger than those junk foods, and with a few of the following good habits, you can avoid tripping and falling into a poor snack choice:

✔ **Pack your lunch.** Packing your lunch most days of the week gives you absolute control over the quality of the food you eat when you need it most. The workday is long and potentially stressful. Taking a break midday to consume high-quality calories sets you up to glide through your afternoon of work and into a pleasant evening. And when you pack your own food, you not only ensure that you're eating well, but you also save money.

✔ **Go out of your way.** One of the easiest ways to avoid the turmoil of temptation is to keep forbidden foods out of sight. If your usual path through the office forces you to look at — or smell — the discarded junk food, microwave meals, or vending machines, chose another path.

✔ **Take it outside.** Feeling overwhelmed by the desire to indulge in the leftover Danish pastry in the break room? Take yourself outside for a walk around the block. The change of scenery and fresh air gives you a renewed perspective.

✔ **Stock up.** Stock up on non-perishable snacks that you can keep in your desk — like coconut chips, dry roasted nuts, fruit-and-nut bars, sardines, sugar-free beef jerky — or bring fresh produce and hard-boiled eggs to keep in your workplace refrigerator for food emergencies.

Chapter 18

Transitioning the Family

*E*ating well, being well, having energy, and carrying that healthy glow is a great feeling. When you start to understand the paradigm that keeps you feeling so good, you don't want to keep it to yourself! You want to share it will those you love. This chapter is dedicated to helping you share your new Paleo lifestyle with your family and helping them make the transition.

You may find yourself considering major changes for your family or only minor ones. This chapter encourages you to think about how to be the strong silent leader, what foods your family is better off without, the right time for treats, how to manage mealtimes, how to build a healthy plate, where to get the good stuff on your family's plate, and how to actually make this process doable and *fun*.

Providing the best environment for your family is what everyone strives for. But what does that really mean? The *best* doesn't mean spending money on a bunch of specialty gadgets, nor does it mean an environment filled with lots of technology or activities. It means providing a *healthy* environment, where kids feel safe, loved, and important. Discovering how to make your kids and your significant other a part of your healthy paradigm is the best possible way to achieve this environment, and you can do all of this with the strategies we provide in this chapter.

Taking the "Kids First" Approach

Knowing that the food children eat influences not only their health but also their behavior makes understanding this chapter all the more important. In the past, people have always been concerned with *how much* their children eat. Now, the focus has shifted to *what* children eat.

If you want your children to flourish in school, have meaningful friendships, and have success in choosing and performing the activities that end up defining them, they have to be well nourished. Just as overfed, undernourished adults can't be at their best potential, neither can children. If you want to encourage your family to have all the tools they need for success, you have to implement healthy nutritional habits.

The following sections cover some basic strategies, such as leading by example and understanding nutrition needs for different ages, for making the conversion to a healthier home. We also discuss the dangers of gluten and dairy for kids, give some tips for sharing the reason for the lifestyle change with your kids, and offer guidance for breaking out the treats.

Leading by example

If you have a child who absolutely won't eat vegetables, reflect for a moment: Do *you* eat vegetables? Do you have healthy eating practices in your home as a matter of course? You can't have rules for children that you don't follow yourself.

When you open the refrigerator in your home, do you have plenty of produce and other healthy foods to choose from? Do your family members see you eating lean proteins, healthy fats, and non-starchy carbohydrates?

Kids download everything you do. They learn from an interesting platform called *modeling*, meaning that they naturally imitate, or mirror, what you do. This is how they learn. Have you ever noticed a daughter who walks just like her mom or a boy who pushes his hair back or maybe sits in a chair just like his dad? What children see and hear creeps into their brain without them even trying or having any awareness.

When kids see you eating healthy foods and feeling good and energized, these patterns are anchored in their brain. They take these patterns in and model after them.

Leading by example, or being a strong *silent* leader, is the most effective way to influence kids. You simply can't bully your way into transformation. When someone peruses change with no heart, it's not lasting change. That's where the theory "they'll come to you when they're ready" holds. If you want other members of your household to embrace change, be a great role model. Have healthy foods available and have *your* food values in order. That's how you can affect change.

My kids look fine, so why should I bother?

Even though your kids may seem fine eating packaged, processed foods or fast food, their cells may be telling another story. Poor eating habits may affect your family in areas that often aren't noticeable but may create issues behind the scenes or set them up for trouble in the future.

Brain power is one of those areas. Researchers in Britain have discovered that feeding your children junk or processed foods can actually lower their IQ. These researchers monitored the diets and general health and well-being of 14,000 children at ages 3, 4½, 7, and again at age 8. They found that a poor diet during the early developmental years could, in fact, lead to a lower IQ by the age of 8.

The problem with fast-food items and junk food is that they lack nutritional value and deliver a high dose of unhealthy fat, calories, sugar, refined salt, and sugary carbs. These foods are robbing kids of essential vitamins and minerals that they need for growth and development. Eating excessive amounts of these foods leads to obesity and malnutrition.

When your kids' nutritional levels keep falling and finally reach the state of malnutrition, you're in trouble. You open the floodgate to sickness and disease. The only way for your kids to boost their immunity and reach their best potential is to have a diet filled with nutrient-dense foods (foods naturally lower in calories and higher in nutrition).

The dietary habits kids pick up in their youth usually stick with them throughout life, unless they consciously do something to interrupt those patterns. So letting your kids eat processed and unhealthy foods can have a lifelong impact. On the other hand, having your kids eat well *just to get into the habit* of healthy eating patterns gives your family a serious head start.

Even if your kids don't have behavior problems, they're not heavy, and their immune systems appear strong, understand the long-term strategy to making the transition to Paleo: to keep your kids healthy and strong *throughout their life* and give them every tool for future success!

Different ages, different stages: Improving nutrition for kids of any age

The best time to introduce your kiddos to nutritious foods is no doubt as young as possible. Actually, when kids are young, they have a huge interest in discovering healthy eating practices. They're intrigued by the human body and how it works and equally as intrigued how to eat in a way that cares for their body in the very best way.

Watching this fascination and enthusiasm peak in your children is a wonderful thing. Children are often interested in cooking with you and talking about the ingredients you use. They're interested in what the labels say and all the things that nutritious foods make them do better (run, play sports, ramp up brain power, and so on).

If you can capture kids' interest in eating healthy when they're young (while in preschool through elementary school), you hit a home run. Even if they stray for some time, choosing healthier options is still *ingrained* in them. Eventually, they come back to the eating principles they know serve them best.

Middle-school kids are no doubt tougher customers. They're not going to go for any old bill of goods you try to sell them. They're the little skeptics. But don't give up. The best way to reach this group is to involve them as much as possible and always have the healthier choices available. Have some household mealtime rules in place (see the later section "Managing Mealtimes") and just keep on keeping on! It will pay off.

When your little kiddo becomes a big kiddo (from about 14 to 18 years old) your role as the silent leader has to really come into play. Leading by example is the best and most effective way to influence this age group. They'll notice that you buy your produce from the farmers' market and that you always have fruits and vegetables on the ready. They'll notice that your meals always consist of lean proteins, healthy fats, and vegetables. They'll notice what's in your cupboards. They'll be aware of the rhythm and vibe your kitchen takes on, and, when they're ready, they'll start asking questions. Better yet, they'll just start doing.

Eliminating gluten and dairy, the dynamic devils

If your child is frequently ill, chronically congested, or suffers from digestive complaints, gluten may be the culprit. Considering that at least 15 percent of the population has a gluten intolerance, cutting out foods with gluten is a good way to keep your family healthy. Wheat, barley, rye, triticale, oats, and most other grains are found in so many food products, making gluten a tough one to snub. Keeping your foods real and unpackaged are your best lines of defense to keep your kids gluten free.

Despite the constant reminder that "milk does a body good" and the number of dairy foods that are wrapped in kid-pleasing packages, milk can be a problem for your family. For some, milk and dairy may cause their body to create mucus, which can cause digestive disturbances, acne, headaches, and other allergies. Some kids may be congested all the time or have a constant runny nose. We provide options in this section for dairy-like foods and calcium that won't cause congestion or other allergic symptoms.

When you decide to make the transition to Paleo in your family, start by checking out some of the recipes in Part III of this book. They're all gluten and dairy free and will definitely start your family off on the right track!

Gluten

The proteins in gluten irritate the intestines, causing discomfort. Following are some of the symptoms kids (and adults) may experience if they're sensitive to gluten:

- ✔ Agitation and mood swings
- ✔ Depression
- ✔ Eczema and other skin rashes
- ✔ Extreme fatigue
- ✔ Headaches
- ✔ Intestinal problems like bloating, diarrhea, and constipation
- ✔ Mouth ulcers
- ✔ Painful joints

Many parents notice a difference in their child's symptoms immediately after cutting down on gluten. You have to be aware, though, that many foods may contain gluten without you even realizing it.

Watch out for these sneaky ingredients that are actually gluten in the flesh:

- ✔ Barley or barley malt extract
- ✔ Dextrimaltose
- ✔ Duram flour
- ✔ Gliadin
- ✔ Kamut
- ✔ Malt vinegar
- ✔ Maltodextrin
- ✔ Maltose
- ✔ Miso
- ✔ Modified starch
- ✔ Natural flavoring
- ✔ Vegetable gum
- ✔ Vegetable starch
- ✔ Whey protein

Also, be on the lookout for these common foods that may contain gluten:

- Broths
- Candy coating
- Imitation seafood
- Some luncheon meats
- Marinades
- Some sausages
- Soy sauce

Don't despair, though; you can still make sandwiches from lettuce wraps, which kids really love. You can also make breads, muffins, and desserts with non-gluten or grain products, such as almond meal coconut flour, and flax meal.

If you really want to use bread for your kids but want to keep out all the nasty ingredients, like grains, cheap sugars, and preservatives (which most breads have in abundance), try looking online for recipes made with almond flour or coconut meal.

Dairy

Like gluten, cow's milk can be another big *trigger food* — a food that causes your body to "trigger a reaction." For example, if you eat cheese and then get a migraine, dairy "triggers" your migraine. Unfortunately, dairy tends to trigger a lot of symptoms in a lot of people. In fact, *dairy is the leading cause of food allergies in children*. If your child has a lot of digestive intolerance, leading to frequent stomach problems, dairy may be the culprit. Many kids have just subtle allergies to cow's milk that perpetuate their nasal congestion and lead to ear infections.

Here are some problems associated with food sensitivity to dairy:

- Allergies
- Childhood-onset (Type 1) diabetes
- Chronic constipation
- Crohn's disease
- Ear infections

You can replace your kids' current dairy products with the following great-tasting substitutes, as an alternative to milk, baking ingredient, and dessert topping:

- Almond milk
- Cashew whipped cream

- Coconut milk
- Flaxseed milk
- Hazelnut milk
- Hemp milk

Some great sources of calcium without dairy include the follwoing:

- Fish (canned sources like canned salmon)
- Leafy greens
- Nut and nut butters (like almond, sesame, and walnut)
- Sea vegetables (like kombu and nori)
- Sesame seeds and sunflower seeds

Teaching kids the "why" behind the "what"

One of the missing keys in the strategies parents use to get their kids to eat healthy is really taking the time to teach them *why* they should eat healthy.

Have you ever gone through the motions of doing something just because? Maybe someone said to do it, maybe it was a role you had to take on for work, or maybe it was just something you got in the habit of doing? Something is usually missing when you do something just because, and that is *heart*. When you do things with heart, the passion to succeed follows.

No matter what age or stage your kids are in, explain some simple facts. You don't have to make a big deal about it; it can even be in passing. As long as you do teach them the *why*. Here are some examples:

- You should be able to pronounce the ingredients on a food label; otherwise, they're probably chemicals that you don't want in your body.
- If too many ingredients are on the label, the foods are too processed and aren't going to give you the nutrients you need. You'll get some energy but no nutrition.
- Fruits and vegetables have antioxidants, which keep your cells super healthy and protect you against getting sick.
- Fruits and vegetables have vitamins and minerals, which make every structure and function of your body work. When you get too low on these vitamins, you get sick easier, and performing in all areas of life as well as you really can is difficult.

✔ Fruits and vegetables have fiber in them, which helps move things along your intestines so your body stays cleansed and not clogged.

✔ Your body needs healthy proteins to build and repair everything in your body, like strong muscles.

✔ Healthy fats make your brain and all your cells work better so you can do everything better. These fats are super important to have.

✔ If you want your cells to flow really nicely, you've got to be hydrated. Your cells really need water so they're not stuck together, which causes you to get tired and worn out.

REMEMBER

Keep your explanations simple — no big words or lengthy lectures — just some simple facts so your children understand why eating healthy foods is important. Explaining the *why* behind the choices you make helps them feel ownership and helps them *want* to have a healthier lifestyle. That's a sure-fire prescription for success!

Providing tasty and nutritious treats

Kids love treats. In fact, many of them would trade you in for a banana split! Even if your kiddo has a hollow leg for sweets, you can manage these cravings in the following ways:

✔ If your kids have a sweet tooth, remember that you're the one in the house with the checkbook and the driver's license. What you say goes. If you don't bring it into the house, it can't be eaten.

✔ Worry about what you *can* control, and don't get crazy about the rest. Teach your kids at home and provide them real foods; they'll begin to make the connection between the foods and sugars they eat and how they make their body feel. They'll discover these positive and negative associations in time with your guidance.

✔ One of the best things you can do when your kids eat sweets is to make sure they're getting real sweets and not a bunch of chemicals or *frankensweets* (fake stuff dressed up to look like cakes and treats). The more refined a sugar is, the worse it is.

✔ The only way you can completely avoid sugar in your kids' diet is to not have any sweeteners or sweet stuff in your household so there's no begging or battles. Remember the rule: What you do, the kids follow. But don't expect your kids to appreciate you removing the sugar from their lives. Your best strategy is to always give a clear explanation as to why you're prohibiting certain sugars in terms that they'll clearly understand.

✔ If you do decide on a treat, such as ice cream, go out and get it instead of stocking it at home. That way when you're home, it's a done deal.

✔ Redefine desserts by making Paleo treats with wholesome ingredients, like fruit and almond and coconut flours. Many of them are simple to put together and really delicious.

✔ Don't fall into the circus animal pattern of rewarding kids with sweets. Don't confuse the fact that food is there to nourish, not to show love or reward.

✔ Let your kids know that some sweets, such as birthday cake at parties or holiday cookies that you bake together, are okay *some of the time*. Make sure they understand the line in the sand and the difference between special occasion treats and everyday real foods.

✔ Trade party bags or Halloween treats for other, more favorable sweets. A movie or some loose coins are often more attractive than candy. The idea of a trade is always enticing.

✔ When dealing with the issue of school sweets, you have to educate at home the best you can. Sometimes, your kiddos will make good choices; other times, they won't. Don't make food and sweets too much of a big deal. Do your work at home, and keep educating. Provide your kids with wholesome meals when you can. Remember that what you focus on grows. Don't put too much focus on sweets. Focus on *clearly defined education*.

✔ Pull the plug on sweet drinks in your home. Don't buy soda or sweet drinks. No sports drinks (unless you need them). Sugary drinks have become a huge problem for kids, and this rule should be an absolute deal breaker with no wiggle room. No liquid sugar! Get your kids used to water and iced herbal teas if they want something else. Just a pitcher of water with some oranges and lemons is usually enough to keep them happy. Hold strong on this one. Explain why; they'll get it.

When considering whether to give the A-Okay on a sugary treat, you have to consider how the sweetener in that food is made and how the body processes it.

These off-limit, toxic sweeteners aren't good for a growing neurological system (or any system for that matter):

✔ Acesulfame-K (Sweet One)

✔ Aspartame (Equal, NutraSweet)

✔ High-fructose corn syrup

✔ Saccharin (Sweet'N Low)

✔ Sucralose (Splenda)

These low-quality, highly refined sweeteners are found in many foods and beverages, so beware! Cutting out sugary drinks considerably reduces the chances of exposing your kids to this garbage.

Kids are exposed to treats at parties, play days, school outings, and holiday gatherings. Maybe you want to keep certain family traditions or recipes around. Although we don't recommend the following sugars, we can give a little wiggle room. However, make sure your kiddos are getting these sugars in their diet *only on rare occasions.*

- ✔ Brown sugar
- ✔ Cane juice, juice crystals, and sugar
- ✔ Coconut nectars, sugar, and crystals
- ✔ Date sugar
- ✔ Raw sugar
- ✔ Turbinado

The top choices (by a landslide) in sweeteners for your kiddos include the following:

- ✔ Dates (you'd be surprised how well these work)
- ✔ Fresh fruit juice (great for baking and dressings)
- ✔ Organic maple syrup
- ✔ Raw honey (although not under the age of 2, due to the risk of botulism, a very serious illness)
- ✔ Ripe bananas

Paleo treats are made with these ingredients, and they taste so good that your kids won't feel like they're missing a thing.

Here's an easy-peasy treat to try: Take some berries and drizzle some honey on top — kids love this. Or just a bowl of berries and coconut milk can do the trick! By the way, you can easily transform fruit into wonderful, gorgeous ice creams and mousses.

If you're giving the green light on sweets, start with some of the recipes in this book. You really can redefine sweets in your house!

Food marketing 101 for kids

Always remember food marketing and its place in a kid's palate. Advertising affects kids' food choices a great deal. In a study conducted by Stanford University, a group of children were offered two identical meals, one in a plain wrapper and one in a package from a popular fast-food chain. Even young children associated a better taste experience with the name-brand selection, suggesting that marketing and expectation have an impact on perceived taste. Remember the bottom line: Teach your kids about food marketing so they understand what's happening and can make intelligent choices.

Managing Mealtimes

Mealtimes are an important part of any family. Although eating together as a family every day isn't always possible, even if you manage it on the weekends, you'll reap the rewards. As we mention earlier in this chapter, children learn by example, and when they see their parents and other family members enjoying healthy foods, they'll be much more inclined to try them, too.

Set up your mealtimes for success. When you do get to have meals together, your family starts seeing mealtimes as an enjoyable family experience, not a chore or a war zone. You can also take advantage of mealtimes to teach your kids expected behavior at the dinner table at home or when dining out. Kids don't come into the world knowing appropriate mealtime behavior — you must teach them.

Avoid distractions, include the kids in the conversation, and focus on any positive interactions. Doing so makes your mealtime a good opportunity to touch on appropriate mealtime behaviors and making smart food choices. The more you manage mealtimes, the healthier the entire family will eat.

The following sections focus on the best meals to start making a healthier transition, how to get your kids to eat more fruit and vegetables, and the basics on building a kid-friendly healthy plate.

Pick a meal, any meal

Not everyone is fortunate enough to have all the tricks of the trade down pat when their kids are toddlers. Of course, this age is the easiest time to make healthy habits stick. No worries, though; you can convert your family's eating habits one meal at a time.

Start your family on the path to putting real foods back in their diet with one meal and work your way toward more. Pick whatever meal works best with the rhythm of your home. The point is to just start somewhere. Breakfast is one of the best meals to start with because it's when your family's the hungriest and willing to try different foods.

When all the foods in your house are healthy, transitioning to healthy foods is easier because your family can have anything in the house when they want to have it.

Always keep hard-boiled eggs on hand. You can eat them on their own or chop them into sausage or bacon for a quick and easy breakfast. Be sure to try the recipes in Part III for some great breakfast ideas.

The 2-plus-1 dinner rule

Dinnertime is a great time for your kids to see you and other family members chowing down on some vegetables. Even if you're still making the transition to Paleo and maybe still focusing on getting breakfast foods down pat, having greens on the table at dinner is always a good idea. Kids *will* notice.

The 2-plus-1 rule goes like this: At every dinner, have *two* cooked vegetables and *one* raw vegetable on the table. Make it a rule, something your family can expect. If you make a dish that includes a vegetable, that counts; if you make spaghetti squash for dinner, that's one vegetable. Just make sure you include a raw vegetable as well, such as snow peas, sugar snap peas, kohlrabi, jicama, cucumbers, carrots, and crisp bell peppers.

What this 2-plus-1 rule does is anchor into a child's mind that vegetables at mealtimes are standard. Therefore, having vegetables becomes normal to them. You can use this time to talk about the different kinds of vegetables (or seasonal vegetables) and encourage them to venture out and try new ones.

Try to prepare fruits and vegetables just before cooking or serving, because nutrient levels begin to diminish as soon as you cut the produce.

The "no biggie" rule

Don't let food create stress in your household. What stress creates in your body is worse than what eating a cupcake does. The key is to have a positive influence without creating stress.

What you focus on grows. So don't focus on the food issues your kiddo may be having 24/7. Don't allow mealtimes to be battle grounds. Control what you can, and then let the rest go.

You influence your family by being a strong leader and keeping a healthy and positive home. Your job is to walk the talk and don't give negative actions/ reactions too much energy. Approach healthy eating like it's a part of who you are and carry that certainty with you. At some point, it will rub off.

The non-negotiable bite

Here's a great rule to help your family venture out and try new flavors: They have to try one bite. That's it — one itty bitty bite.

So if want your children to try a certain vegetable, have it on the table at mealtimes. Your kids can scrunch their nose up and stick their tongue out all they want, but they've gotta give it a try. If they try it and discover that they don't like it, let them know that's okay with you. At least they tried.

Keep in mind that a rejection is often not a true indication of dislike. Reintroduce them to the vegetable at another point, and the results may be different. Also, dressing the vegetables up to look differently entices kids' palates leaps and bounds. (See the section "Making foods look fun," later in this chapter.)

The point in the non-negotiable bite rule is to get your family's taste buds (and brain) used to real foods. Every time they try a vegetable, their body creates neurological pathways. These pathways create habits, making eating healthy second nature. Think of it this way: With every tiny bite, you take a small chunk out of their veggie resistance and one step closer to balanced mealtimes.

Building a kid-friendly plate

What we eat so should our kids. What's healthy for us is healthy for them. Knowing how to build a healthy plate is the cornerstone of healthy eating. Understanding that a healthy plate, shown in Figure 18-1, includes vegetables, some fruit, a little protein, good-for-you fats, and healthy starches not only makes your kids healthier by leaps and bounds, but it also sets the stage for a lifetime of health. They'll be "in the know" when it comes to creating health, and that's a gift.

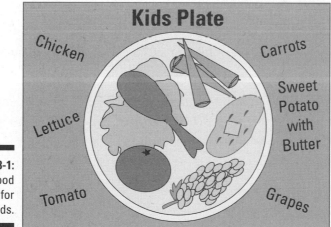

Figure 18-1: Superfood plate for kids.

As you put together your kids' plate, be sure to steer away from the following foods, which don't do anything good for the health of your kids:

- ✔ **French fries:** Rich in trans fats, refined salt, and carcinogens, the French fries you buy in most places are made by poor cooking methods and include rancid, unhealthy fats.

- ✔ **Artificially sweetened foods and drinks:** What most people don't realize is that the body responds to these substances by triggering the brain to release insulin in response to the brain receiving a sweet message. Your body will lay down insulin anyway, so why expose it to the artificial stuff that can create havoc?

- ✔ **Foods that contain trans fat:** These foods are filled with artificial harmful substances that are very unhealthy.

- ✔ **Foods with high-fructose corn syrup:** This liquid corn promotes altered cycles in the body and is a toxin.

Don't *ever* talk calories with your kids. If your child needs to eat more, the messages from the brain determine hunger. When your children experience a true physiological need for calories and when they're truly hungry, they'll eat. If they need to lose weight, talk to them about eating better for health. Health should *always* be the focus. Don't focus on bad foods or make a big deal about it. Control what you can, and do your best to teach your kids how to make choices outside of the home.

The end goal is to have your kids eating real foods that are rich in every nutrient under the sun, including lean proteins, healthy fats and oils, low-starch vegetables, healthy carb-dense vegetables, fruits, nuts, seeds and their butters. These foods truly are superfoods.

Fruits and vegetables

A portion size of fruits and vegetables for kids differs from adults and is smaller than you may think. A portion size is the amount a child can hold in one hand, and as her hand grows, so should the size of the portion. For school-age kids, a portion is about half a cup. Try to incorporate the following amounts in your kids' diet:

- ✔ Three to five (kid-sized handfuls) servings of vegetables a day
- ✔ Two to four (kid-sized handfuls) servings of fruit a day

Healthy carbs

Be sure to include some dense sources of healthy carbohydrates for your kids. Kids are so active and usually need more of a refuel than adults. Here are some healthy carb suggestions:

- ✔ Beets
- ✔ Butternut squash

- Carrots
- Kohlrabi
- Parsnips
- Pumpkin
- Raw cassava
- Raw jicama
- Spaghetti squash
- Sweet potatoes
- Taro root
- Winter squash
- Yams

Healthy fats

Kids older than 2 years of age should get about 30 percent of their daily calories from fat. Here are some great healthy fats for your kids:

- Bacon
- Coconut milk or shredded coconut
- Eggs
- Fatty fish (salmon, trout, or mackerel)
- Flax milk
- Grass-fed butter
- Guacamole dips
- Healthy oils
- Nut butters
- Nuts
- Seeds

Make up a trail mix of shredded coconut, nuts, and seeds and throw in some dark chocolate, which has some valuable nutrients as well.

Protein

Kids need about 10 to 15 percent (about three servings per day) of their diet to come from protein. The more they're growing (growth spurts) and the more active they are, the more building blocks they need. Animal proteins are better tailored to meet the needs of infants and growing children than are plant proteins, which is why nature provides human milk for babies.

Convincing Your Significant Other

The best thing you can do to get your partner involved is to show — don't tell — how amazing and delicious living Paleo can be. Doing so requires you to be a strong leader and lead by example above and beyond all else. First, give your absolute best, most compelling pitch as to why trying Paleo for 30 days is so important. If your partner accepts your pitch, do what you can to support him or her. Be enthusiastic to help during the transition, because you know that after 30 days, your partner will be onboard.

If your significant other doesn't want to try Paleo, your only course of action is to be a strong leader. Show by example how much energy you have and how much better you feel. Prepare some Paleo recipes from Part III and let your partner see how simple it is to stay onboard. Show him or her that Paleo meals are simple and delicious and won't make you heavy, bloated, constipated, or get your blood sugar all out of whack. Eating can actually make you feel better, not worse.

Let your significant other see how your body, mind, and spirit transform for the positive. If, after you do all of this, your significant other still decides that trying to live Paleo is just not something he or she is willing to do, you have one card to play: Accept your partner for who he or she is — crappy food and all. Don't get resentful or frustrated; the stress hormones counter balance your great strides and efforts. It simply isn't worth what it does to you internally.

The best thing you can do is keep on keeping on. Create the best life you can and keep the best attitude you can. That's what in your control.

Part V
The Part of Tens

The 5th Wave   By Rich Tennant

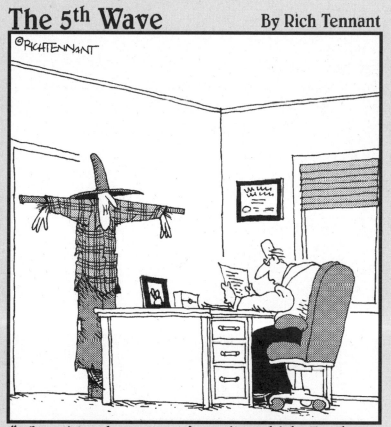

"Your blood pressure's a little high. Is there any way you can incorporate some aerobic activity into your daily schedule?"

In this part . . .

In this final section, we list ten foods to always have in the kitchen. We also show you ten excellent exercises that require no equipment.

Chapter 19

Ten Foods to Always Have in the Kitchen

Giving up some of your favorite foods and old routines can be challenging. People have an emotional attachment to food that runs even deeper than their nutritional needs, and they like to follow familiar patterns. Eating the same thing for breakfast every morning as part of a routine is comforting and gets you out the door on time. But the best way to guarantee success with your new Paleo lifestyle is to develop new routines, new habits, and new favorite foods. If you identify a short list of must-have foods that satisfy your nutritional needs and your appetite, stock your kitchen with them so you can avoid feelings of deprivation.

To stock your kitchen the right way, you want a variety of protein sources, fruits and vegetables that you can eat raw or cooked, and an array of high-quality fats for cooking and eating.

The foods and tips in this chapter cover all the nutritional bases, and they all taste great, too. With these staples on hand, you can make meals and snacks that leave you feeling energized and satisfied, emotionally and physically.

Cage-Free, Organic Eggs

Great any time of day, eggs are a terrific source of fast protein. Keep a dozen hard-boiled in the refrigerator for egg salad or deviled eggs made with Homemade Mayonnaise (see Chapter 14). After a long day, breakfast for dinner can be comforting — simple scrambled eggs or a vegetable omelet does the trick.

Organic, Grass-Fed Ground Beef

With a few pounds of grass-fed ground beef in the refrigerator, you're only about ten minutes away from a delicious dinner. Browned and seasoned with garlic and spices, ground beef is like a blank canvas that you can turn into just about any ethnic-inspired meal. Stir-fry it with vegetables and Chinese five-spice powder for an Asian-inspired dinner. Shape it into a burger patty and pile it on top of a big all-American salad. Make easy Thai wraps by rolling cooked ground beef with thinly sliced cucumber, carrot, and jalapeño in a lettuce leaf and then sprinkle with lime juice. Plus you can always make meatballs.

To ensure that your grass-fed beef stays tender, cook it on medium to medium-high heat, never very high heat.

Sardines Packed in Olive Oil

These little fish are the perfect on-the-go food. Lunch is less than five minutes away when you crack open a can of boneless, skinless sardines and arrange them on a plate with a red bell pepper cut into strips, a cucumber cut into coins, and a carrot cut into sticks — with a side of fresh fruit. With a pleasing amount of oil and a not-too-fishy taste, the sardines are a power food, and the leftover oil from the can is perfect for dipping raw veggies.

If you're squeamish about sardines, definitely look for the boneless, skinless variety, rather than the whole fish. Boneless and skinless, the sardines have the texture and appearance of a small fish fillet, rather than an actual fish.

Cauliflower

Cauliflower may be the most versatile vegetable in the kitchen, so you should always have a head (or two!) in the refrigerator. You can grate it in a food processor and sauté it with fat and spices to make Cauliflower Rice or boil it in broth and mash with coconut milk to transform it into Mashed Cauliflower (both recipes are in Chapter 12). Cauliflower also adds a big crunch when chopped raw in salads, and it becomes crisp-tender when roasted in the oven with a sprinkle of sea salt and crushed garlic.

Collard Greens

When people talk about how delicious and nutritious leafy greens can be, they usually mention kale as the superstar. But collard greens are also an excellent choice. Easier to clean and cook than kale, they're packed with similar nutrients. The leaves are large and flat — and a little sturdier than kale. Collard greens tenderize during steaming without becoming too mushy. You can braise them in a coconut milk curry, wrap them around meat fillings and bake in tomato sauce, or sauté them in coconut oil with seasonings to make a vitamin-packed side dish. Collard greens are mild enough to taste great at breakfast with eggs and leftover protein.

Frozen, Unsweetened Berries

Low in fructose and high in antioxidants, blueberries, blackberries, and raspberries are loaded with nutrition and flavor. And thanks to frozen varieties, you can enjoy them all year long. Try them halfway defrosted, drizzled with coconut milk for dessert or as a special weekend breakfast alongside an omelet. Because they're not too sweet, they don't wake up the sugar demon, but they're sweet enough to feel like a treat.

Sweet Potatoes

Roasted whole, cut into dice and sautéed, or mashed with a little cinnamon and nutmeg, sweet potatoes are packed with sweet flavor and nutrition. They're an excellent choice for a snack after a demanding workout and are equally at home for breakfast, lunch, and dinner.

Need a cooked sweet potato in a hurry? Wash the whole potato, poke it a few times with a fork, wrap in a paper towel, and microwave for 7 to 9 minutes, until tender to the touch.

Full-Fat Coconut Milk

Equally at home in sweet and savory dishes, coconut milk is an excellent replacement for heavy cream or yogurt in curries and creamy sauces. It's also luscious when whipped into a creamy cloud and served over fresh fruit. Organic brands are best — and always choose the full-fat version. ("Light" coconut milk is merely the full-fat kind watered down.) Be sure to check the ingredient list: Guar gum is okay, but avoid brands that include sulfites or added sugar.

For richer, creamier curries — and when making Whipped Coconut Cream (Chapter 12) — don't shake the can of coconut milk before opening. As it sits, the cream rises to the top. Just scoop out the thickened coconut milk and discard the leftover liquid.

Organic, Unsweetened Coconut Flakes

Eaten on their own as a snack (like the Cocoa-Cinnamon Coconut Chips recipe in Chapter 13) or sprinkled into and on top of dishes, coconut flakes add another dimension of flavor and texture. They're delicious, little wisps of good-for-you fat that are equally good on savory and sweet dishes. Try tossing a few on top of Thai curries or sprinkling them on a bowl of a Tropical Mango Parfait (also in Chapter 13).

Unrefined Coconut Oil

For cooking, organic unrefined coconut oil is a great choice. It lends a somewhat buttery flavor to dishes and can be used at medium to medium-high temperatures without oxidizing (which means it remains good for you, even if you turn up the heat). Because coconut oil is saturated, it's solid at cooler temperatures and is a good stand-in for butter in Paleo baked treats. You can use clarified butter or ghee for cooking and baking, too, but coconut has many nutritional benefits and the silky taste can't be beat.

If you don't like the flavor of coconut oil, you may choose to use expeller-pressed refined coconut oil instead. It's refined through mechanics, not chemicals, so it's safe to eat.

Chapter 20

Ten Effective No-Equipment Exercises

In This Chapter

▶ Freeing yourself from exercise excuses

▶ Discovering effective exercises for when you're on the go

▶ Reaping the benefits of high-intensity movements

▶ Recharging your body with (non-liquid) energy boosters

You gotta move! It's as simple as that. The value of exercising is so high that making it a priority is super smart for your health and well-being. The key to looking and feeling healthy is understanding that your body needs exercise and movement to fuel you with energy. In fact, exercise is the best anti-aging pill around! It can also minimize the risk of stroke, heart attack, diabetes, and cancer. Making this one lifestyle change will have a major impact on reducing your risk of slow, progressing chronic diseases, and it will improve your quality of life.

When you make something meaningful to you a priority, you find ways to get it done. Even though you may have a hectic life, you can fit some quick movement throughout your day with the exercises we discuss in this chapter. You can use these exercises as your springboard to move your body in short bursts throughout the day, or you can stack a couple of these movements together for a quick, high-intensity workout. If you're super busy or traveling or you can't get to your favorite place to work out, these ten no-equipment exercises will do the trick!

Burpees

The burpee is a staple movement. You can find this exercise in just about every fitness trainer's toolbox in some form or another. It's a great way to get a full-body workout in just a couple of short, swift movements, and it's a great cardiovascular workout to boot. Try to do ten of these guys without breathing super heavy afterward — we dare you!

Burpees combine a squat, a plank, and a vertical leap:

1. Begin in a standing position.

2. Drop into a squat position with your hands on the ground.

3. Extend your feet back in one quick motion to assume the plank position.

4. Return to the squat position in one quick motion.

5. Jump straight in the air as high as you can.

To scale your burpees to a more challenging variation, perform a push-up (or double push-ups) when you're in the plank position.

Sit-Ups

What happened to the old-fashioned sit-up? Although nowadays it may be less popular, the sit-up is great for hip flexors and the deep muscles of your abdomen. It builds core strength, which you use in everything you do in your modern-day living.

Here are the steps to a proper sit-up:

1. Bend your knees and place the balls of your feet and heels on the ground.

2. Place your hands on opposing shoulders so your arms are crossed over your chest.

3. Tighten your abdominal muscles by drawing your belly button to your spine.

4. Keep your heels on the ground and your toes flat to the ground, and slowly and gently lift your head first, followed by your shoulder blades. Come all the way up, touching your armpits to your knees.

5. Slowly bring your torso down to the floor and keep a slight yet relaxed arch.

If you have back pain, do sit-ups with an exercise ball to minimize back strain, and go easy!

Walking Lunges

If you're motivated by having a better butt, more shapely legs, and a smaller waist, you definitely want in on this exercise. Walking lunges are one of our favorite exercises for lifting and firming everything below the torso. Be sure to fit this exercise into your workout rotation!

Walking lunges are similar to regular walking, but you just add a lunge:

1. Stand tall holding your hands at your hips.

2. Take a step, tighten your abdominal muscles to give you more spinal stability, and bend forward with your foot, bending both knees so that your front knee is aligned over your ankle and the back knee comes close to the floor, with your back heel lifted off the floor.

3. Before your back knee touches the floor, push up with your back leg, forcing the weight of your body through your front heel, at the same time bringing your back foot together with your front foot.

   At first, your lunges may be more of a dip, but as you progress, you'll find yourself easing into deeper lunges.

4. Continue the previous steps, alternating legs.

If you have knee problems, this exercise may cause some strain. To avoid injury, be sure you don't overextend your front knee past your front foot.

Air Squats

Embrace the burn! These squats give you a fit and firm bottom, tummy, and thighs, and they're actually really fun to do. Air squats are a traveler's dream because you can do them alone, and they provide a nice morning pick-me-up.

Because squatting is an essential functional movement, be sure to throw a couple of these exercises into your routine as often as you can.

1. Begin by standing with your legs apart.

2. Bend down and squat, making sure your thighs and calves connect. Your knees should always be out and over the feet. The hips should dip down farther than the knees. At the same time, push your arms straight out in front of you at shoulder height with hands straight out, palms down, and fingers together.

3. Make sure your weight is distributed evenly as you push back up into a standing position.

4. Return your arms to your sides. (Be sure to fully complete one squat before beginning the next.)

You can use a medicine ball to make sure you're squatting down far enough. Your butt should skim the top of the ball each time you squat.

Step-Ups

Step-ups are a great way to strengthen your thighs and knees. They add great muscle tone and definition to your legs. Remember when "step" classes were all the rage? They caught on fast and furious because the constant repetitive motion of stepping up and down did a great job at creating shapely strong legs and an uplifted bottom. Step-ups are also a great way to develop your explosive cardiovascular potential.

1. Standing in front of a bench or staircase, place your foot flat on the stair or bench. Push into your heel and bring your other foot up to the step, but don't put any weight on that foot — just tap your toe.

2. Keeping your first foot planted flat on the stair or bench, place the other foot gently back down to the floor. Come up and down eight to ten times, just tapping the toe of your other foot on the step.

3. Repeat on the other side.

Be careful not to add strain on the knee joint by lunging too far forward. Your knee shouldn't extend past the toes on the leg you're keeping still.

Dips

Dips are an oldie but a goodie. They never left the gym scene because they work as good as any exercise out there to build and shape triceps. If you want shapely arms with defined triceps, dips are a great way to get there! Dips also work your chest, shoulders, and biceps to get your entire upper body toned. This movement is a great balance to all the lower body workouts.

1. Sit on the edge of a bench or chair. Place your hands on either side of your hips, fingers gripping forward over the edge of the seat. Plant both feet on the floor and scoot your hips forward off the seat.

2. Bend your arms, lowering your body. Keep your torso straight and hips as close to the bench as possible. Use your arm muscles to control your decent.

3. Stop when your shoulders are level with your elbows or just before. Your elbows should stay directly over your hands throughout the movement.

4. Straighten your arms by pressing yourself back up to the start position. You can use your legs as necessary, but try to keep the power coming from your arms.

Jumping Jacks

This exercise needs no introduction. The first fitness ads that ever existed were of folks doing jumping jacks. They worked then, and they work now. This classic exercise is a full-body exercise that gives you a cardiovascular workout and tones everything from soup to nuts. Not only can you do jumping jacks anywhere, but you can also totally control the intensity.

1. Begin by standing with your feet together and arms at your side.

2. Bend your knees and jump, moving your feet apart, making sure they're wider than your shoulders. At the same time, raise your arms over your head. Make sure you're on the balls of your feet when you land.

3. Keep your knees bent while you jump, again bringing your feet together and your arms at your sides. When you're done, your weight should be on your heels.

Plank Hold

We're not gonna lie. This exercise doesn't tickle. But if you want an exercise that gives you a super strong core and a rock-solid trunk and spine, the plank hold is the exercise for you. Doing this exercise creates a very stable framework for your body, helping protect you from injury. The plank hold will keep you looking good, too!

1. Lay down, face down, on the floor. Place your forearms on the mat with your shoulders aligned directly over your elbows. Clasping your hands in front of you makes this a little easier.

2. Extend your legs behind you and rest on your toes. Don't lift your hips toward the ceiling, and don't arch your back. You should have a straight line between your shoulders and toes.

3. Tighten your stomach muscles and hold as long as you can. If you feel your back start to cave from fatigue, take a minute then regroup and go at it again! The better you get at this, the longer you'll be able sustain the hold without fatiguing. Challenge yourself to go a little longer each time.

Walking and Running

The great thing about walking and running is that they have no limitations. You can enjoy their benefits in the busiest of cities or in the sprawling countryside. Also, you can easily adjust the intensity to scale these exercises to your liking.

To make sure you get the best experience, warm your muscles with some dynamic range of motion (see Chapter 6). Start slow and easy if you're hitting the pavement as a newbie. Healthy progression is essential when exercising and allows you to sustain your exercising without having to take time off for little injuries or setbacks.

For more advanced running, you can add bursts to your workout by going as hard and as fast as you can for 6 to 60 seconds, followed by about 1½ minutes of rest. You can add two or more of these bursts to up the intensity of your run as you progress (see Chapter 6 for details).

Qi Gong K-27 Energy Buttons

K-27 stands for *kidney meridian number 27,* which describes the pathway of energy used in Eastern medicine that flows from the balls of the feet to the collarbone. This pathway is an important area of energy flow throughout the body. You can stimulate these points to give yourself a pick-me-up whenever you need it. Rubbing these points sends a signal to the brain, telling it to get the flow of energy moving along this pathway and help you extend your energy limits. You can expect to experience more energy, clearer thinking, and better immunity.

You may think this exercise looks ridiculously easy, but it really works. And you'll no longer need those sugary energy drinks after doing this exercise — trust us! To stimulate the K-27 energy buttons, just do the following:

1. Place your fingers on your collarbone (clavicle). Use both hands.

2. Follow your collarbone inward until you reach the corner, and drop down and outward a bit to the indent below the collarbone. You found the K-27 points. (The K-27 point is located just below the collarbone, close to the middle of the body.)

3. Massage these points in a rotating motion for about 20 seconds. You can do both sides simultaneously or one at a time.

This technique is a great tool to use before taking a test. Stimulating these buttons helps you think clearly and oxygenates the brain so you can access more brain power!

Index

Apple & Mac

iPad 2 For Dummies,
3rd Edition
978-1-118-17679-5

iPhone 4S For Dummies,
5th Edition
978-1-118-03671-6

iPod touch For Dummies,
3rd Edition
978-1-118-12960-9

Mac OS X Lion
For Dummies
978-1-118-02205-4

Blogging & Social Media

CityVille For Dummies
978-1-118-08337-6

Facebook For Dummies,
4th Edition
978-1-118-09562-1

Mom Blogging
For Dummies
978-1-118-03843-7

Twitter For Dummies,
2nd Edition
978-0-470-76879-2

WordPress For Dummies,
4th Edition
978-1-118-07342-1

Business

Cash Flow For Dummies
978-1-118-01850-7

Investing For Dummies,
6th Edition
978-0-470-90545-6

Job Searching with Social
Media For Dummies
978-0-470-93072-4

QuickBooks 2012
For Dummies
978-1-118-09120-3

Resumes For Dummies,
6th Edition
978-0-470-87361-8

Starting an Etsy Business
For Dummies
978-0-470-93067-0

Cooking & Entertaining

Cooking Basics
For Dummies, 4th Edition
978-0-470-91388-8

Wine For Dummies,
4th Edition
978-0-470-04579-4

Diet & Nutrition

Kettlebells For Dummies
978-0-470-59929-7

Nutrition For Dummies,
5th Edition
978-0-470-93231-5

Restaurant Calorie Counter
For Dummies,
2nd Edition
978-0-470-64405-8

Digital Photography

Digital SLR Cameras &
Photography For Dummies,
4th Edition
978-1-118-14489-3

Digital SLR Settings
& Shortcuts
For Dummies
978-0-470-91763-3

Photoshop Elements 10
For Dummies
978-1-118-10742-3

Gardening

Gardening Basics
For Dummies
978-0-470-03749-2

Vegetable Gardening
For Dummies,
2nd Edition
978-0-470-49870-5

Green/Sustainable

Raising Chickens
For Dummies
978-0-470-46544-8

Green Cleaning
For Dummies
978-0-470-39106-8

Health

Diabetes For Dummies,
3rd Edition
978-0-470-27086-8

Food Allergies
For Dummies
978-0-470-09584-3

Living Gluten-Free
For Dummies,
2nd Edition
978-0-470-58589-4

Hobbies

Beekeeping
For Dummies,
2nd Edition
978-0-470-43065-1

Chess For Dummies,
3rd Edition
978-1-118-01695-4

Drawing For Dummies,
2nd Edition
978-0-470-61842-4

eBay For Dummies,
7th Edition
978-1-118-09806-6

Knitting For Dummies,
2nd Edition
978-0-470-28747-7

Language &
Foreign Language

English Grammar
For Dummies,
2nd Edition
978-0-470-54664-2

French For Dummies,
2nd Edition
978-1-118-00464-7

German For Dummies,
2nd Edition
978-0-470-90101-4

Spanish Essentials
For Dummies
978-0-470-63751-7

Spanish For Dummies,
2nd Edition
978-0-470-87855-2

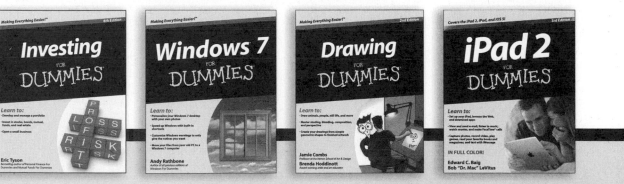

Math & Science

Algebra I For Dummies,
2nd Edition
978-0-470-55964-2

Biology For Dummies,
2nd Edition
978-0-470-59875-7

Chemistry For Dummies,
2nd Edition
978-1-1180-0730-3

Geometry For Dummies,
2nd Edition
978-0-470-08946-0

Pre-Algebra Essentials
For Dummies
978-0-470-61838-7

Microsoft Office

Excel 2010 For Dummies
978-0-470-48953-6

Office 2010 All-in-One
For Dummies
978-0-470-49748-7

Office 2011 for Mac
For Dummies
978-0-470-87869-9

Word 2010
For Dummies
978-0-470-48772-3

Music

Guitar For Dummies,
2nd Edition
978-0-7645-9904-0

Clarinet For Dummies
978-0-470-58477-4

iPod & iTunes
For Dummies,
9th Edition
978-1-118-13060-5

Pets

Cats For Dummies,
2nd Edition
978-0-7645-5275-5

Dogs All-in One
For Dummies
978-0470-52978-2

Saltwater Aquariums
For Dummies
978-0-470-06805-2

Religion & Inspiration

The Bible For Dummies
978-0-7645-5296-0

Catholicism For Dummies,
2nd Edition
978-1-118-07778-8

Spirituality For Dummies,
2nd Edition
978-0-470-19142-2

Self-Help & Relationships

Happiness For Dummies
978-0-470-28171-0

Overcoming Anxiety
For Dummies,
2nd Edition
978-0-470-57441-6

Seniors

Crosswords For Seniors
For Dummies
978-0-470-49157-7

iPad 2 For Seniors
For Dummies, 3rd Edition
978-1-118-17678-8

Laptops & Tablets
For Seniors For Dummies,
2nd Edition
978-1-118-09596-6

Smartphones & Tablets

BlackBerry For Dummies,
5th Edition
978-1-118-10035-6

Droid X2 For Dummies
978-1-118-14864-8

HTC ThunderBolt
For Dummies
978-1-118-07601-9

MOTOROLA XOOM
For Dummies
978-1-118-08835-7

Sports

Basketball For Dummies,
3rd Edition
978-1-118-07374-2

Football For Dummies,
2nd Edition
978-1-118-01261-1

Golf For Dummies,
4th Edition
978-0-470-88279-5

Test Prep

ACT For Dummies,
5th Edition
978-1-118-01259-8

ASVAB For Dummies,
3rd Edition
978-0-470-63760-9

The GRE Test For
Dummies, 7th Edition
978-0-470-00919-2

Police Officer Exam
For Dummies
978-0-470-88724-0

Series 7 Exam
For Dummies
978-0-470-09932-2

Web Development

HTML, CSS, & XHTML
For Dummies, 7th Edition
978-0-470-91659-9

Drupal For Dummies,
2nd Edition
978-1-118-08348-2

Windows 7

Windows 7
For Dummies
978-0-470-49743-2

Windows 7
For Dummies,
Book + DVD Bundle
978-0-470-52398-8

Windows 7 All-in-One
For Dummies
978-0-470-48763-1

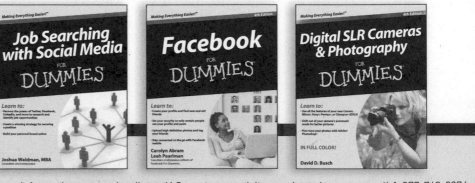

Available wherever books are sold. For more information or to order direct: U.S. customers visit www.dummies.com or call 1-877-762-2974.
U.K. customers visit www.wileyeurope.com or call (0) 1243 843291. Canadian customers visit www.wiley.ca or call 1-800-567-4797.
Connect with us online at www.facebook.com/fordummies or @fordummies